Simultaneous Systems of Differential Equations and Multi-Dimensional Vibrations

Mathematics and Physics for Science and Technology

Series Editor: L.M.B.C. Campos
Director of the Center for Aeronautical
and Space Science and Technology
Lisbon University

Volumes in the series:

For more information about this series, please visit: https://www.crcpress.com/Mathematics-and-Physics-for-Science-and-Technology/book-series/CRCMATPHYSCI

Mathematics and Physics for Science and Technology

Volume IV

Ordinary Differential Equations with Applications to Trajectories and Vibrations

Book 7

Simultaneous Systems of Differential Equations and Multi-Dimensional Vibrations

By

L.M.B.C. Campos

Director of the Center for Aeronautical
and Space Science and Technology
Lisbon University

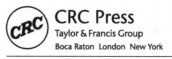

CRC Press
Taylor & Francis Group
Boca Raton London New York

CRC Press is an imprint of the
Taylor & Francis Group, an **informa** business

CRC Press
Taylor & Francis Group
6000 Broken Sound Parkway NW, Suite 300
Boca Raton, FL 334 87-2742

International Standard Book Number-13: 978-0-367-13721-2 (Hardback)

Library of Congress Cataloging-in-Publication Data

Names: Campos, Luis Manuel Braga da Costa, author.
Title: Simultaneous differential equations and multi-dimensional vibrations/
Luis Manuel Braga da Campos.
Description: First edition. | Boca Raton, FL : CRC Press/Taylor & Francis
Group, 2018. | Includes bibliographical references and index.
Identifiers: LCCN 2018049440| ISBN 9780367137212 (hardback : acid-free paper)
| ISBN 9780429030253 (ebook)
Subjects: LCSH: Vibration--Mathematical models. | Oscillations–Mathematical
models. | Differential equations. | Equations, Simultaneous. | Engineering
mathematics.
Classification: LCC TA355 .C28 2018 | DDC 531/.320151535–dc23
LC record available at https://lccn.loc.gov/2018049440

DOI: 10.1201/9780429030253

Visit the Taylor & Francis Web site at
http://www.taylorandfrancis.com

and the CRC Press Web site at
http://www.crcpress.com

to Leonor Campos

Contents

Diagrams, Notes, and Tables

Diagrams

Notes

Tables

Preface

Volume IV (*Ordinary Differential Equations with Applications to Trajectories and Oscillations*) is organized like the preceding three volumes of the series *Mathematics and Physics Applied to Science and Technology*: (volume III) *Generalized Calculus with Applications to Matter and Forces*; (volume II) *Transcendental Representations with Applications to Solids and Fluids*; and (volume I) *Complex Analysis with Applications to Flows and Fields*. The first book, *Linear Differential Equations and Oscillators*; the second book, *Non-Linear Differential Equations and Dynamical Systems*; and the third book, *Higher-Order Differential Equations and Elasticity* of volume IV, correspond, respectively, to books four to six of the series, and consist of chapters 1 to 6 of volume IV. The present book, *Simultaneous Differential Equations and Multidimensional Vibrations*, is the fourth book of volume IV and the seventh book of the series; it consists of chapters 7 and 8 of volume IV.

Chapters 1, 3, and 5 focus on single differential equations, starting with (i) linear differential equations of any order with constant or homogeneous coefficients; and continuing with (ii) non-linear first-order differential equations, including variable coefficients and (iii) non-linear differential second-order and higher-order equations. Chapter 7 discusses simultaneous systems of ordinary differential equations, and focuses mostly on the cases that have a matrix of characteristic polynomials, namely linear systems with constant or homogeneous power coefficients. The method of the matrix of characteristic polynomials also applies to simultaneous systems of linear finite difference equations with constant coefficients.

Chapters 2 and 4 focus on, respectively, linear and non-linear oscillators described by second-order differential equations, like the elastic bodies without stiffness in the chapter 6; the elastic bodies with stiffness in chapter 6 lead to fourth-order differential equations equivalent to coupled second-order systems. Chapter 8 considers linear multi-dimensional oscillators with any number of degrees of freedom, including damping, forcing, and multiple resonance. The discrete oscillators may be extended from a finite number of degrees-of-freedom to infinite chains. The continuous oscillators correspond to waves in homogeneous or inhomogeneous media, including elastic, acoustic, electromagnetic, and water surface waves. The combination of propagation and dissipation leads to the equations of mathematical physics.

Organization of the Contents

Volume IV consists of ten chapters: (i) the odd-numbered chapters present mathematical developments; (ii) the even-numbered chapters contain physical applications; (iii) the last chapter is a set of 20 detailed examples of (i) and (ii). The chapters are divided into sections and subsections, for example, chapter 7, section 7.1, and subsection 7.1.1. The formulas are numbered by chapters in curved brackets; for example, (8.2) is equation 2 of chapter 8. When referring to volume I the symbol I is inserted at the beginning, for example: (i) chapter I.36, section I.36.1, subsection I.36.1.2; (ii) equation (I.36.33a). The final part of each chapter includes: (i) a conclusion referring to the figures as a kind of visual summary; (ii) the notes, lists, tables, diagrams, and classifications as additional support. The latter (ii) appear at the end of each chapter, and are numbered within the chapter (for example, diagram—D7.2, note—N8.10, table—T7.4); if there is more than one diagram, note, or table, they are numbered sequentially (for example, notes—N7.1 to N7.55). The chapter starts with an introductory preview, and related topics may be mentioned in the notes at the end. The sections "Series Preface," and "Mathematical Symbols" from the first book of volume IV are not repeated. The sections "Physical Quantities," "References," and "Index" focus on the contents of the present fourth book of volume IV.

Acknowledgments

The fourth volume of the series justifies renewing some of the acknowledgments made in the first three volumes. Thank you to those who contributed more directly to the final form of this volume: Ms. Ana Moura, L. Sousa, and S. Pernadas for help with the manuscripts; Mr. J. Coelho for all the drawings; and at last, but not least, to my wife, my companion in preparing this work.

About the Author

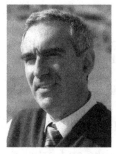

L.M.B.C. Campos was born on March 28, 1950, in Lisbon, Portugal. He graduated in 1972 as a mechanical engineer from the Instituto Superior Tecnico (IST) of Lisbon Technical University. The tutorials as a student (1970) were followed by a career at the same institution (IST) through all levels: assistant (1972), assistant with tenure (1974), assistant professor (1978), associate professor (1982), chair of Applied Mathematics and Mechanics (1985). He has served as the coordinator of undergraduate and postgraduate degrees in Aerospace Engineering since the creation of the programs in 1991. He is the coordinator of the Scientific Area of Applied and Aerospace Mechanics in the Department of Mechanical Engineering. He is also the director and founder of the Center for Aeronautical and Space Science and Technology.

In 1977, Campos received his doctorate on "waves in fluids" from the Engineering Department of Cambridge University, England. Afterwards, he received a Senior Rouse Ball Scholarship to study at Trinity College, while on leave from IST. In 1984, his first sabbatical was as a Senior Visitor at the Department of Applied Mathematics and Theoretical Physics of Cambridge University, England. In 1991, he spent a second sabbatical as an Alexander von Humboldt scholar at the Max-Planck Institut fur Aeronomic in Katlenburg-Lindau, Germany. Further sabbaticals abroad were excluded by major commitments at the home institution. The latter were always compatible with extensive professional travel related to participation in scientific meetings, individual or national representation in international institutions, and collaborative research projects.

Campos received the von Karman medal from the Advisory Group for Aerospace Research and Development (AGARD) and Research and Technology Organization (RTO). Participation in AGARD/RTO included serving as a vice-chairman of the System Concepts and Integration Panel, and chairman of the Flight Mechanics Panel and of the Flight Vehicle Integration Panel. He was also a member of the Flight Test Techniques Working Group. Here he was involved in the creation of an independent flight test capability, active in Portugal during the last 30 years, which has been used in national and international projects, including Eurocontrol and the European Space Agency. The participation in the European Space Agency (ESA) has afforded Campos the opportunity to serve on various program boards at the levels of national representative and Council of Ministers.

His participation in activities sponsored by the European Union (EU) has included: (i) 27 research projects with industry, research, and academic institutions; (ii) membership of various Committees, including Vice-Chairman of the Aeronautical Science and Technology Advisory Committee; (iii) participation on the Space Advisory Panel on the future role of EU in space. Campos has been a member of the Space Science Committee of the European Science Foundation, which works with the Space Science Board of the National Science Foundation of the United States. He has been a member of the Committee for Peaceful Uses of Outer Space (COPUOS) of the United Nations. He has served as a consultant and advisor on behalf of these organizations and other institutions. His participation in professional societies includes member and vice-chairman of the Portuguese Academy of Engineering, fellow of the Royal Aeronautical Society, Astronomical Society and Cambridge Philosophical Society, associate fellow of the American Institute of Aeronautics and Astronautics, and founding and life member of the European Astronomical Society.

Campos has published and worked on numerous books and articles. His publications include 10 books as a single author, one as an editor, and one as a co-editor. He has published 152 papers (82 as the single author, including 12 reviews) in 60 journals, and 254 communications to symposia. He has served as reviewer for 40 different journals, in addition to 23 reviews published in *Mathematics Reviews*. He is or has been member of the editorial boards of several journals, including *Progress in Aerospace Sciences, International Journal of Aeroacoustics, International Journal of Sound and Vibration,* and *Air & Space Europe.*

Campos's areas of research focus on four topics: acoustics, magnetohydrodynamics, special functions, and flight dynamics. His work on acoustics has concerned the generation, propagation, and refraction of sound in flows with mostly aeronautical applications. His work on magnetohydrodynamics has concerned magneto-acoustic-gravity-inertial waves in solar-terrestrial and stellar physics. His developments on special functions have used differintegration operators, generalizing the ordinary derivative and primitive to complex order; they have led to the introduction of new special functions. His work on flight dynamics has concerned aircraft and rockets, including trajectory optimization, performance, stability, control, and atmospheric disturbances.

The range of topics from mathematics to physics and engineering fits with the aims and contents of the present series. Campos's experience in university teaching and scientific and industrial research has enhanced his ability to make the series valuable to students from undergraduate level to research level.

Campos's professional activities on the technical side are balanced by other cultural and humanistic interests. Complementary non-technical interests include classical music (mostly orchestral and choral), plastic arts (painting, sculpture, architecture), social sciences (psychology and biography), history (classical, renaissance and overseas expansion) and technology (automotive, photo, audio). Campos is listed in various biographical publications, including *Who's Who in the World* since 1986, *Who's Who in Science and Technology* since 1994, and *Who's Who in America* since 2011.

Physical Quantities

The location of first appearance is indicated, for example "2.7" means "section 2.7," "6.8.4" means "subsection 6.8.4," "N8.8" means "note 8.8," and "E10.13.1" means "example 10.13.1."

1 Small Arabic Letters

b — width of a water channel: N7.12

c — phase speed of waves: N8.1

c_e — speed of transversal waves in an elastic string: N7.9

c_{em} — speed of electromagnetic waves: N7.15

c_ℓ — speed of longitudinal waves in an elastic rod: N7.11

c_s — adiabatic sound speed: N7.16

c_t — speed of torsional waves along an elastic rod: N7.10

c_w — speed of water waves along a channel: N7.13

$\vec{e}_i$ — non-unit base vector: N8.8

f_r — reduced external force: 8.2.1

g — determinant of the covariant metric tensor: N8.8

g_ℓ — reduced modal force: 8.1.1

g_{ij} — covariant metric tensor: N8.8

g^{ij} — contravariant metric tensor: N8.8

h — depth of water channel: N7.12

h_i — friction force vector: 8.1.1

   —scale factors: N8.8

j_i — restoring force vector: 8.1.1

k — wavenumber: N7.25, N8.2

k_{rs} — resilience matrix: 8.1.2

ℓ — lengthscale for horns: N7.28

m_{rs} — mass matrix: 8.2.1

q_ℓ — modal coordinates: 8.2.4

z — specific impedance: N7.47

2 Capital Arabic Letters

A — cross-sectional area of a horn: N7.16

— admittance: 8.9.1

A_n — modal amplitudes: 8.8.5

B_{mn} — terms in the modal matrix: 8.8.5

E_v — kinetic energy: 6.8.5

F_ℓ — reduced external force: 8.2.1

G_ℓ — modal forces: 8.2.9

$J^\pm$ — invariants of acoustic horns: N7.28

K — reduced wavenumber: N7.29

$\vec{K}$ — enhanced wavenumber: N7.33

L_A — lengthscale of variation of the cross-sectional area: N7.17

L_b — lengthscale of variation of the width of a water channel: N7.12

L_c — lengthscale of variation of the torsional stiffness: N7.10

L_E — lengthscale of change of the Young modulus: N7.11

L_T — lengthscale of change of tension: N7.9

L_ε — lengthscale of variation of the dielectric permittivity: N7.15

L_μ — lengthscale of variation of the magnetic permeability: N7.15

M_n— mass of n-th element of a radioactive disintegration chain: 8.7.1

M_{rs} — modal matrix: 8.2.13

N — number of particles: 5.5.17

N_{rs} — undamped modal matrix: 8.2.14

P — reduced pressure perturbation spectrum: N7.23

P_{2N} — dispersion polynomial: 8.2.2

P_{ij} — dispersion matrix: 8.2.2

$Q_{r\ell}$ — transformation matrix: 8.2.7

R — electrical resistance: 8.9.2

— reflection coefficient: N7.47

S — surface adsorption coefficient: N7.48

S_{ij} — scattering matrix: N7.53

T — transmission coefficient: N7.51

V — reduced velocity perturbation spectrum: N7.23

Y — inductance: 8.9.1

Z — impedance: 8.9.1

$\tilde{Z}$ — overall impedance: N7.52

Z_0 — impedance of a plane sound wave: N7.47

3 Small Greek Letters

α — diffusivity: N8.1

β — amplification/attenuation factor: N7.50

—potential: N8.1

δ_{ij} — identity matrix: 8.1.4

λ_ℓ — modal dampings: 8.2.5

λ_{rs} — damping matrix: 8.2.1

μ_{rs} — kinematic friction matrix: 8.1.3

ν_n — disintegration rate of the mass of the n-th element in a chain: 8.7.1

σ — mass density per unit length: N7.8

ω_ℓ —modal frequencies: 8.2.4

$\bar{\omega}_\ell$ — oscillation frequency of modes: 8.2.6

ω_{rs}^2 — oscillation matrix: 8.2.1

4 Capital Greek Letters

Φ — primal wave variable: N7.19

Φ_m — mechanical potential energy: 8.1.2

Ψ — dual wave variable: N7.19

Ψ_m — dissipation by mechanical friction: 8.1.2

7

Simultaneous Differential Equations

An ordinary differential equation of order N relates one independent and one dependent variable, with a set of derivatives of the latter with regard to the former up to and including the order N. In the case of a system of simultaneous differential equations, there are M dependent variables and only one dependent variable (section 7.1). The derivatives of the former with regard to the latter appear in a set of simultaneous equations, which cannot be separated for each dependent variable (at least without some manipulation).

The simplest case of a system of M simultaneous ordinary differential equations is an autonomous system (section 7.1) in which the first-order derivative of each of the M dependent variables is an explicit function of all the dependent variables, and does not involve any derivatives. The autonomous system of ordinary differential equations is related to the problem of finding the family of curves tangent to a given continuous vector field (section 7.2), which always has a solution. In contrast, the problem of finding a family of hypersurfaces orthogonal to a given continuous vector field leads to a differential of first order in M variables, which has (does not have) a solution (sections 3.8–3.9 and notes 3.1–3.15) if the differential is exact or has an integrating factor (is inexact and has no integrating factor). Any system of M simultaneous ordinary differential equations can be transformed to an autonomous system (section 7.1); this leads to a method to eliminate a system of M simultaneous ordinary differential equations in M dependent variables into a single ordinary differential equation of order N for one of the dependent variables (section 7.3). This specifies the order N of the system of M simultaneous ordinary differential equations that equals (is less than) the sum of the higher-order derivatives in all M equations if the system is independent (redundant).

The most important class of single (simultaneous) ordinary differential equation(s) is the linear case with constant coefficients [sections 1.3–1.5 (7.4–7.5)] to which can be reduced the case of power coefficients [sections 1.6–1.8 (7.6–7.7)]. In all of the cases, the solution is determined by the roots of a single characteristic polynomial. For a single linear ordinary differential equation with constant coefficients, the characteristic polynomial is the differential operator acting on the dependent variable (section 1.3). In the case of a simultaneous system of M equations with M dependent variables, there is (section 7.4) an $M \times M$ matrix of linear operators with constant coefficients, and its determinant specifies the characteristic polynomial of the

1

system of simultaneous differential equations, whose order N is the degree of the characteristic polynomial. The solutions corresponding to single or multiple, real or complex roots, are similar for a single (set of simultaneous) differential equation(s), and each dependent variable is a linear combination of them, with coefficients determined by the initial conditions; the number of independent and compatible initial conditions needed to specify a unique solution is equal the order of the single (set of simultaneous) differential equation(s). This implies that in the solution of a linear simultaneous system of M ordinary differential equations with constant (homogeneous) coefficients without forcing [section 7.4 (7.5)]: (i) each of the M dependent variables is a linear combination of N linearly independent particular integrals specified by the roots of the characteristic polynomial; (ii) there are N arbitrary constants of integration, for example, those in the first dependent variable; (iii) the coefficients in all other dependent variables involve the same N arbitrary constants of integration, in a way that is compatible with substitution back into the system of simultaneous ordinary differential equations.

The case of a single (set of simultaneous) linear ordinary differential equation(s) with constant coefficients and a forcing term, can be considered using [sections 1.4–1.5 (7.5)] the characteristic polynomial directly or as an inverse operator. A characteristic polynomial also exists for a single (set of simultaneous) linear ordinary differential equation(s) with power coefficients, leading to similar methods of solution [sections 1.6–1.8 (7.6–7.7)]. The characteristic polynomial also exists for a single (set of simultaneous) linear finite difference equation(s), again leading to similar methods of solution [section(s) 1.9 (7.8–7.9)].

7.1 Reduction of General to Autonomous Systems

A general system of M simultaneous ordinary differential equations (subsection 7.1.2) can be reduced to an autonomous system of differential equations (subsection 7.1.1).

7.1.1 Autonomous System of Differential Equations

A **generalized autonomous system of order M** of ordinary differential equations (standard CXXI) has one independent variable x, and M dependent variables (7.1a) whose first-order derivatives (7.1b) depend explicitly only on all the dependent variables and the dependent variable:

$$m = 1,...,M: \qquad y'_m(x) \equiv \frac{dy_m}{dx} = Y_m(x;y_1,....,y_M); \qquad (7.1a, b)$$

This excludes the appearance of any derivatives of any order on the right-hand side (r.h.s.) of (7.1b). *An ordinary differential equation (1.1a, b) of order N with independent (dependent) variable x(y), which is explicit in the highest-order derivative (7.2):*

$$y^{(N)}(x) = G\left(x; y, y', ..., y^{(N-1)}\right),\qquad(7.2)$$

can be transformed into (standard CXXI) an autonomous system of order N:

$$r = 1, ..., M-1:\qquad y_r(x) \equiv y^{(r)}(x), \qquad y'_{N-1}(x) = G\left(x; y_1, ..., y_{N-1}\right),\qquad(7.3a\text{–}c)$$

by: (i) defining N − 1 new dependent variables (7.3a, b) as the derivatives of the dependent variable up to the order N − 1; (ii) rewriting the original differential equation (7.2) in autonomous form (7.3c). For example, the third-order differential equation (7.4a) explicit for the third-order derivative:

$$y''' = F\left(x; y, y', y''\right):\qquad y' \equiv y_1, \quad y'_1 \equiv y_2 = y'', \quad y'_2 = y''' = F\left(x; y, y_1, y_2\right),$$
$$(7.4a\text{–}d)$$

can be reduced to the autonomous system (7.4b–d) also of order 3. The preceding method of reduction to an autonomous system of differential equations applies both [subsection 7.1.1 (7.1.2)] to a single (set of simultaneous) differential equation(s) of any order(s).

7.1.2 General System of Simultaneous Differential Equations

A set of *M* differential equations with one independent variable *x* and *M* dependent variables is **decoupled** if like (7.2):

$$m = 1, ..., M:\qquad F_m\left(x; y_m, y'_m, y''_m, ..., y_m^{(N_m)}\right) = 0,\qquad(7.5a, b)$$

each dependent variable (7.5a) satisfies an ordinary differential equation (7.5b) of order N_m involving only the same dependent variable and its derivatives of order up to N_m; in this case each of the *M* differential equations (7.5b) can be solved separately from the others. This is not the case if each differential equation involves more than one dependent variable and/or its derivatives:

$$m, s = 1, ..., M; \quad N_{m,s} \in |N:\qquad 0 = F_s\left(x; y_m, y'_m, y''_m, ..., y_m^{(N_{m,s})}\right).\qquad(7.6a\text{–}c)$$

*The **general simultaneous system** of M (7.6a) ordinary differential equations (7.6c) relates (standard CXII) the independent variable x to all (7.6b) dependent* *variables y_s and their derivatives up to the order $N_{m,s}$. Assume that the system (7.6a–c) can be solved explicitly (7.7d) for the highest-order derivative (7.7c) of each dependent variable (7.7a):*

$$m,r = 1,...,M; \quad r \neq m: \quad y_m^{(N_{m,m})}(x) = G_s\left(x; y_m, y_m', ..., y_m^{(N_{m,m}-1)}; y_r, y_r', ..., y_r^{(N_{m,r})}\right),$$

$$(7.7a\text{–}d)$$

with the remaining dependent variables (7.7b) and their derivatives also appearing. The corresponding autonomous system:

$$m = 1,...,M; \quad s_m = 1,2,...,N_{m,n} - 1 \equiv t_m: \quad y_{m,s_m}(x) = y_m^{(s_m)}(x), \quad (7.8a\text{–}c)$$

$$N = \sum_{m=1}^{M} N_{m,m}: \quad y_{m,t_m}' = G_m\left(x; y_m, y_{m,1}, ..., y_{m,t_m}; y_{r,1}, ..., y_{r,t_r}\right) \quad (7.8d, e)$$

has: (i) extra variables (7.8a–c) for a total (7.8d); (ii) all equations (7.8c, e) have an autonomous form. For example, the pair of simultaneous ordinary differential equations of orders 2(1) explicit in the highest-order derivatives (7.9a, b):

$$y'' = F(x; y, y'; z), \qquad z' = G(x; z; y, y'), \qquad (7.9a, b)$$

is equivalent to the autonomous system (7.10a–c) of order 3:

$$y' = y_1, \qquad y_1' = y'' = F(x; y, y_1; z), \qquad z' = G(x; z; y, y_1). \quad (7.10a\text{–}c)$$

The implicit autonomous system of differential equations (7.1a, b) has a simple geometrical interpretation (section 7.2).

7.2 Tangents, Trajectories, and Paths in N-Dimensions

An autonomous system of N first-order coupled differential equations specifies a family of curves in a space of N dimensions (subsection 7.2.1), which may lie on the intersection of $M \leq N$ hypersurfaces (subsection 7.2.3). The simplest cases $N = 2(N = 3)$ are [subsection 7.2.2 (7.2.4)] plane curves (space curves specified by the intersection of two surfaces). Thus, the consideration of hypercurves (hypersurfaces) tangent (orthogonal) to a continuous N-dimensional vector field leads to an autonomous system of N differential equations [a first-order differential in N variables (notes 3.1–3.15)] that always has (may not have) a solution.

7.2.1 *N*-Dimensional Hypercurve Specified by Tangent Vectors

Denoting by (7.11b) the coordinates in an *N*-dimensional space (7.11a) and by a parameter such as time (*t*), a regular curve has parametric equations (7.11c), where the coordinates are functions of the parameter with a continuous first-order derivative, and specify a **trajectory**:

$$n, m = 1, ..., N: \qquad x_n(t) \in C^1(a \leq t \leq b): \qquad \frac{dx_n}{dt} = X_n(x_m), \qquad (7.11a\text{--}c)$$

in the autonomous system of first-order differential equations (7.11c). The independent variable *t* does not appear explicitly, as it is designated an **implicit autonomous system** (standard CXXIII). The differentiation of the coordinates with regard to time (7.11c) specifies a continuous (7.12a) tangent vector field (Figure 7.1), not necessarily of unit length, since a metric (notes III.9.35–III.9.45) need not exist; if the dependent variables x_n are spatial coordinates and the parameter *t* is time, then the vector field defined by the derivatives (7.11c) is the velocity. Eliminating the parameter (7.12b) leads to a set of $(N-1)$ simultaneous ordinary differential equations (7.12c):

$$X_n(x_1, ..., x_N) \in C(|R^N): \qquad dt = \frac{dx_1}{X_1} = \frac{dx_2}{X_2} = ... = \frac{dx_n}{X_n}, \qquad (7.12a\text{--}c)$$

whose solution (7.13b) specifies the **path** as the intersection of $(N-1)$ hypersurfaces (7.13a):

$$m = 1, ..., N-1: \qquad f_m(x_1, x_2, ..., x_N) = C_m, \qquad (7.13a, b)$$

where $C_1, ..., C_{N-1}$ are arbitrary constants. Note that the trajectory (7.11a–c) [path (7.13a, b)] correspond to the same curve with (without) a parameter that specifies its direction, say increasing time for the direction along the trajectory. Thus, (standard CXXIV) *an implicit autonomous system of N dimensional equations (7.11a–c) specifies a family of regular curves (7.13a, b) with N − 1*

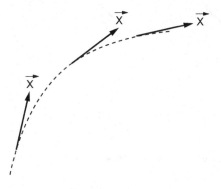

FIGURE 7.1
A continuous vector field leads to an autonomous system of ordinary differential equations whose solution is the tangent curve.

parameters $C_1,...,C_{N-1}$, which are tangent (Figure 7.1) to a given continuous vector field (7.12a). The simplest cases are the plane $N = 2$ (three-dimensional space $N = 3$), where a continuous vector field specifies a family of tangent curves (section 7.2.2) with one (two) parameters.

7.2.2 Families of Curves in the Plane or in Space

In the two-dimensional case, the trajectory (7.14a):

$$\left\{\frac{dx}{dt},\frac{dy}{dt}\right\} = X,Y(x,y), \qquad \frac{dy}{dx} = \frac{Y}{X}, \qquad f(x,y) = C, \qquad \text{(7.14a–b)}$$

specifies a differential equation (7.14b), whose solution (7.14c) is a one-parameter family of which are curves tangent (Figure 7.1) to the vector field of components $\{X,Y\}$.

In the three-dimensional case:

$$\left\{\frac{dx}{dt},\frac{dy}{dt},\frac{dz}{dt}\right\} = X,Y,Z(x,y,z), \qquad \text{(7.15a)}$$

the system of two equations (7.15b):

$$\frac{dx}{X} = \frac{dy}{Y} = \frac{dz}{Z}, \qquad f,g(x,y,z) = C_1,C_2, \qquad \text{(7.15b, c)}$$

specifies two families of surfaces (7.15a), whose intersection determines (Figure 7.2) a family of curves with two parameters C_1, C_2, which are tangent to the vector field of components $\{X,Y,Z\}$.

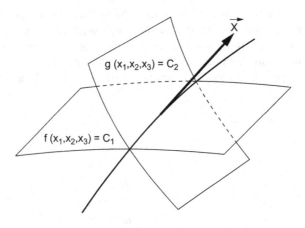

FIGURE 7.2
The tangent curve to a continuous vector field (Figure 7.1) in three dimensions may be obtained as the intersection of two surfaces.

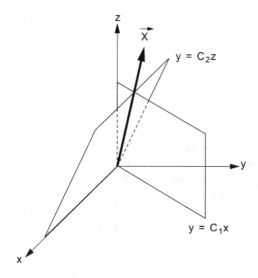

FIGURE 7.3
A particular case of Figure 7.2 is a radial vector field tangent to a straight line passing through the origin, which is the intersection of two planes, each passing through a distinct coordinate axis.

For example, a radial vector field (7.16a):

$$\{X,Y,Z\}=\{x,y,z\}, \qquad \frac{dx}{x}=\frac{dy}{y}=\frac{dz}{z}, \qquad \text{(7.16a, b)}$$

specifies a system of equations (7.16b), whose solution (7.17a):

$$\log C_1 + \log x = \log y = \log z + \log C_2, \qquad y = C_1\,x, C_2\,z, \qquad \text{(7.17a, b)}$$

is the intersection of two families of planes (7.17b), orthogonal to the (x,y) and (x,z) planes and passing through the origin, which specify (Figure 7.3) an arbitrary straight line through the origin. In the general case of a space of N dimensions, a curve is the intersection of $N-1$ hypersurfaces with linearly independent normal vectors, and lies (subsection 7.2.3) in a subspace of dimension $1 \le M \le N$.

7.2.3 N-Dimensional Curve Lying on the Intersection of M Hypersurfaces

If $\lambda_1,...,\lambda_n$ are arbitrary functions, then (7.12c) implies:

$$\frac{dx_1}{X_1}=...=\frac{dx_N}{X_N}=\frac{\lambda_1\,dx_1+...+\lambda_N\,dx_N}{\lambda_1\,X_1+...+\lambda_N\,X_N}. \qquad \text{(7.18)}$$

For example, if the $\lambda_1, ..., \lambda_N$ can be so chosen that the denominator of (7.18) vanishes (7.19a):

$$\sum_{n=1}^{N} \lambda_n X_n = 0: \qquad 0 = \sum_{n=1}^{N} \lambda_n dx_n = d\Phi, \qquad \Phi(x_1, ..., x_N) = C, \qquad \text{(7.19a–c)}$$

then the numerator also vanishes (7.19b). If it is an exact differential, it specifies an integral (7.19c). If M independent integrals can be obtained, then they can be used to eliminate M variables, reducing the system (2) to one with a lesser number $N - M$ of variables, which may be simpler to solve. In the latter case, the integral curve lies on the intersection of M hypersurfaces, spanning a subspace of dimension M, and leaving $N - M$ coordinates free. An example is a continuous vector field in three dimensions for which the two-parameter family of tangent curves is the intersection of two one-parameter families of surfaces (subsection 7.2.4).

7.2.4 Space Curves as the Intersection of Two Surfaces

As an example, consider the family of curves in three-dimensional space (7.20b) tangent to the vector field (7.20a):

$$\{X, Y, Z\} = \{z(x+y), z(x-y), x^2 + y^2\}: \qquad \frac{dx}{z(x+y)} = \frac{dy}{z(x-y)} = \frac{dz}{x^2 + y^2}.$$

$$\text{(7.20a, b)}$$

Then using the identities:

$$y X + x Y - z Z = 0 = x X - y Y - z Z, \qquad \text{(7.21a, b)}$$

leads to the relations:

$$y\, dx + x\, dy - z\, dz = 0 = x\, dx - y\, dy - z\, dz, \qquad \text{(7.22a, b)}$$

that specify the integrals:

$$2xy - z^2 = C_1, \qquad x^2 - y^2 - z^2 = C_2, \qquad \text{(7.23a, b)}$$

of the system (7.20b). The section of the surface (7.23a) by planes y = const or by planes x = const are parabolas, and the section by planes z = const are hyperbolas, so the surface is a parabolic hyperboloid. The section of the surface (7.23b) by planes $y = $ const or $z = $ const are hyperbolas. The section of the surface by planes $x = $ const exist only for $|x| > |C_2|^{1/2}$, and are circles, that is, the surface is an hyperboloid of revolution with two sheets and axis along the x-axis. The intersection of the parabolic hyperboloid (7.23a) and the hyperboloid of revolution (7.23b) specify a doubly-parametric $[C_1, C_2]$ family of curves, satisfying (7.20b), which is tangent to the vector field (7.20a).

As another example, consider the system (7.24b) corresponding to the vector field (7.24a):

$$\{X, Y, Z\} = \left\{2x, -4x, \frac{4x^2}{y + 2x}\right\}: \quad \frac{dx}{1} = \frac{dy}{-2} = \frac{y + 2x}{2x}dz, \quad y + 2x = C_1, \quad \text{(7.24a, b)}$$

for which one integral (7.24c) is immediate. In order to find another integral, substitute the first integral (7.24c) into the system (7.24b), leading to (7.25a):

$$2x\, dx = (y + 2x)dz = C_1\, dz, \qquad C_2 = x^2 - C_1 z = x^2 - (y + 2x)z. \quad \text{(7.25a–c)}$$

The surface (7.25b) is a parabolic cylinder with generators parallel to the y-axis, and (7.24b) is a plane parallel to the z-axis, so that their intersection, which is the solution of (7.24b), is a parabola lying on this plane (Figure 7.4), and is tangent to the vector field (7.24a). The solution of the autonomous system of differential equations (7.12c) by the method (7.18) leads (7.19a) to first-order differentials in several variables (notes 3.11–3.16) suggesting the next comparison (subsection 7.2.5).

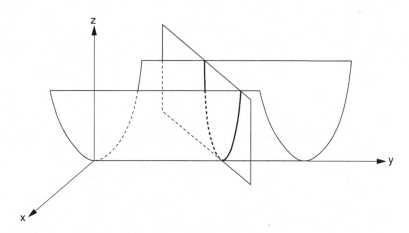

FIGURE 7.4
Another particular case of Figure 7.2 is the vector field tangent to the curve of intersection of a parabolic cylinder with a plane oblique to its axis.

7.2.5 Hypersurfaces Orthogonal to a Vector Field

Given a continuous vector field (7.26b) in N-dimensions (7.26a):

$$n,s = 1,...,N; \quad X_n(x_s) \in C(|R^N|): \quad \frac{dx_n}{dt} - X_n = 0 = \sum_{N=1}^{N} X_n \, dx_n, \qquad (7.26a\text{–}d)$$

the autonomous system of differential equations (7.26b, c) ≡ (7.11c; 7.12a) [first-order differential (7.26b, d) ≡ (3.267b)] specifies [standard CXXIV (CXXV)] a family of hypercurves (hypersurfaces) tangent (orthogonal) to the vector field [Figure 7.1 (3.7)], that always exist (section 9.1) [may or may not exist (notes 3.1–3.15)]. Concerning the existence of orthogonal hypersurfaces three cases arise. First, if the first-order differential (7.27a) ≡ (3.278b) is exact (7.27b) ≡ (3.278c), then (Figure 7.5) the family of hypersurfaces (7.27c) ≡ (3.278e) is orthogonal to the vector field:

$$0 = \sum_{n=1}^{N} X_n \, dx_n = d\Phi: \quad \Phi(x_n) = C \quad \Leftrightarrow \quad X_n \in C^1(|R^N|): \quad \nabla \wedge \vec{X} = 0; \qquad (7.27a\text{–}e)$$

the necessary and sufficient condition for a vector field with continuous first-order derivatives (7.27d) ≡ (3.278a) is that the curl (7.27e) ≡ (3.278d) is zero. Second, if the first-order differential (7.26d) is not exact but has an integrating factor λ that renders it exact by multiplication (7.28a) ≡ (3.284b), then there is an orthogonal family of hypersurfaces (7.28b) ≡ (7.284c):

$$0 = \lambda \sum_{n=1}^{N} X_n \, dx_n = d\Phi \quad \Leftrightarrow \quad \Phi(x_n) = C \quad \Leftrightarrow \quad \vec{X}.\left(\nabla \wedge \vec{X}\right) = 0, \qquad (7.28a\text{–}d)$$

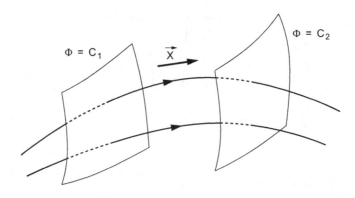

FIGURE 7.5
The Stokes theorem involves a regular surface D with area element dS_{mn} equal to the area dS multiplied by the unit normal N_{nm}, whose closed regular boundary ∂D is a curve with tangential displacement dx_n equal to the arc length ds multiplied by the unit tangent vector T_n.

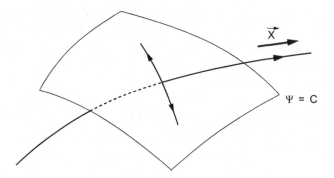

FIGURE 7.6
Given a continuous vector field: (i) there is always a tangent curve (Figure 7.1); (ii) there may or may not exist a family of orthogonal surfaces (Figure 7.6).

the necessary and sufficient condition for a continuously differentiable vector field (7.27d) is that it is orthogonal to its curl (7.28d) ≡ *(3.284a). Third, if the first-order differential is inexact and has no integrating factor (7.29a)* ≡ *(3.291d), then (Figure 7.6) on any set of (7.29b)* ≡ *(3.292a) hypersurfaces (7.29c)* ≡ *(3.292b) with linearly independent normal vectors (7.29d)* ≡ *(3.292c) there exist curves orthogonal to the vector field:*

$$\bar{X}.\left(\nabla \wedge \bar{X}\right) \neq 0: \quad r = 1,...., N-2, \quad \Psi_r(x_n) = const, \quad Ra\left(\frac{\partial \Psi_r}{\partial x_n}\right) = N-2.$$

$$(7.29a\text{--}d)$$

The autonomous system of differential equations (7.1a–c) can be used: (i) to prove the existence, unicity, and regularity of solutions of fairly general classes of differential equations (section 9.1); (ii) to establish the stability or instability of dynamical systems specified by simultaneous ordinary differential equations (section 9.2); (iii) to determine the order of a simultaneous system of ordinary differential equations (section 7.3). The derivation of some of these results uses the Stokes Theorem (Figure 7.7) stating that (7.30d) the

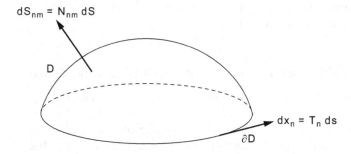

FIGURE 7.7
In the case where a continuous vector field does not have a family of orthogonal surfaces (Figure 7.6) there is on any surface a family of curves orthogonal to the vector field (Figure 7.7).

flux of the curl of a continuously differentiable vector field (7.30a) across a regular surface D with unit normal bivector N_{nm} and area element (7.30b) equals the circulation of the vector along the closed regular boundary ∂D with unit tangent vector T_n and displacement (7.30c).

$$X_n(x_m) \in C^1\left(|R^N\right): \quad ds_{nm} = N_{nm}ds, \quad dx_n = T_n ds;$$

$$\int_D (\partial_m X_n - \partial_n X_m) ds_{nm} = \int_{\partial D} T_n \, dx_n. \tag{7.30a–d}$$

The proof of the Stokes Theorem (its generalizations) uses vector (tensor) calculus [section III.5.7 (notes III.9.19–III.9.51)]. The reduction to an autonomous system of differential equations (section 7.1) can be used to establish the order of any system of ordinary differential equations (section 7.3).

7.3 Order of a Simultaneous System of Differential Equations

The order of a simultaneous system of ordinary differential equations is defined as *the highest of the orders of the decoupled ordinary differential equations satisfied by each of the dependent variables* (subsection 7.3.1). The transformation to an autonomous system (subsection 7.1.2) leads to a procedure to eliminate all dependent variables but one (subsection 7.3.1), thus, specifying the order of the original simultaneous system (subsection 7.3.2). Alternative but less general methods to determine the order of a system of simultaneous ordinary differential equations apply in particular cases, for example, using first integrals to introduce arbitrary constants of integration and reduce the ordinary of the system (subsection 7.3.3). Knowledge of the order is essential to determine the number of independent and compatible initial conditions to ensure unicity of solution.

7.3.1 Definition of Order for Simultaneous Differential Equations

The **order** of a simultaneous system of ordinary differential equation (7.6c) with one independent x and M dependent y_m variables (7.6a, b) is defined as the highest (7.31a) of the orders of the system of M decoupled ordinary differential equations (7.31b) obtained by elimination for each of the variables:

$$N = \max(N_1,....,N_M): \qquad F_m\left(x; y_m, y'_m,...., y_m^{(N_m)}\right) = 0, \tag{7.31a, b}$$

assuming that such elimination is possible. A simultaneous system of M ordinary differential equations (7.6a–c) that can be solved explicitly for the higher-order derivatives of each dependent variable (7.7a–d) can be transformed (7.8a–e) to an autonomous system (7.1a, b) of order Q so it's sufficient to eliminate the latter to find the order.

Consider the first equation (7.32a) of the autonomous system (7.1b) of order Q:

$$y_1' \equiv \frac{dy_1}{dx} = Y_1(x; y_1, y_2, \ldots, y_Q). \tag{7.32a}$$

Differentiating (7.32a) with regard to x leads to (7.32b):

$$y_1'' = \frac{dy_1}{dx} = \frac{\partial Y_1}{\partial x} + \sum_{q=1}^{Q} \frac{\partial Y_1}{\partial y_q} \frac{dy_q}{dx} = \frac{\partial Y_1}{\partial x} + \sum_{q=1}^{Q} \frac{\partial Y_1}{\partial y_q} Y_q(x; y_1, \ldots, y_Q) \equiv F_1(x; y_1, \ldots, y_Q),$$

$$\tag{7.32b–d}$$

where (7.1b) was used in (7.32c) to obtain a function (7.32d) involving only the independent and dependent variables and without derivatives. The procedure is applied N_1 times:

$$n = 2, \ldots, N_1: \qquad y_1^{(n)}(x) \equiv \frac{d^n y_1}{dx^n} = F_n(x; y_1, \ldots, y_Q), \tag{7.33a, b}$$

until it is possible to eliminate all dependent variables $y_2, y_3, \ldots, y_M$ other than y_1 among the N_1 equations (7.31; 7.33a, b) leading to a decoupled ordinary differential equation of order N_1 for y_1:

$$G\left(x; y_1(x), y_1'(x), \ldots, y_1^{(N_1)}(x)\right) = 0. \tag{7.34}$$

Proceeding in the same way with all dependent variables leads to (7.30b), which determines the order of the system. Not more than $M - 1$ equations are needed to eliminate $M - 1$ variables, and thus, none of the N_m can exceed Q.

Thus, *a simultaneous system of M simultaneous ordinary differential equations with one independent x and M dependent $(y_1, \ldots, y_m)$ variables (7.6a–c), which is solvable for the highest-order derivative in each of the dependent variables (7.7a–d) can be transformed (7.8a–e) to an autonomous system (7.1a–c) in Q variables. The autonomous system (7.1a–c) can be (7.34) eliminated to a decoupled ordinary differential equation of order N_1 for the dependent variable y_1; using the preceding method in the same way for all dependent variables $y_1, \ldots, y_Q$ leads to a set of Q decoupled ordinary differential equations (7.31b) of orders N_m. The highest order (7.31a) is the order (standard CCXXVI) of the system N, which cannot exceed Q leading to two* *cases: (i) if elimination for at least one dependent variable y_m leads to the maximum possible order $N_m = Q$, then the system is of order N and **independent**; (ii) if elimination for all dependent variables leads to a lower order $N < Q$ the system is **redundant** with a degree of redundancy $Q - N$.* The process of transformation of a simultaneous system of ordinary differential to find its order via the elimination of the corresponding autonomous system is illustrated next (subsection 7.3.2).

7.3.2 Transformation from a Simultaneous to a Decoupled System

As an example, consider the coupled system of two non-linear simultaneous ordinary differential equations (7.35c, d) with dependent variables y, z:

$$\{y', z'\} \equiv \left\{ \frac{dy}{dx}, \frac{dz}{dx} \right\}: \qquad y'' + z'y + y^2 = 0 = z' + zy', \qquad (7.35a\text{--}d)$$

where prime denotes (7.35a, b) derivative with regard to the independent variable x. Since the highest-order derivatives are y'' in (7.35c) and z' in (7.35d) the order of the system cannot exceed $2 + 1 = 3$, but could be lower if the equations (7.35c, d) are redundant. It is shown next that the order of the system has the maximum value 3 and thus, the equations (7.35c, d) are independent. The first step is to transform (7.35c, d) into an autonomous differential system (7.36a–c):

$$y' \equiv y_1, \qquad z' = -y_1 z, \qquad y_1' = y'' = -y^2 - z'y = -y^2 + y_1 y z, \qquad (7.36a\text{--}c)$$

with three dependent variables (y, z, y_1). The second step is to obtain two higher-order derivatives of y, beyond (7.36a), that is: (i) the second-order derivatives is given by (7.36c) $\equiv$ (7.37a), which is equivalent to (7.37a) $\equiv$ (7.37b):

$$y'' = -y^2 + y'yz \quad \Leftrightarrow \quad y'yz = y'' + y^2; \qquad (7.37a, b)$$

(ii) the third-order derivative of y is obtained (7.38a) by differentiation of (7.36c) $\equiv$ (7.37a):

$$y''' = -2yy' + yzy_1' + y_1 yz' + y_1 zy' \qquad (7.38a)$$

$$= -2y_1 y - y^3 z + y_1 y^2 z^2 - y_1^2 yz + y_1^2 z, \qquad (7.38b)$$

$$= -2y'y - y^3 z + y'y^2 z^2 - y'^2 yz + y'^2 z, \qquad (7.38c)$$

and on substitution of (7.36a, b) leads to (7.38b) and (7.38c).

The third step is to eliminate (y_1, z) among the three equations (7.36a; 7.36c; 7.38b), which is equivalent to eliminating z between the two equations (7.37b; 7.38c); the result is a relation between y and its derivatives, that is, a decoupled ordinary differential equation for y. The latter can be obtained by multiplication (7.38c) by $y_1 y = y'y$ leading to (7.39a):

$$y''' y' y = -2y'^2 y^2 - (y^3 + y'^2 y - y'^2) y' y z + y(y' y z)^2 \tag{7.39a}$$

$$= -2y'^2 y^2 - (y^3 + y'^2 y - y'^2)(y'' + y^2) + y(y'' + y^2)^2, \tag{7.39b}$$

and substitution of (7.37b) yields (7.39b). The latter (7.39b) ≡ (7.39c):

$$0 = y''' y' y - y''^2 y - y''(y^3 - y'^2 y + y'^2) + y'^2 y^2 (1+y), \tag{7.39c}$$

is a non-linear ordinary differential equation of order 3. Since this is the maximum possible order: (i) the two coupled ordinary differential equation (7.35c, d) are independent; (ii) the system (7.35c, d) is of order 3; (iii) it is not necessary to eliminate for the other variable z. The proof the coupled system of ordinary differential equations (7.35c, d) is of order 3 can be made in an alternative way (subsection 7.3.3) distinct from (subsection 7.3.2) the general method (subsection 7.3.1).

7.3.3 Constants of Integration and Depression of the Order

In the particular case of the coupled system of ordinary differential equations (7.35c, d) the proof that it is of the third order can alternatively be made as follows: (i) rewriting (7.35d) ≡ (7.40a) leads to the first integral (7.40b) relating the two dependent variables (y, z) and involving (7.40c), an arbitrary constant C:

$$-y' = \frac{z'}{z} = (\log z)', \qquad \log C - y = \log z, \quad z = Ce^{-y}; \tag{7.40a–c}$$

(ii) substitution of (7.40c) in (7.35c) ≡ (7.41a) leads to a decoupled second-order differential equation (7.41b) ≡ (7.41c) for y, involving an arbitrary constant C:

$$y'' + y^2 = -yz' = -y(Ce^{-y})' = Cy'ye^{-y}; \tag{7.41a–c}$$

(iii) this is equivalent to a third-order decoupled ordinary differential equation for y without any arbitrary constant, as follows by eliminating C.

The third step (iii) is performed as follows: (iii-1) differentiation of (7.41c) leads to (7.42):

$$y''' + 2y'y = Ce^{-y}\left[y''y + y'^2\left(1-y\right)\right];$$ (7.42)

(iii-2) elimination of the arbitrary constant between (7.41c) and (7.42) leads to (7.43):

$$\frac{y'' + y^2}{y'y} = Ce^{-y} = \frac{y''' + 2y'y}{y''y + y'^2\left(1-y\right)};$$ (7.43)

(iii-3) the latter can be rewritten as (7.43) ≡ (7.44):

$$\left(y''' + 2y'y\right)y'y = \left(y'' + y^2\right)\left[y''y + y'^2\left(1-y\right)\right],$$ (7.44)

which is a third-order decoupled ordinary differential equation for y equivalent to (7.44) ≡ (7.39c) ≡ (7.39b). Step (iii) of the proof is quite general as it concerns the elimination of arbitrary constants of integration in the general integral of an ordinary differential equation (subsection 1.1.2) and shows that the incorporation of one arbitrary constant of integration is equivalent to a **first integral** depressing the order of the differential equation by unity. More generally, *an ordinary differential equation of order N is equivalent to an ordinary differential equation of order N − P involving* $0 \le P \le N$ *arbitrary constants of integration corresponding to (standard CXXVII) first integrals. The particular case P = N is the general integral*, since no derivatives remain. The determination of the order of a simultaneous system of ordinary linear differential equations can be made as part of the solution in the cases of constant (homogeneous) coefficients [sections 7.4–7.5 (7.6–7.7)]. In these two cases, as well as for systems of simultaneous linear finite difference equations (sections 7.8–7.9) the elimination for single decoupled equations (section 7.3) is not necessary. The order of the system and its solution can be obtained by extending the method of characteristic polynomials (sections 1.3–1.9) to matrices (sections 7.4–7.9).

7.4 Linear Simultaneous System with Constant Coefficients

The general simultaneous system of M ordinary differential equations with M dependent variables and one independent variable (subsection 7.4.1) reduces in the linear case (subsection 7.4.2) to a matrix system; if the coefficients are all constant, the determinant of the matrix specifies the characteristic polynomial (subsection 7.4.3), whose degree N is the order of the system indicating whether it is degenerate or non-degenerate (subsection 7.4.4). The roots of the characteristic polynomial may be simple (multiple) and [subsection 7.4.5 (7.4.6)] specify N linearly independent particular integrals called the natural integrals, whose linear combination specifies the general integral for each of the dependent variables (subsection 7.4.7). The N constants of integration are determined by N independent initial conditions, (subsection 7.4.9), and all of the remaining coefficients follow from the compatibility of the system of simultaneous differential equations (subsection 7.4.8). The general integral for single (multiple) roots the characteristic polynomial [subsections 7.4.8–7.4.9 (7.4.10)] transform a non-diagonal to a diagonal (banded) system [subsection 7.4.13 (7.4.14)]. The mixed cases of the transformation (subsection 7.4.11) lead to diagonal block banded systems (subsection 7.4.12).

7.4.1 Linear Simultaneous System with Variable Coefficients

A simultaneous system of M ordinary differential equations (7.6c) with one dependent variable x and M dependent variables $(y_1,....,y_M)$ is **linear** (standard CXXVIII) if there are no power or products of the dependent variables or their derivatives, implying that it must be of the form:

$$m = 1,....,M: \qquad \sum_{r=1}^{M}\left\{P_{m,r}\left(\frac{d}{dx}\right)\right\}y_r(x) = B_m(x), \qquad (7.45a, b)$$

without (with) **forcing** if all B_m vanish (at least one does not vanish). The operators in (7.45b) are polynomials of ordinary derivatives of any degree (7.46a) with coefficients (7.46b) that may involve the independent variable x but not any of the dependent variable or its derivatives:

$$N_{m,r} \in | N: \qquad P_{m,r}\left(\frac{d}{dx}\right) = \sum_{k=0}^{N_{m,r}}A_{m,r,k}(x)\frac{d^k}{dx^k}. \qquad (7.46a, b)$$

Two particular cases (7.47) [(7.48)] are [standard CXXIX (CXXX)] **the constant (homogeneous) coefficients**:

$$P_{m,r}\left(\frac{d}{dx}\right) = \sum_{k=0}^{N_{m,r}}A_{m,r,k}\frac{d^k}{dx^k}, \qquad (7.47)$$

$$P_{m,r}\left(\frac{d}{dx}\right) = \sum_{k=0}^{N_{m,r}}A_{m,r,k}\,x^k\,\frac{d^k}{dx^k}; \qquad (7.48)$$

In the latter, (7.48), each derivative of order k is multiplied by the same power k of the independent variable x. In the sequel, the following are considered: (i) the general integral of a simultaneous system of unforced linear ordinary differential equations (7.45a, b) with $B_m = 0$ in the cases (7.46a, b) of constant (7.47) [homogeneous (7.48)] coefficients [section 7.4 (7.6)]; (ii) the complete integral of the forced system (section 1.2) adds a particular integral of the forced system [section 7.5 (7.7)]. The starting point (subsection 7.4.2) is the general integral of a simultaneous system of linear unforced ordinary differential equations with constant coefficients.

7.4.2 Linear Forced System with Constant Coefficients

In the presence of forcing the simultaneous system of linear ordinary differential equations (7.45a, b) with constant coefficients (7.47) equations can be written alternatively and equivalently: (i) in the algebraic form (7.49b):

$$D \equiv \frac{d}{dx} : \qquad B_m(x) = \sum_{r=1}^{M} P_{m,r}(D) y_r(x) = \sum_{r=1}^{M} \sum_{k=0}^{N_{m,r}} A_{m,r,k} \frac{d^k y_r}{dx^k}, \qquad (7.49\text{a–c})$$

involving (7.49c) the polynomials P_{ms} of degree N_{ms} of ordinary derivatives (7.49a); (ii) in the matrix form (7.50) with **the matrix of polynomials of ordinary derivatives** P_{mr}, which applies to the vector of dependent variables $y_r(x)$ and equated to **the forcing vector** $B_m(x)$:

$$
\begin{bmatrix}
P_{1,1}(D) & P_{1,2}(D) & \cdots & P_{M,1}(D) \\
P_{2,1}(D) & P_{2,2}(D) & \cdots & P_{M,2}(D) \\
\vdots & \vdots & \ddots & \vdots \\
P_{M,1}(D) & P_{M2}(D) & \cdots & P_{M,M}(D)
\end{bmatrix}
\begin{bmatrix}
y_1(x) \\
y_2(x) \\
\vdots \\
y_M(x)
\end{bmatrix}
=
\begin{bmatrix}
B_1(x) \\
B_2(x) \\
\vdots \\
B_M(x)
\end{bmatrix}.
$$

$$(7.50)$$

In the case of constant coefficients (7.49a–c), the polynomials in (7.50) commute (7.51c) with any other polynomial (7.51b):

$$m, r, s, q = 1, \dots, M:$$

$$Q_{sq}(D) = \sum_{k=0}^{N_{s,q}} B_{s,q,k}\, D^k : P_{m,r}(D) Q_{s,q}(D) y(x) = Q_{s,q}(D) P_{m,r}(D) y(x), \qquad (7.51\text{a–c})$$

and the system (7.50) can be solved for $y_1(x), \dots, y_M(x)$ as if the polynomials $P_{m,r}(D)$ were constants, leading to ordinary differential equations, which have (3.14) solutions of the form e^{ax}, in the unforced case. For example, the system of two linear unforced ordinary differential equations with constant coefficients, dependent variables y, z and independent variable x:

$$y'' + cz'' + z - y = 0 = z' + y' + y,$$
(7.52a, b)

where c is a constant, can be written:

$$D \equiv \frac{d}{dx}: \qquad \begin{bmatrix} D^2 - 1 & cD^2 + 1 \\ D + 1 & D \end{bmatrix} \begin{bmatrix} y(x) \\ z(x) \end{bmatrix} = 0,$$
(7.53a, b)

involving a 2×2 matrix (7.53b) of polynomials of ordinary derivatives (7.49a) with constant coefficients.

7.4.3 Characteristic Polynomial of a Simultaneous System

The general integral of the system of simultaneous differential equations (7.49a–c) with constant coefficients (7.50) can be obtained without performing any algebraic eliminations. For example, the unforced case (7.54):

$$\begin{bmatrix} P_{1,1}\left(\frac{d}{dx}\right) & P_{1,2}\left(\frac{d}{dx}\right) & \cdots & P_{M,1}\left(\frac{d}{dx}\right) \\ P_{2,1}\left(\frac{d}{dx}\right) & P_{2,2}\left(\frac{d}{dx}\right) & \cdots & P_{M,2}\left(\frac{d}{dx}\right) \\ \vdots & \vdots & \ddots & \vdots \\ P_{M,1}\left(\frac{d}{dx}\right) & P_{M2}\left(\frac{d}{dx}\right) & \cdots & P_{M,M}\left(\frac{d}{dx}\right) \end{bmatrix} \begin{bmatrix} y_1(t) \\ y_2(t) \\ \vdots \\ y_M(t) \end{bmatrix} = 0,$$
(7.54)

corresponds to $(7.54) \equiv (7.55a, b)$:

$$B_m(x) = 0: \qquad \sum_{r=1}^{M} P_{m,r}(D)y_r = 0; \qquad y_r(x) = E_r e^{ax},$$
(7.55a–c)

the system of linear simultaneous unforced ordinary differential equations with constant coefficients (7.55b). When eliminated (section 7.3) for any of the dependent variables $y_r(x)$ leads to a single linear ordinary differential equation with constant coefficients (1.54) that has solutions of the form of exponentials of the independent variable x (1.56a). The exponentials of the independent variable x in (7.55c) have the same parameter a and different coefficients E_r for each dependent variable $y_r(x)$. The ordinary derivative (7.53a) applied to (7.55c) is equivalent (7.56a) to multiplication by a:

$$D(e^{ax}) \equiv \frac{d}{dx}(e^{ax}) = a e^{ax}, \qquad \{P_{m,r}(D)\} e^{ax} = e^{ax} P_{m,r}(a), \qquad (7.56a, b)$$

and the same applies to a polynomial of derivatives (7.56b). Substituting (7.55c) in (7.55b) and using (7.56b) leads to (7.57a–c):

$$m,r = 1,...,M: \quad 0 = \sum_{s=1}^{M} P_{m,r}(D) E_r\, e^{ax} = e^{ax} \sum_{r=1}^{M} E_r\, P_{m,r}(a); \quad e^{ax} \neq 0, \qquad (7.57a\text{–}d)$$

since the exponential (7.57d) does not vanish, follow the linear homogeneous system of equations (7.57c) $\equiv$ (7.58b):

$$(E_1,...,E_M) \neq (0,...,0): \quad 0 = \sum_{r=1}^{M} E_r\, P_{m,r}(a), \quad P_N(a) \equiv Det\{P_{m,r}(a)\} = 0,$$

$$(7.58a\text{–}c)$$

where the constants are not all zero (7.58a); otherwise a trivial solution is obtained in (7.55c). Thus, the determinant of the coefficients must vanish (7.58c), specifying **the characteristic polynomial,** whose degree N is the **order** of the system of simultaneous linear ordinary differential equations with constant coefficients (7.49a–c) $\equiv$ (7.50), that is: (i) the number of linearly independent normal integrals; (ii) that coincides with the number of arbitrary constants of integration; (iii) and the number of independent and compatible initial conditions. *The system of **simultaneous** linear unforced ordinary differential equations with constant coefficients (7.54) $\equiv$ (7.55a, b) is (standard CXXXI) **non-degenerate (degenerate)** if the characteristic polynomial (7.58c) has the (has less than the) maximum possible degree (7.59b) [(7.59c)]:*

$$\bar{N} \equiv \sum_{m=1}^{M} \max(N_{m,r}): \qquad N \begin{cases} = \bar{N} & non\text{-}degenerate, \\ < \bar{N} & degenerate, \end{cases} \qquad (7.59a\text{–}c)$$

where the maximum is (7.55a) the sum of the highest degrees of the polynomials applied to each dependent variable.

7.4.4 Non-Degenerate and Degenerate Differential Systems

For example, the system (7.52a, b) ≡ (7.53a, b) has a characteristic polynomial:

$$
\begin{vmatrix} D^2 - 1 & cD^2 + 1 \\ D + 1 & D \end{vmatrix} = (D^2 - 1)D - (cD^2 + 1)(D+1) = (1-c)D^3 - cD^2 - 2D - 1.
$$

(7.60)

Since the highest-order derivative in (7.52a) [(7.52b)] is 2(1), the maximum possible order is $\bar{N} = 3$. The characteristic polynomial (7.60) ≡ (7.61b) is of degree $N = 3 = \bar{N}$, and the system (7.52a, b) is non-degenerate if (7.61a) is met:

$$c \neq 1: \qquad\qquad P_3(D) = (1-c)D^3 - cD^2 - 2D - 1; \qquad\qquad \text{(7.61a, b)}$$

$$c = 1: \qquad\qquad P_2(D) = -D^2 - 2D - 1, \qquad\qquad \text{(7.62a, b)}$$

the exception is the case (7.62a) when the characteristic polynomial (7.62b) is of degree $N = 2 < 3 = \bar{N}$ and the system (7.52a, b) is degenerate. The system (7.52a, b) can be eliminated for y:

$$
0 = y''' + cz''' + z' - y' = y''' - c\left(y' + y\right)'' - y' - y - y'
$$

$$
= (1-c)y''' - cy'' - 2y' - y = \left\{(1-c)D^3 - cD^2 - 2D - 1\right\}y(x) = \left\{P_3(D)\right\}y(x),
$$

(7.63)

confirming that the characteristic polynomial is of degree 3 in (7.63) ≡ (7.61b) ≡ (7.60) in the non-degenerate case (7.61a) and reduces (7.62b) to degree 2 in the degenerate case (7.62a). The natural integrals (7.55c) are specified by the roots a of the characteristic polynomial (7.58c) that [subsection 7.4.5 (7.4.6)] may be simple (multiple).

7.4.5 Distinct Roots of the Characteristic Polynomial

As in (1.54; 1.56a) *if the characteristic polynomial (7.58c) of degree N has all roots (7.64c) distinct (7.64a, b), the N linearly independent particular integrals of the system (7.54) ≡ (7.55a, b) of simultaneous unforced linear ordinary differential equations with constant coefficients are (standard CXXXII) the natural integrals (7.64d):*

$$
P_N(a_n) = 0 \neq P'(a_n): \qquad P_N(a) = A \prod_{n=1}^{N}(a - a_n), \qquad q_n(x) = \exp(a_n x). \qquad \text{(7.64a–d)}
$$

For example, for the system (7.52a, b) with (7.65a) simplifies to (7.65b, c):

$$c = 0: \qquad\qquad y'' + z - y = 0 = z' + y' + y, \qquad\qquad \text{(7.65a–c)}$$

or alternatively in matrix form (7.66):

$$\begin{bmatrix} D^2 - 1 & 1 \\ D + 1 & D \end{bmatrix} \begin{bmatrix} y(x) \\ z(x) \end{bmatrix} = 0; \qquad\qquad \text{(7.66)}$$

the corresponding characteristic polynomial (7.60) is of degree 3 (7.67a) ≡ (7.67b):

$$P_3(D) = D^3 - 2D - 1 = (D+1)(D^2 - D - 1), \qquad\qquad \text{(7.67a, b)}$$

with roots (7.68a):

$$a_{1-3} = -1, \quad \frac{1 \pm \sqrt{5}}{2}: \quad q_1(x) = e^{-x}, \quad q_{\pm}(x) = e^{x/2} \exp\left(\pm \frac{\sqrt{5}}{2} x \right), \qquad \text{(7.68a–c)}$$

leading to the three linearly independent natural integrals (7.68b, c), or alternatively, any linear combination, such as (7.69a–c):

$$q_1(x) = e^{-x}, \qquad q_{2,3}(x) = e^{x/2} \cosh, \sinh\left(\frac{\sqrt{5}}{2} x \right) = \frac{1}{2}\left[q_+(x) \pm q_-(x) \right].$$

$$\text{(7.69a–c)}$$

Next, multiple roots of the characteristic polynomial (subsection 7.4.6) are considered.

7.4.6 Multiple Roots of the Characteristic Polynomial

As (1.91a, b) for a single unforced linear ordinary differential equation with constant coefficients (subsection 1.3.6), a root of the characteristic polynomial (7.70c) with (7.70a) multiplicity α in (7.70b) corresponds to α linearly independent (7.70c) natural integrals (7.70d):

$$R_{N-\alpha}(a_0) \neq 0: \quad P_N(a) = (a - a_0)^\alpha R_{N-\alpha}(a); \quad \beta = 1, \ldots, \alpha: \quad q_\beta(t) = x^{\beta-1} \exp(a_0 x),$$

$$\text{(7.70a–d)}$$

Thus, *if the characteristic polynomial (7.58c) of degree N of the system of simultaneous unforced linear ordinary differential equations (7.54) ≡ (7.55a, b) with constant coefficients has S distinct roots (7.71b) with multiplicities (7.71a), the corresponding (standard CXXXIII) linearly independent natural integrals are (7.71c, d):*

$$\sum_{s=1}^{S}\alpha_s = N; \quad P_N(a) = A\prod_{s=1}^{S}(a - a_s)^{\alpha_s} : \beta_s = 1,....,\alpha_s : \quad q_{s,\beta_s}(x) = x^{\beta_s - 1}\exp(a_s\,x).$$

$$(7.71\text{a–d})$$

For example, in the case (7.72a) the system (7.52a, b) simplifies to (7.72b, c):

$$c = 1: \qquad\qquad y'' + z'' + z - y = 0 = z' + y' + y, \qquad\qquad (7.72\text{a–c})$$

or alternatively, in matrix form (7.73):

$$\begin{bmatrix} D^2 - 1 & D^2 + 1 \\ D + 1 & D \end{bmatrix}\begin{bmatrix} y(x) \\ z(x) \end{bmatrix} = 0; \qquad\qquad (7.73)$$

from (7.73) follows the characteristic polynomial (7.74a–c):

$$P_2(D) = D(D^2 - 1) - (D + 1)(D^2 + 1) = -D^2 - 2D - 1 = -(D + 1)^2, \qquad (7.74\text{a–c})$$

which has the double root (7.75a):

$$a_{1,2} = -1: \qquad q_1(x) = e^{-x}, \qquad\qquad q_2(x) = e^{-x}x, \qquad\qquad (7.75\text{a–c})$$

corresponding to the natural integrals (7.75b, c).

7.4.7 General Integral and Linearly Independent Particular Integrals

The general integral of the simultaneous linear unforced system of M differential equations (7.54) ≡ (7.55a, b) with constant coefficients is given by: (i) for one dependent variable, for example, the first:

$$y_1(x) = \sum_{n=1}^{N} C_n\,q_n(x), \qquad\qquad (7.76)$$

it is a linear combination of linearly independent normal integrals, involving N arbitrary constants of integration; (ii) the remaining $(M - 1)$ dependent variables (7.77a) involve no new arbitrary constants of integration, that is, they are given by a linear combination of normal integrals (7.77b):

$$\gamma = 2,\dots,M: \qquad\qquad y_\gamma(x) = \sum_{n=1}^{N} F_{\gamma n} C_n q_n(x), \qquad\qquad (7.77a, b)$$

where the constant coefficients $F_{\gamma n}$ are determined by compatibility of the system (7.54). *The preceding results may be summarized as follows: a simultaneous linear unforced system of M ordinary differential equations in M variables (7.54) with constant coefficients (7.49a–c) has order N equal to the degree of the characteristic polynomial (7.58c), which is the determinant of the matrix of polynomials in (7.54). The simple roots (7.64a–c) [roots of multiplicity α in (7.70a, b)] lead to a set of N linearly independent natural integrals (7.64c) [(7.70c, d)] each satisfying a decoupled ordinary differential equation, namely (7.78a) for simple roots [(7.78b, c) for roots of multiplicity α]:*

$$\left\{\frac{d}{dx} - a_m\right\} q_m(x) = 0; \qquad \beta = 1,\dots,\alpha: \qquad \left\{\frac{d}{dx} - a_m\right\}^\beta q_{m,\beta}(x) = 0. \qquad (7.78a\text{--}c)$$

The general integral (standard CXXXIV) is a linear combination of normal integrals namely: (i) for distinct roots of the characteristic polynomial (7.64a–d) the general integral is:

$$m = 1,\dots,M; n = 1,\dots,N: \qquad y_m(x) = \sum_{N=1}^{N} C_n F_{m,n} \exp(a_n x); \qquad (7.79a\text{--}c)$$

(ii) for multiple roots of the characteristic polynomial (7.71a–d) the general integral is:

$$y_m(x) = \sum_{s=1}^{S} \exp(a_s x) \sum_{\beta_S=1}^{\alpha_S} x^{\beta_S - 1} C_{s,\beta_S} F_{m,s,\beta_S}. \qquad (7.80)$$

In (7.79c) [(7.80)] there are N arbitrary constants of integration C_n $\left(C_{s,\beta_S}\right)$, *which is the same number as the degree of the characteristic polynomial and the order of the simultaneous differential system; the N constants of integration are determined (standard CXXXV) by N independent and compatible* **boundary conditions**. *The coefficients $F_{m,n}$ in (7.79c) [F_{m,s,β_S} in (7.80)] form a N x M matrix determined by compatibility of the system (7.54) $\equiv$ (7.55a, b) for example, (7.81a, b) [(7.81c–e)] may be specified at will:*

$$m = 1,\dots,M: \qquad F_{1,m} = 1; \quad s = 1,\dots,S; \quad \beta_s = 0,\dots,\alpha_S - 1: \quad F_{1,s,\beta_S} = 1, \qquad (7.81a\text{--}e)$$

and all others follow by substitution in (7.54) as (standard CXXXVI) **compatibil-ity conditions**. The process of determination of the general integral of the unforced system (7.54) is illustrated next for simple (multiple) roots [subsec-tions 7.4.8–7.4.9 (7.4.10)] of the characteristic polynomial (7.67a, b) [(7.74a–c)].

7.4.8 General Integral for Distinct Roots

In the case of the characteristic polynomial (7.67a, b), corresponding to the system (7.65a–c) ≡ (7.66), the three roots (7.68a) lead to the natural integrals (7.68b, c) or (7.69a–c). A linear combination specifies the general integral:

$$y(x) = C_1 e^{-x} + e^{x/2} \left[C_2 \cosh\left(\frac{\sqrt{5}}{2} x \right) + C_3 \sinh\left(\frac{\sqrt{5}}{2} x \right) \right], \tag{7.82}$$

for the first dependent variable, where (C_1, C_2, C_3) are arbitrary constants. The second dependent variable is a linear combination of the same natu-ral integrals (7.69a–c), but there cannot exist more arbitrary constants, so the coefficients are determined by compatibility with the system (7.65b, c). For example, from (7.82) follows (7.83)

$$y''(x) = C_1 e^{-x} + e^{x/2} \left[\left(\frac{3}{2} C_2 + \frac{\sqrt{5}}{2} C_3 \right) \cosh\left(\frac{\sqrt{5}}{2} x \right) + \left(\frac{3}{2} C_3 + \frac{\sqrt{5}}{2} C_2 \right) \sinh\left(\frac{\sqrt{5}}{2} x \right) \right], \tag{7.83}$$

which substituted in (7.65b) specifies the second dependent variable:

$$z(x) = y - y'' = -e^{x/2} \left[\left(\frac{1}{2} C_2 + \frac{\sqrt{5}}{2} C_3 \right) \cosh\left(\frac{\sqrt{5}}{2} x \right) + \left(\frac{1}{2} C_3 + \frac{\sqrt{5}}{2} C_2 \right) \sinh\left(\frac{\sqrt{5}}{2} x \right) \right]. \tag{7.84}$$

The three arbitrary constants are determined by three independent and compatible boundary conditions (subsection 7.4.9).

7.4.9 Arbitrary Constants and Boundary Conditions

For example, from (7.82) follows:

$$y'(x) = -C_1 e^{-x} + e^{x/2} \left[\left(\frac{1}{2} C_2 + \frac{\sqrt{5}}{2} C_3 \right) \cosh\left(\frac{\sqrt{5}}{2} x \right) + \left(\frac{1}{2} C_3 + \frac{\sqrt{5}}{2} C_2 \right) \sinh\left(\frac{\sqrt{5}}{2} x \right) \right], \tag{7.85}$$

which is used in the boundary conditions:

$$\{1,0,0\}=\{y(0),y'(0),z(0)\}=\left\{C_1+C_2,\frac{1}{2}C_2+\frac{\sqrt{5}}{2}C_3-C_1,-\frac{1}{2}C_2-\frac{\sqrt{5}}{2}C_3\right\},$$

(7.86a, b)

leading to:

$$C_1=0,\qquad C_2=1-C_1=1,\qquad C_3=-\frac{1}{\sqrt{5}}C_2=-\frac{1}{\sqrt{5}}. \qquad (7.87a\text{–}c)$$

Substituting (7.87a–c) in (7.82; 7.84), it follows that:

$$y(x)=e^{x/2}\left[\cosh\left(\frac{\sqrt{5}}{2}x\right)-\frac{1}{\sqrt{5}}\sinh\left(\frac{\sqrt{5}}{2}x\right)\right], \qquad (7.88a)$$

$$z(x)=\frac{e^{x/2}}{2}\left(\sqrt{5}-\frac{1}{\sqrt{5}}\right)\sinh\left(\frac{\sqrt{5}}{2}x\right), \qquad (7.88b)$$

or equivalently in matrix form (7.89a) ≡ (7.89b):

$$
\begin{bmatrix} y(x) \\ z(x) \end{bmatrix}=
\begin{bmatrix} 0 & 1 & -\dfrac{1}{\sqrt{5}} \\[2ex] 0 & 0 & \dfrac{1}{2}\left(\sqrt{5}-\dfrac{1}{\sqrt{5}}\right) \end{bmatrix}
\begin{bmatrix} e^{-x} \\[1ex] e^{x/2}\cosh\left(x\,\sqrt{5}/2\right) \\[1ex] e^{x/2}\sinh\left(x\,\sqrt{5}/2\right) \end{bmatrix}
$$

$$
=\begin{bmatrix} 0 & 1 & -\dfrac{1}{\sqrt{5}} \\[2ex] 0 & 0 & \dfrac{1}{2}\left(\sqrt{5}+\dfrac{1}{\sqrt{5}}\right) \end{bmatrix}
\begin{bmatrix} q_1(x) \\[1ex] q_2(x) \\[1ex] q_3(x) \end{bmatrix},
$$

(7.89a, b)

is the general integral (7.88a, b) ≡ (7.89a) ≡ (7.89b) of the system of two coupled linear unforced ordinary differential equations with constant coefficients (7.65a–c) ≡ (7.66) of order 3 satisfying the boundary conditions (7.86a).

7.4.10 General Integral with Multiple Roots

In the case of the characteristic polynomial, (7.62a, b) ≡ (7.74a–c), corresponding to the system, (7.72a–c) ≡ (7.73), the double root (7.75a) leads to the natural
integrals (7.75b, c), whose linear combination specifies the two dependent
variables (7.90a, b):

$$y(x) = e^{-x}(C_1 + C_2 x), \qquad z(x) = e^{-x}(C_3 + C_4 x). \qquad (7.90a, b)$$

There are only two arbitrary constants, (C_1, C_2) in (7.90a), with (C_3, C_4) in
(7.90b), specified by compatibility with (7.72b, c). For example, substituting
(7.90a, b) in the first (last two) terms of (7.72c) leads to (7.91a) [(7.91b, c)]:

$$z'(x) = e^{-x}(C_4 - C_3 - C_4 x), \qquad (7.91a)$$

$$-y'(x) - y(x) = e^{-x}(-C_2 + C_1 + C_2 x - C_1 - C_2 x) = -C_2 e^{-x}. \qquad (7.91b, c)$$

From (7.72c) follows (7.91a) = (7.91c), which specifies (C_3, C_4) in terms (7.92a, b)
of (C_1, C_2):

$$C_4 = 0, \quad C_3 = C_2; \qquad z(x) = C_2 e^{-x}. \qquad (7.92a\text{–}c)$$

Substituting (7.92a, b) in (7.90b) specifies the second dependent variable
(7.92c). It can be checked that (7.90a; 7.92c) satisfy (7.72b, c) for arbitrary values
of the constants of integration. The constants of integration are determined
from two independent and compatible boundary conditions, for example,
(7.93a) leads to (7.93b):

$$\{1, -1\} = \{y(0), z(0)\} = \{C_1, C_2\}. \qquad (7.93a, b)$$

Substituting (7.93a, b) in (7.90a; 7.92c) it follows that (7.94a, b):

$$y(x) = e^{-x}(1 - x), \qquad z(x) = -e^{-x}, \qquad (7.94a, b)$$

or alternatively, in matrix form (7.95a, b):

$$\begin{bmatrix} y(x) \\ z(x) \end{bmatrix} = \begin{bmatrix} 1 & -1 \\ -1 & 0 \end{bmatrix} \begin{bmatrix} e^{-x} \\ xe^{-x} \end{bmatrix} = \begin{bmatrix} 1 & -1 \\ -1 & 0 \end{bmatrix} \begin{bmatrix} q_1(x) \\ q_2(x) \end{bmatrix}, \qquad (7.95a, b)$$

is the general integral, (7.94a, b) ≡ (7.95a) ≡ (7.95b), of the system of two coupled linear unforced ordinary differential equations (7.72b, c) satisfying the
two boundary conditions (7.93a).

7.4.11 Natural Integrals and Diagonal or Banded System

If all roots of the natural characteristic polynomial (7.58c) of the $M \times M$ matrix system (7.54) are distinct (7.64a–c) the N normal integrals (7.64d) satisfy a decoupled system of N ordinary linear differential equations of first order with the roots as coefficients (7.78a) $\equiv$ (7.96a, b):

$$n = 1,\dots,N: \quad \frac{dq_n}{dx} = a_n\, q_n:$$

$$
\begin{bmatrix}
a_1 & 0 & 0 & \cdots & 0 \\
0 & a_2 & 0 & \cdots & 0 \\
\vdots & \vdots & & \ddots & \vdots \\
0 & 0 & \cdots & & a_N
\end{bmatrix}
\begin{bmatrix}
q_1(x) \\
q_2(x) \\
\vdots \\
q_N(x)
\end{bmatrix}
=
\begin{bmatrix}
dq_1/dx \\
dq_2/dx \\
\vdots \\
dq_N/dx
\end{bmatrix}
; \qquad (7.96\text{a–c})
$$

*which is equivalent (standard CXXXVII) to the $N \times N$ **diagonal system** (7.96c); thus, the transformation from simultaneous $(y_1,\dots,y_M)$ to natural $(q_1,\dots,q_N)$ dependent variables diagonalizes the system (7.54), leading to a complete decoupling. If a root of the characteristic polynomial (7.70a, b) has multiplicity α, the corresponding (standard CXXXVIII) normal integrals (7.70c, d) satisfy (7.97a–c):*

$$\frac{dq_\beta}{dx} = \frac{d}{dx}\left[x^{\beta-1}\exp(ax)\right] = \exp(ax)\left[x^{\beta-1}a + (\beta-1)x^{\beta-2}\right] = a\,q_\beta(x) + (\beta-1)q_{\beta-1}(x),$$

$$(7.97\text{a–c})$$

*and in this case, the diagonal element a_0 is replaced by a **two-banded matrix**:*

$$
\begin{bmatrix}
a & 0 & 0 & \cdots & 0 & 0 \\
1 & a & 0 & \cdots & 0 & 0 \\
0 & 2 & a & & 0 & 0 \\
\vdots & \vdots & & \ddots & \vdots & \vdots \\
0 & 0 & \cdots & & \alpha-1 & a
\end{bmatrix}
\begin{bmatrix}
q_1(x) \\
q_2(x) \\
q_3(x) \\
\vdots \\
q_\alpha(x)
\end{bmatrix}
=
\begin{bmatrix}
dq_1/dx \\
dq_2/dx \\
dq_3/dx \\
\vdots \\
dq_\alpha/dx
\end{bmatrix}
, \qquad (7.97\text{d})
$$

along the diagonal of the multiple root (7.97d), so that there is partial decoupling.

7.4.12 Block-Banded Diagonal System

For example, the characteristic polynomial (7.98a) of degree $N = 6$ with a simple $N_1 = 0$ root a_1, a double $N_2 = 2$ root a_2, and a triple $N_3 = 3$ root a_3:

$$P_6(a) = \sum_{n=1}^{6} A_n a^n = A_6 (a - a_1)(a - a_2)^2 (a - a_3)^2, \qquad (7.98a, b)$$

leads to set of six normal integrals:

$$q_1(x) = \exp(a_1 x); \quad q_{2,3}(x) = \{1, x\} \exp(a_2 x), \quad q_{4,5,6}(x) = \{1, x, x^2\} \exp(a_3 x),$$

$$(7.99a\text{–}c)$$

which satisfy:

$$
\begin{bmatrix}
a_1 & 0 & 0 & 0 & 0 & 0 \\
0 & a_2 & 0 & 0 & 0 & 0 \\
0 & 1 & a_2 & 0 & 0 & 0 \\
0 & 0 & 0 & a_3 & 0 & 0 \\
0 & 0 & 0 & 1 & a_3 & 0 \\
0 & 0 & 0 & 0 & 2 & a_3
\end{bmatrix}
\begin{bmatrix}
q_1(x) \\
q_2(x) \\
q_3(x) \\
q_4(x) \\
q_5(x) \\
q_6(x)
\end{bmatrix}
=
\begin{bmatrix}
dq_1 / dx \\
dq_2 / dx \\
dq_3 / dx \\
dq_4 / dx \\
dq_5 / dt \\
dq_6 / dx
\end{bmatrix},
\qquad (7.100)
$$

where the 6×6 matrix is divided into 1×1, 2×2, and 3×3 **diagonal blocks bands** of the type (7.97d), respectively, for the roots (a_1, a_2, a_3) of multiplicity (1, 2, 3) of the characteristic polynomial (7.98a, b). *A general unforced (7.54) linear simultaneous system of differential equations whose characteristic polynomial (7.58c) has distinct multiple roots (7.71a–c) leads to natural integrals (7.71d) that form (standard CXXXVIII) a block-banded diagonal diagonal system, like the example (7.98a, b; 7.99a–c; 7.100).* The natural integrals of the characteristic polynomial (7.67a, b) [(7.74a–c)] with three distinct roots (one double root) serves as an example of the transformation from a non-diagonal simultaneous (7.50) to a diagonal decoupled (banded minimally simultaneous) system of linear system ordinary differential equations [subsection 7.4.13 (7.4.14)].

7.4.13 Diagonalization of a Square System

For example, the third-order system (7.65a–c) ≡ (7.66) corresponds (7.53a) to **the non-diagonal matrix:**

$$
c = 0: \qquad
\begin{bmatrix}
\dfrac{d^2}{dx^2} - 1 & 1 \\[2mm]
\dfrac{d}{dx} + 1 & \dfrac{d}{dx}
\end{bmatrix}
\begin{bmatrix}
y(x) \\[2mm]
z(x)
\end{bmatrix}
= 0.
\qquad\text{(7.101a, b)}
$$

Since the characteristic polynomial (7.67a, b) has three distinct roots (7.68a), the normal integrals (7.68b) satisfy the diagonal system (7.102):

$$
\begin{bmatrix}
dq_1 / dx \\[2mm]
dq_+ / dx \\[2mm]
dq_- / dx
\end{bmatrix}
=
\begin{bmatrix}
-1 & 0 & 0 \\[2mm]
0 & \dfrac{1+\sqrt{5}}{2} & 0 \\[2mm]
0 & 0 & \dfrac{1-\sqrt{5}}{2}
\end{bmatrix}
\begin{bmatrix}
q_1(x) \\[2mm]
q_+(x) \\[2mm]
q_-(x)
\end{bmatrix}.
\qquad\text{(7.102)}
$$

The diagonalization from (7.101b) to (7.102) corresponds, in general, to (7.82) [(7.84)] leading: (i) to (7.103a) [(7.104a)] by (7.69a, b):

$$
y(x) = C_1\, q_1(x) + C_2 q_1(x) + C_3 q_3(x) = C_1 q_1(x) + \frac{C_2 + C_3}{2}\, q_+(x) + \frac{C_2 - C_3}{2}\, q_-(x);
$$

$$
\text{(7.103a, b)}
$$

$$
z(x) = -\left(\frac{1}{2}C_2 + \frac{\sqrt{5}}{2}C_3\right) q_2(x) - \left(\frac{1}{2}C_3 + \frac{\sqrt{5}}{2}C_2\right) q_3(x)
$$

$$
\text{(7.104a, b)}
$$

$$
= -\frac{1+\sqrt{5}}{4}(C_2 + C_3) q_+(x) - \frac{1-\sqrt{5}}{4}(C_2 - C_3)\, q_+(x);
$$

(ii) to (7.103b) [(7.104b)] by (7.69a, c).

Introducing the new alternative arbitrary constants (7.105a) leads from (7.103b) [(7.104b)] to (7.105b) [(7.105c)]:

$$
C_\pm \equiv \frac{C_2 \pm C_3}{2}: \qquad y(x) = C_1\, q_1(x) + C_+\, q_+(x) + C_-\, q_-(x),
$$

$$
\text{(7.105a–c)}
$$

$$
z(x) = -\frac{1+\sqrt{5}}{2} C_+\, q_+(x) - \frac{1-\sqrt{5}}{2} C_-\, q_-(x),
$$

which corresponds to the transformation from the natural variables (7.68b, c) to the dependent variables (7.105b, c) ≡ (7.106):

$$
\begin{bmatrix} y(x) \\ z(x) \end{bmatrix} = \begin{bmatrix} C_1 & C_+ & C_- \\ 0 & -\dfrac{1+\sqrt{5}}{2}C_+ & -\dfrac{1-\sqrt{5}}{2}C_- \end{bmatrix} \begin{bmatrix} q_1(x) \\ q_+(x) \\ q_-(x) \end{bmatrix}, \qquad (7.106)
$$

in general. In the particular case of the boundary conditions (7.86a), the constants (7.105a) are given (7.87a–c) by (7.107a) and simplify the transformation (7.106) to (7.107b):

$$
C_\pm = \frac{1}{2}\left(1\mp\frac{1}{\sqrt{5}}\right): \begin{bmatrix} y(x) \\ z(x) \end{bmatrix}
$$

$$
= \begin{bmatrix} 1 & \dfrac{1}{2}\left(1-\dfrac{1}{\sqrt{5}}\right) & \dfrac{1}{2}\left(1+\dfrac{1}{\sqrt{5}}\right) \\ 0 & \dfrac{1}{4}\left(\dfrac{1}{\sqrt{5}}-\sqrt{5}\right) & \dfrac{1}{4}\left(\sqrt{5}-\dfrac{1}{\sqrt{5}}\right) \end{bmatrix} \begin{bmatrix} q_1(x) \\ q_+(x) \\ q_-(x) \end{bmatrix}. \qquad (7.107a\text{–}c)
$$

Substitution of (7.105b, c) in the boundary conditions, (7.86a) ≡ (7.108a), leads to (7.108b):

$$
\{1,0,0\} = \{y(0), y'(0), z(0)\}
$$

$$
= \left\{ C_1 + C_+ + C_-, -C_1 + \frac{1+\sqrt{5}}{2}C_+ + \frac{1-\sqrt{5}}{2}C_-, -\frac{1+\sqrt{5}}{2}C_+ - \frac{1-\sqrt{5}}{2}C_- \right\};
$$

$$
(7.108a, b)
$$

the solution of (7.108b) is (7.109a–c):

$$
C_1 = 0, \quad C_- = 1 - C_+, \quad C_+ = -\frac{1-\sqrt{5}}{1+\sqrt{5}}C_- = \frac{\left(1-\sqrt{5}\right)^2}{4}C_- = \frac{3-\sqrt{5}}{2}(1-C_+);
$$

$$
(7.109a\text{–}c)
$$

solving (7.109c) for C_+ confirms the value (7.109c) ≡ (7.110a) ≡ (7.107a):

$$
C_+ = \frac{3-\sqrt{5}}{5-\sqrt{5}} = \frac{\left(3-\sqrt{5}\right)\left(5+\sqrt{5}\right)}{20} = \frac{10-2\sqrt{5}}{20} = \frac{1}{2} - \frac{1}{2\sqrt{5}}, \qquad (7.110a, b)
$$

and (7.109b) ≡ (7.110a) ≡ (7.107a) confirm the value of C_-.

7.4.14 Transformation from a Non-Diagonal to a Banded System

For example, the second-order system (7.72a–c) ≡ (7.73) corresponds (7.53a) to the non-diagonal matrix:

$$c = 1: \qquad \begin{bmatrix} \dfrac{d^2}{dx^2} - 1 & \dfrac{d^2}{dx^2} + 1 \\[3mm] \dfrac{d}{dx} + 1 & \dfrac{d}{dx} \end{bmatrix} \begin{bmatrix} y(x) \\[3mm] z(x) \end{bmatrix} = 0. \qquad (7.111)$$

Since the characteristic polynomial (7.74c) has a double root (7.75a), the natural integrals (7.75b, c) satisfy:

$$\frac{dq_1}{dx} = -e^{-x} = -q_1(x), \qquad \frac{dq_2}{dx} = e^{-x}(1-x) = q_1(x) - q_2(x), \qquad (7.112a, b)$$

corresponding to the banded system:

$$\begin{bmatrix} dq_1 / dx \\[3mm] dq_2 / dx \end{bmatrix} = \begin{bmatrix} -1 & 0 \\ 1 & -1 \end{bmatrix} \begin{bmatrix} q_1(x) \\[3mm] q_2(x) \end{bmatrix}. \qquad (7.113)$$

The transformation from a non-diagonal system (7.111) to a banded system (7.113) corresponds to (7.90a; 7.92c) ≡ (7.114):

$$\begin{bmatrix} y(x) \\[3mm] z(x) \end{bmatrix} = \begin{bmatrix} C_1 & C_2 \\ C_2 & 0 \end{bmatrix} \begin{bmatrix} q_1(x) \\[3mm] q_2(x) \end{bmatrix}, \qquad (7.114)$$

in general, simplifying to (7.115):

$$\begin{bmatrix} y(x) \\[3mm] z(x) \end{bmatrix} = \begin{bmatrix} 1 & -1 \\ -1 & 0 \end{bmatrix} \begin{bmatrix} q_1(x) \\[3mm] q_2(x) \end{bmatrix}, \qquad (7.115)$$

for the boundary conditions (7.93a, b).

7.5 Integrals of Forced and Unforced Systems

The complete integral [section 1.2.6 (7.5.7)] of a single (simultaneous system of) linear forced ordinary differential equation(s) with variable coefficients [subsection 1.2.1 (7.4.1)] consists of the sum of: (i) the general integral [subsection 1.2.4 (section 7.4)] of the unforced equation(s), which contains all of the necessary constants of integration; (ii) any particular integral of the forced equation(s) [subsection 1.2.5 (section 7.5)], the simpler the better. In the case of a single (simultaneous system of) linear ordinary differential equation(s) with constant coefficients the characteristic polynomial (matrix of polynomials of derivatives) specifies: (i) the general integral of the unforced system [section 1.4 (7.4); (ii) the forcing by exponential, circular, and hyperbolic sines and cosines and their products [subsection 1.5 (subsections 7.5.1–7.5.5); (iii) the forcings involving powers by using inverse polynomials (matrices of polynomials) of derivatives [section 1.5 (subsections 7.5.6–7.5.7)]. Since the methods are similar (sections 1.4–1.5) a shorter account is given concerning a particular integral of a simultaneous system of linear ordinary differential equations with constant coefficients with forcing by: (i) exponentials (subsection 7.5.1), including non-resonant and resonant cases [subsection 7.5.3] and single and multiple resonances (subsection 5.7.2); (ii) the product of exponentials by circular or hyperbolic cosines and sines (subsections 7.5.4–7.5.5); (iii) powers or polynomials (subsections 7.5.6–7.5.7). The principle of superposition applies to simultaneous systems of linear differential equations and allows addition of particular integrals (subsection 7.5.8).

7.5.1 Forcing of a Simultaneous System by an Exponential

Consider a simultaneous system of linear ordinary differential equations with constant coefficients (7.49a–c) ≡ (7.50) with exponential (7.116b) forcing terms (7.116a):

$$B_m(x) = G_m e^{bx}: \qquad \sum_{r=1}^{M}\left\{P_{m,r}\left(\frac{d}{dx}\right)\right\}y_m(x) = G_m e^{bx}. \qquad (7.116a, b)$$

The solution is sought as a similar exponential (7.117a) with coefficients H_r to be determined (7.117b) by substitution into (7.116b):

$$y_r(x) = H_r e^{bx}: \qquad G_m e^{bx} = \sum_{r=1}^{M}P_{m,r}(D)H_r e^{bx} = e^{bx}\sum_{r=1}^{M}P_{m,r}(b)H_r, \qquad (7.117a, b)$$

where (7.56b) was used. Using also (7.57d) ≡ (7.118a) from (7.117b) follows a linear inhomogeneous system of equations (7.118b):

$$e^{bx} \neq 0: \qquad\qquad G_m = \sum_{r=1}^{M} P_{m,r}(b) H_r. \qquad\qquad (7.118a, b)$$

The matrix of polynomials of derivatives $P_{m,r}$, multiplied by the matrix of co-factors $\bar{P}_{\ell,m}$, equals (7.119a, b), the identity matrix times the determinant, which is (7.58c) the characteristic polynomial in (7.119c):

$$m, r, \ell = 1, ..., M: \quad \sum_{m=1}^{M} \bar{P}_{\ell,m}(b) P_{m,r}(b) = \delta_{\ell r} \, Det\left[P_{m,r}(b) \right] = \delta_{\ell r} \, P_N(b). \qquad (7.119a\text{–}c)$$

Substitution of (7.119b, c) allows inversion of (7.118b):

$$\sum_{m=1}^{M} \bar{P}_{\ell,m}(b) \, G_m = \sum_{m=1}^{M} \bar{P}_{\ell,m}(b) \sum_{r=1}^{M} P_{m,r} \, H_r = \sum_{r=1}^{M} P_N(b) \delta_{\ell r} \, H_r = P_N(b) H_\ell, \qquad (7.120)$$

expressing the unknown H_r in (7.120) in terms of the known G_m. In the **non-resonant** case, when b is not a root of the characteristic polynomial (7.121a), it can be divided in (7.120) and substituting H_r in (7.117a):

$$P_N(b) \neq 0: \qquad\qquad y_r(x) = \frac{e^{bx}}{P_N(b)} \sum_{m=1}^{M} \bar{P}_{\ell,m}(b) \, G_m, \qquad\qquad (7.121a, b)$$

specifies the particular integral (7.121b). The case when b is a simple (multiple) root of the characteristic polynomial leads to simple (multiple) resonant forcing (subsection 7.5.2).

7.5.2 Single and Multiple Resonant Forcing

In the **resonant case** when b is a root of multiplicity α of the characteristic polynomial (7.122a) the particular integral is (7.122b):

$$P_N(b) = P_N'(b) = ... = P_N^{(\alpha-1)}(b) = 0 \neq P_N^{(\alpha)}(b):$$

$$y_r(x) = \left[P_N^{(\alpha)}(b) \right]^{-1} \sum_{m=1}^{M} G_m \frac{\partial^\alpha}{\partial b^\alpha} \left[e^{bx} \bar{P}_{r,m}(b) \right], \qquad (7.122a, b)$$

as follows (subsection 1.4.2) by L'Hôspital rule, (I.19.35) ≡ (1.140): (i) the characteristic polynomial in the denominator of (7.121b) has a root (7.122a) of multiplicity α; (ii) from the numerator of (7.121b) can be subtracted a linear combination of particular integrals (7.70a–d) of the unforced equation (7.54), leading also to a root of multiplicity α; (iii) thus, (7.121b) becomes an indeterminacy of type 0:0 with zeros of equal multiplicity α in the numerator and denominator; (iv) the indeterminacy is lifted by L'Hôspital rule (section 1.9.8) by differentiating (I.19.34) separately the numerator and denominator α times leading from (7.121b) to (7.122b). Note that in (7.122b): (i) the denominator is the lowest-order derivative of the characteristic polynomial that does not vanish (7.122a), that is, the order of differentiation α coincides with the multiplicity of the root; (ii) in the numerator the Leibnitz rule, (I.13.31) ≡ (7.123), may be applied:

$$\frac{\partial^\alpha}{\partial b^\alpha}\left\{e^{bx}\,\bar{P}_{r,m}(b)\right\}=\sum_{\gamma=0}^{\alpha}\left(\begin{array}{c}\alpha\\\gamma\end{array}\right)\bar{P}_{r,m}^{(\alpha-\gamma)}(b)\frac{\partial^\gamma}{\partial b^\gamma}\left(e^{bx}\right),\qquad(7.123)$$

showing that the forced particular integral (7.122d):

$$y_r(x)=\frac{e^{bx}}{P_N^{(\alpha)}(b)}\sum_{\gamma=0}^{\alpha}\frac{\alpha!\,x^\gamma}{\gamma!(\alpha-\gamma)!}\sum_{m=0}^{M}G_m\,\bar{P}_{r,m}^{(\alpha-\gamma)}(b),\qquad(7.124)$$

involves the product of exponentials by power $e^{bx}x^\gamma$ up to one degree $\gamma=\alpha$ higher than $\gamma=0,1,...,\alpha-1=\beta$ in the unforced particular integrals (7.70a–d). It has been shown that *the simultaneous system of linear ordinary differential equations with constant coefficients (7.49a–c) ≡ (7.50) and exponential forcing (7.116a) has (standard CXXXIX) particular integral (7.121b) [(7.122b)] in the non-resonant (resonant) case when b is not a root (7.121a) [is a root (7.122a) of multiplicity α] of the characteristic polynomial (7.58c) and $\bar{P}_{r,m}$ denote the co-factors (7.119a–c) of the matrix of polynomials. The simple (multiple) resonance corresponds to a simple (7.125a, b) [multiple (7.122a, b) ≡ (7.124)] root of the characteristic polynomial:*

$$P_N(b)=0\neq P_N'(b):\qquad y_r(x)=\frac{e^{bx}}{P_N'(b)}\sum_{m=1}^{M}G_m\left[\bar{P}_{r,m}'(b)+x\bar{P}_{r,m}(b)\right].\qquad(7.125a,b)$$

Next are given examples of both non-resonant (7.114a, b) and resonant (7.115a, b) exponential forcing (subsection 7.5.3).

7.5.3 Non-Resonant and Resonant Forcing by an Exponential

The coupled system of linear ordinary differential equations with constant coefficients (7.52a, b) in the degenerate case (7.72a–c) with exponential forcing terms:

$$y''+z''+z-y=e^{bx},\qquad\qquad z'+y'+y=2e^{bx},\qquad(7.126a,b)$$

is equivalent in matrix form to:

$$\begin{bmatrix} D^2 - 1 & D^2 + 1 \\ D+1 & D \end{bmatrix} \begin{bmatrix} y(x) \\ z(x) \end{bmatrix} = e^{bx} \begin{bmatrix} 1 \\ 2 \end{bmatrix};$$ (7.127)

the matrix of polynomials of derivatives is (7.128a):

$$P_{m,r}(D) = \begin{bmatrix} D^2 - 1 & D^2 + 1 \\ D+1 & D \end{bmatrix}, \quad \bar{P}_{r,\ell}(D) = \begin{bmatrix} D & -D^2 - 1 \\ -D-1 & D^2 - 1 \end{bmatrix},$$

(7.128a, b)

specifying the matrix of co-factors (7.128b) and the determinant specifying the characteristic polynomial (7.74a–c) with double root (7.75a). Substitution in (7.121b) leads for all non-resonant cases (7.129a) to the particular integral (7.129b):

$$b \neq -1: \quad \begin{bmatrix} y(x) \\ z(x) \end{bmatrix} = -\frac{e^{bx}}{(b+1)^2} \begin{bmatrix} b & -b^2 - 1 \\ -b-1 & b^2 - 1 \end{bmatrix} \begin{bmatrix} 1 \\ 2 \end{bmatrix}$$

(7.129a, b)

$$= \frac{e^{bx}}{(b+1)^2} \begin{bmatrix} 2b^2 - b + 2 \\ -2b^2 + b + 3 \end{bmatrix}.$$

In the case of resonance (7.130a) should be used (7.122b) for a root (7.122a) of multiplicity $\alpha = 2$, leading to (7.130b):

$$b = -1: \quad \begin{bmatrix} y(x) \\ z(x) \end{bmatrix} = \frac{1}{P_2''(-1)} \lim_{b \to -1} \frac{\partial^2}{\partial b^2} \left\{ e^{bx} \begin{bmatrix} b & -b^2 - 1 \\ -b-1 & b^2 - 1 \end{bmatrix} \begin{bmatrix} 1 \\ 2 \end{bmatrix} \right\}$$

$$= -\frac{1}{2} \lim_{b \to -1} \frac{\partial^2}{\partial b^2} \left\{ e^{bx} \begin{bmatrix} b - 2b^2 - 2 \\ 2b^2 - b - 3 \end{bmatrix} \right\}$$

$$= \frac{e^{-x}}{2} \lim_{b \to -1} \left\{ x^2 \begin{bmatrix} 2 - b + 2b^2 \\ 3 + b - 2b^2 \end{bmatrix} + 2x \begin{bmatrix} 4b - 1 \\ 1 - 4b \end{bmatrix} + \begin{bmatrix} 4 \\ -4 \end{bmatrix} \right\},$$

(7.130a, b)

which simplifies to:

$$y(x) = e^{-x} \left(\frac{5}{2} x^2 - 5x + 2 \right), \qquad z(x) = e^{-x}(5x - 2); \qquad (7.131a, b)$$

this is a particular integral of:

$$x'' + y'' + z - y = e^{-x}, \qquad z' + y' + y = 2e^{-x}, \qquad (7.132a, b)$$

that is, $(7.126a, b) \equiv (7.127)$ with $(7.130a)$ yields $(7.132a, b)$.

7.5.4 Forcing by the Product of an Exponential by a Sine or Cosine

As an extension of (7.116b; 7.121a, b), it follows that: *a particular integral of the linear system of simultaneous ordinary differential equations with constant coefficients (7.45a, b) $\equiv$ (7.50) with forcing term: (i) a product of an exponential and hyperbolic sine or cosine or cosine (7.133a):*

$$B_m(x) = G_m e^{bx} \cosh, \sinh(cx) = \frac{1}{2}G_m\left[e^{(b+c)x} \pm e^{(b-c)x}\right], \qquad (7.133a)$$

$$y_r(x) = \frac{1}{2}\sum_{m=1}^{M}G_m\left[\frac{e^{(b+c)x}}{P_N(b+c)}\,\bar{P}_{r,m}(b+c) \pm \frac{e^{(b-c)x}}{P_N(b-c)}\,\bar{P}_{r,m}(b-c)\right], \qquad (7.133b)$$

is given (standard CXL) by (7.133b); (ii) a product of an exponential and a circular sine or cosine (7.134a) is given (standard CXLI) by (7.134b):

$$B_m(x) = G_m e^{bx} \cos, \sin(gx) = \frac{1}{\{2, 2i\}}G_m\left\{e^{(b+ig)x} \pm e^{(b-ig)x}\right\}, \qquad (7.134a)$$

$$y_r(x) = \frac{1}{\{2, 2i\}}\sum_{m=1}^{M}G_m\left[\frac{e^{(b+ig)x}}{P_N(b+ig)}\,\bar{P}_{r,m}(b+ig) \pm \frac{e^{(b-ig)x}}{P_N(b-ig)}\,\bar{P}_{r,m}(b-ig)\right],$$

$$(7.134b)$$

which simplifies to (7.135d) for (7.135a–c) real a, b, and real polynomials $P_{m,r}$:

$$b, g, P_{m,r} \in | R: \qquad B_m(x) = G_m e^{bx} \operatorname{Re}, \operatorname{Im}(e^{igx}), \qquad (7.135a–d)$$

$$y_r(x) = \sum_{m=1}^{M}G_m x^b \operatorname{Re}, \operatorname{Im}\left\{e^{igx}\frac{\bar{P}_{r,m}(b+ig)}{P_N(b+ig)}\right\}; \qquad (7.135e)$$

(iii) a product of an exponential by a hyperbolic and a circular cosine or sine (7.136e):

$$b, c, g, P_{m,r} \in | R: \qquad B_m(x) = G_m e^{bx} \cosh, \sinh(cx)\cos, \sin(gx)$$

$$(7.136a–e)$$

$$= \frac{1}{2}G_m \operatorname{Re}, \operatorname{Im}\left\{e^{(b+c+ig)x} \pm e^{(b-c+ig)x}\right\},$$

$$y_r(x) = \frac{e^{bx}}{2} \sum_{m=1}^{M} G_m \, \mathrm{Re},$$

$$\mathrm{Im}\left\{ \frac{e^{(ig+c)x}}{P_N(b+c+ig)} \bar{P}_{r,m}(b+c+ig) \pm \frac{e^{(ig-c)x}}{P_N(b-c+ig)} \bar{P}_{r,m}(b-c+ig) \right\},$$

(7.136f)

is given (standard CXLII) by (7.136f) for real b, c, g and real matrix of polynomials of derivatives (7.136a–d). In (7.133b)/(7.134b)/(7.135d)/(7.136b) it was assumed that $b \pm c / b \pm ic / b + ic / b \pm c + ig$ are not roots of the characteristic polynomial; otherwise the corresponding term has to be modified as in the passage from (7.121a, b) to (7.122a, b) ≡ (7.124). The example given next (subsection 7.5.5) corresponds to (7.135a, b) with a cosine.

7.5.5 Forcing by Hyperbolic or Circular Cosines or Sines

As an example, consider the coupled system of linear ordinary differential equations with constant coefficients (7.72b, c) forced by the product of an exponential and a circular cosine (7.137a, b):

$$y'' + z'' + z - y = 2e^x \cos(2x) = 2\mathrm{Re}\left\{ \exp\left[(1+2i)x\right] \right\}, \qquad (7.137a)$$

$$z' + y' + y = e^x \cos(2x) = \mathrm{Re}\left\{ \exp\left[(1+2i)x\right] \right\}. \qquad (7.137b)$$

Since $b = 1 + 2i \neq -1$ in (7.138a, b), this is a non-resonant case, so (7.121a, b) should be used, with (7.128b) and taking the real part in (7.135a–c) leads to (7.138b):

$$\begin{bmatrix} y(x) \\ z(x) \end{bmatrix} = \lim_{b \to 1+2i} \mathrm{Re}\left\{ -\frac{e^{bx}}{(b+1)^2} \begin{bmatrix} b & -b^2-1 \\ -b-1 & b^2-1 \end{bmatrix} \begin{bmatrix} 2 \\ 1 \end{bmatrix} \right\}$$

$$= \lim_{b \to 1+2i} \mathrm{Re}\left\{ \frac{e^{bx}}{(b+1)^2} \begin{bmatrix} 1-2b+b^2 \\ 3+2b-b^2 \end{bmatrix} \right\}$$

(7.138a, b)

$$= \mathrm{Re}\left\{ \frac{e^{(1+2i)x}}{(2+2i)^2} \begin{bmatrix} -1-4\,i+(1+2i)^2 \\ 5+2i-(1+2\,i)^2 \end{bmatrix} \right\}$$

$$= \frac{e^x}{8} \mathrm{Re}\left\{ \frac{e^{2ix}}{i} \begin{bmatrix} -4 \\ 8-2i \end{bmatrix} \right\} = \frac{e^x}{4} \mathrm{Re}\left\{ e^{2ix} \begin{bmatrix} 2i \\ -1-4i \end{bmatrix} \right\},$$

which is equivalent to:

$$y(x) = -\frac{e^x}{2}\sin(2x), \qquad z(x) = e^x\left[\sin(2x) - \frac{1}{4}\cos(2x)\right], \qquad (7.139a, b)$$

as a particular integral of (7.137a, b).

7.5.6 Inverse Matrix of Polynomials of Derivatives

A particular integral of the simultaneous forced linear system of ordinary differential equations with constant coefficients (7.49a–c) ≡ (7.50) is formally given by (7.140):

$$\frac{1}{P_N(D)}\sum_{m=1}^{M}\overline{P}_{\ell,m}(D)B_m(x) = \frac{1}{P_N(D)}\sum_{m=1}^{M}\overline{P}_{\ell,m}(D)P_{m,r}(D)y_r(x) = \sum_{r=1}^{M}\delta_{\ell r}\,y_r(x) = y_\ell(x),$$

$$(7.140)$$

where the inversion of matrices (7.119a–c) applied to ordinary derivatives (7.53a) was used; there is a formal similarity between (7.120) ≡ (7.140) replacing the constant b by an ordinary derivative (7.53a). The formal particular integral:

$$y_r(x) = \frac{1}{P_N(D)}\sum_{m=1}^{M}\overline{P}_{r,m}(D)B_m(x), \qquad (7.141)$$

uses an inverse characteristic polynomial of derivatives (section 1.5). Thus, *the simultaneous linear forced system of ordinary differential equations with constant coefficients (7.49a–c) ≡ (7.50) has (standard CXLIII) a particular integral (7.141) where: (i) appears the matrix of co-factors (7.119a–c) of the matrix of polynomials in (7.50); (ii) the inverse of the characteristic polynomial (7.58c) is interpreted (section 1.5) as a series of derivatives applied to the forcing functions $B_m(x)$ that must converge (1); (iii) if the forcing functions $B_m(x)$ are polynomials with degrees b_m, then all derivatives of order $k > b_m$ vanish and no convergence issues arise.* An example of polynomial forcing is considered next (subsection 7.5.7).

7.5.7 Power Series Expansion of Inverse Polynomial Operator

The coupled linear system of ordinary differential equations with constant coefficients (7.72b, c) with forcing by power of the independent variable (7.142a, b):

$$y'' + z'' + z - y = x, \qquad z' + y' + y = x^2, \qquad (7.142a, b)$$

can be written in the form emphasizing the matrix of polynomials of derivatives:

$$D \equiv \frac{d}{dx}: \qquad \begin{bmatrix} D^2 - 1 & D^2 + 1 \\ D + 1 & D \end{bmatrix} \begin{bmatrix} y(x) \\ z(x) \end{bmatrix} = \begin{bmatrix} x \\ x^2 \end{bmatrix}; \qquad (7.143a, b)$$

this suggests the formal solution (7.141) using the characteristic polynomial (7.74c) and the matrix of co-factors (7.128b) of the matrix of polynomials of derivatives of derivatives (7.128a):

$$\begin{bmatrix} y(x) \\ z(x) \end{bmatrix} = \frac{1}{(1+D)^2} \begin{bmatrix} -D & 1+D^2 \\ 1+D & 1-D^2 \end{bmatrix} \begin{bmatrix} x \\ x^2 \end{bmatrix}$$

$$\qquad\qquad (7.144)$$

$$= \frac{1}{(1+D)^2} \begin{bmatrix} -1 + x^2 + 2 \\ x+1+ x^2 - 2 \end{bmatrix} = \frac{1}{(1+D)^2} \begin{bmatrix} x^2 + 1 \\ x^2 + x - 1 \end{bmatrix}.$$

Since on the right-hand side (r.h.s.) of (7.144) appear polynomials of degree 2, the derivatives of higher order ≥ 3 vanish, and the inverse of the characteristic polynomial needs to be expanded explicitly only to $O(D^2)$ using: (i) the geometric series (I.21.62c) $\equiv$ (7.145a):

$$\frac{1}{1+D} = 1 - D + D^2 + O(D^3); \qquad (7.145a)$$

$$\frac{1}{(1+D)^2} = (1 - D + D^2)^2 + O(D^3) = (1-D)^2 + 2D^2 (1-D) + O(D^3)$$

$$\qquad\qquad (7.145b)$$

$$= 1 - 2D + 3D^2 + O(D^3),$$

(ii) its square, (7.145b) $\equiv$ (I.25.40c), which corresponds to a binomial series. Substituting (7.145b) in (7.144) gives:

$$\begin{bmatrix} y(x) \\ z(x) \end{bmatrix} = \left[1 - 2D + 3D^2 + O(D^3) \right] \begin{bmatrix} x^2 + 1 \\ x^2 + x - 1 \end{bmatrix} = \begin{bmatrix} x^2 + 1 - 4x + 6 \\ x^2 + x - 1 - 4x - 2 + 6 \end{bmatrix},$$

$$\qquad\qquad (7.146)$$

as the particular integrals:

$$y(x) = x^2 - 4x + 7, \qquad\qquad z(x) = x^2 - 3x + 3, \qquad (7.147a, b)$$

of (7.142a, b) $\equiv$ (7.143a, b).

7.5.8 Principle of Superposition and Addition of Particular Integrals

The principle of superstition (subsection 1.2.1) applies both to single (simultaneous systems of) linear ordinary differential equation(s) and allows: (i) linear combinations of linearly independent particular integrals in the general integral of the unforced system (section 7.4); (ii) addition of particular integrals corresponding to distinct forcings in the complete integral (section 7.5). As an example, the complete integral of the coupled system of forced system of forced linear ordinary differential equations with constant coefficients (7.148a, b) is considered:

$$y'' + z'' + z - y = e^{3x} + e^{-x} + 2e^x \cos(2x) + x, \tag{7.148a}$$

$$z' + y' + y = 2e^{3x} + 2e^{-x} + e^x \cos(2x) + x^2, \tag{7.148b}$$

consisting of: (i) the general integral (7.90a; 7.92c) of the unforced degenerate system (7.52a, b; 7.72a) ≡ (7.72b, c) ≡ (7.73) of order 2 involving two arbitrary constants $(C_1, C_1) \equiv (A, B)$:

$$\bar{y}(x) = e^{-x}(A + Bx) + \frac{17}{16}e^{3x} + e^{-x}\left(\frac{5}{2}x^2 - 5x + 2\right) - \frac{e^x}{2}\sin(2x) + x^2 - 4x + 7,$$
$$\tag{7.149a}$$

$$\bar{z}(x) = e^{-x}B - \frac{3}{4}e^{3x} + e^{-x}(5x - 2) + e^{-x}\left[\sin(2x) - \frac{1}{4}\cos(2x)\right] + x^2 - 3x + 3;$$
$$\tag{7.149b}$$

(ii) plus the particular integrals of the forced system, namely (7.129a, b) with $b = 3$ for the exponential non-resonant forcing (7.126a, b) ≡ (7.127), plus (7.131a, b) for the exponential resonant forcing (7.132a, b), plus (7.139a, b) for the forcing by the product of an exponential by a circular cosine (7.137a, b), plus (7.147a, b) for the forcing by powers (7.142a, b) ≡ (7.143a, b). Thus, *(7.149a, b) is (standard CXLIV) the complete integral of (7.148a, b). Also, two independent and compatible boundary conditions (7.93a) [≡ (7.150a)] applied to the general (7.90a; 7.92c) [complete (7.149a, b)] integral of the unforced (7.72b, c) [forced (7.147a, b)] system of coupled linear ordinary differential equations with constant coefficients lead to: (i) the arbitrary constants (7.93b) [(7.150b)]:*

$$\{1, -1\} = \{\bar{y}(0), \quad \bar{z}(0)\} = \left\{A + \frac{161}{16}, \quad B\right\}, \quad \{A, B\} = \left\{-\frac{145}{16}, -1\right\}, \tag{7.150a–c}$$

in the unique solution (7.94a, b) ≡ (7.95a) [(7.149a, b; 7.150c)]. In (7.149a, b) the particular integrals of the forced differential system, such as $e^{-x}(e^{-x}x)$, should not be included in the arbitrary constants of integration $A(B)$ because this could be inconsistent with the compatibility relations between the dependent variables y and z.

7.6 Natural Integrals for Simultaneous Homogeneous Systems

The characteristic polynomial (matrix of polynomials of derivatives) applies to a single (simultaneous system of) linear differential equation(s) with: (i) constant coefficients [sections 1.3–1.5 (7.4–7.5)] using ordinary derivatives; (ii) power coefficients [sections 1.6–1.7 (7.6–7.7)] using homogeneous derivatives. Concerning the simultaneous linear system of ordinary differential equations with homogeneous coefficients (subsection 7.6.1), in the unforced (section 7.6) case: (i) the system involves a matrix of polynomials of homogeneous derivatives (subsection 7.6.2); (ii) its determinant specifies the characteristic polynomial (subsection 7.6.3); (iii) the simple (multiple) root(s) of the characteristic polynomial lead to (subsection 7.6.4) the natural integrals, which are powers (multiplied by logarithms) and specify the exponent(s); (iv) the general integral is a linear combination of the natural integrals (subsection 7.6.5) whose coefficients are arbitrary constants of integration for one dependent variable; (v) the remaining dependent variables are also linear combinations of the natural integrals, with coefficients determined by compatibility conditions (subsection 7.6.6) arising from the simultaneous differential system; (vi) the arbitrary constants of integration are determined by an equal number of independent and compatible boundary conditions (subsection 7.6.7); (vii–viii) the dependent variables satisfy a non-diagonal system whereas (subsection 7.6.8) the natural integrals satisfy a diagonal uncoupled (two-banded diagonal minimally coupled) system for simple (multiple) roots of the characteristic polynomial (subsection 7.6.9).

7.6.1 Linear System of Homogeneous Derivatives

A simultaneous linear system of ordinary differential equations (7.45a, b) involves: (i) in the case of constant coefficients (7.47) a matrix (7.151b) of ordinary derivatives (7.151a):

$$D \equiv \frac{d}{dx}: \qquad P_{m,r}(D) = \sum_{k=1}^{N_{m,r}} A_{m,r,k} D^k; \qquad (7.151a, b)$$

$$\delta \equiv x\frac{d}{dx}: \qquad \sum_{k=1}^{N_{m,r}} A_{m,r,k} x^k D^k \equiv Q_{m,r}(\delta), \qquad (7.152a, b)$$

(ii) in the case of homogeneous coefficients (7.48) a matrix (7.152b) of homogeneous derivatives (7.152a) specified by:

$$Q_{m,r}(\delta) = \sum_{k=1}^{N_{m,r}} A_{m,r,k}\, \delta(\delta-1)...\delta(\delta-k+1), \qquad (7.153)$$

using the relation (1.304) ≡ (7.154b):

$$F \in D^k(|R): \qquad F^{(k)}(x) \equiv x^k \, D^k \, F(x) = \{\delta(\delta-1)....\delta(\delta-k+1)\} F(x), \qquad \text{(7.154a, b)}$$

which applies to a k-times differentiable function (7.154a). The proof of (7.154a, b) can be made either by (i) induction (subsection 1.6.5) or by (ii) the alternative method that is indicated next.

The proof of (7.154a, b) can be made in five steps: (i) the homogeneous derivative has the properties (7.155a, b):

$$\delta(x^a) = \left(x\frac{d}{dx}\right) x^a = a x^a, \qquad \delta^k x^a = \left(x\frac{d}{dx}\right)^k x^a = a^k x^a ; \qquad \text{(7.155a, b)}$$

(ii) choosing as function (7.154a) the power (7.156a) leads to (7.156b):

$$F(x) = x^a: x^k \, D^k x^a = a(a-1)....(a-k+1) x^a = \delta(\delta-1)....(\delta-k+1) x^a ;$$
$$\text{(7.156a, b)}$$

(iii) thus, (7.154b) is proved for a power (7.156b); (iv) a k-times differentiable function, (7.154a) ≡ (7.157a), has a MacLaurin series (I.23.34a) ≡ (7.157b):

$$F \in D^k(|R): \qquad F(x) = \sum_{\ell=0}^{k} \frac{x^k}{k!} F^{(k)}(0) + o(x^k); \qquad \text{(7.157a, b)}$$

(v) since the property (7.154b) applies to a power (7.156b) and hence, to each term of (7.157b), it also applies to the function (7.154a) ≡ (7.157a) to within higher order terms.

The proof by induction (subsection 1.6.5) does not require the use of the Taylor series; the power (7.156a, b) is the simplest example of (7.154a, b). There are analogous properties of the ordinary (7.151a) [homogeneous (7.152a)] derivatives with regard to the exponential (7.158a, b) [power (7.155a)]:

$$D(e^{ax}) \equiv \frac{d}{dx}(e^{ax}) = a e^{ax}, \qquad D^k(e^{ax}) = \frac{d^k}{dx^k}(e^{ax}) = a^k e^{ax}, \qquad \text{(7.158a, b)}$$

which extend to polynomials of ordinary (7.158c) [homogeneous (7.158d)] derivatives:

$$\{P_N(D)\} e^{ax} = e^{ax} P_N(a), \qquad \{P_N(\delta)\} x^a = x^a P_N(a), \qquad \text{(7.158c, d)}$$

and are used in the sequel (subsection 7.6.2).

7.6.2 Matrix of Polynomials of Homogeneous Derivatives

The simultaneous linear system (7.45a, b) of ordinary differential equations with homogeneous coefficients (7.45a, b; 7.48) ≡ (7.159):

$$B_m(x) = \sum_{r=1}^{M} \sum_{k=0}^{N_{m,r}} A_{m,r,k}\, x^k \frac{d^k y_r}{dx^k}, \tag{7.159}$$

can be written (standard CXLV) alternatively: (i) in terms (7.160a) of polynomials (7.153; 7.154a, b) of homogeneous derivatives (7.152a):

$$B_m(x) = \sum_{r=1}^{M} \sum_{k=0}^{N_{m,r}} A_{m,r,k}\, \delta(\delta-1)....\delta(\delta-k+1) y_r(x) = \sum_{r=1}^{M} Q_{m,r}(\delta) y_r(x); \tag{7.160a, b}$$

*(ii) equivalently, (7.160b) ≡ (7.161), using a **matrix of polynomials of homogeneous derivatives** applied to the vector of dependent variables $y_r(x)$ and equated to the forcing vector $B_m(x)$:*

$$
\begin{bmatrix}
Q_{1,2}(\delta) & Q_{1,2}(\delta)... Q_{1,M}(\delta) \\
Q_{1,2}(\delta) & Q_{2,2}(\delta)... Q_{2,M}(\delta) \\
\vdots & \vdots \quad \vdots \ \ddots \quad \vdots \\
Q_{M,2}(\delta) & Q_{M,2}(\delta)... Q_{M,M}(\delta)
\end{bmatrix}
\begin{bmatrix}
y_1(x) \\
y_2(x) \\
\vdots \\
y_M(x)
\end{bmatrix}
=
\begin{bmatrix}
B_1(x) \\
B_2(x) \\
\vdots \\
B_M(x)
\end{bmatrix}. \tag{7.161}
$$

As an example, consider the coupled unforced linear system of ordinary differential equations with homogeneous coefficients, with dependent variables y, z and dependent variable x:

$$x^2 y'' - x y' + x z' + y - z = 0 = 2 x y' + x z' - 2 y; \tag{7.162a, b}$$

the corresponding matrix form using (7.154b) homogeneous (7.152a) instead of ordinary (7.151a) derivatives is (7.163a) ≡ (7.163b):

$$
0 =
\begin{bmatrix}
x^2 D^2 - x\,D + 1 & x D - 1 \\
2\,x\,D - 2 & x\,D
\end{bmatrix}
\begin{bmatrix}
y(x) \\
z(x)
\end{bmatrix}, \tag{7.163a}
$$

$$
=
\begin{bmatrix}
\delta(\delta-1) - \delta + 1 & \delta - 1 \\
2\delta - 2 & \delta
\end{bmatrix}
\begin{bmatrix}
y(x) \\
z(x)
\end{bmatrix}, \tag{7.163b}
$$

$$= \begin{bmatrix} (\delta-1)^2 & \delta-1 \\ 2(\delta-1) & \delta \end{bmatrix} \begin{bmatrix} y(x) \\ z(x) \end{bmatrix}, \tag{7.163c}$$

which simplifies to (7.163c).

7.6.3 Unforced System and Characteristic Polynomial

Consider the unforced (7.164a) simultaneous linear system of ordinary differential equations, (7.159) $\equiv$ (7.160a, b), with homogeneous coefficients (7.164b):

$$B_m(x) = 0: \qquad\qquad 0 = \sum_{r=1}^{M} Q_{m,r}(\delta) y_r(x), \tag{7.164a, b}$$

or alternatively in matrix form (7.165):

$$\begin{bmatrix} Q_{1,1}(\delta) & Q_{1,2}(\delta) & \cdots & Q_{1,M}(\delta) \\ Q_{2,1}(\delta) & Q_{2,2}(\delta) & \cdots & Q_{2,M}(\delta) \\ \vdots & \vdots & \vdots & \ddots & \vdots \\ Q_{M,1}(\delta) & Q_{M,2}(\delta) & \cdots & Q_{M,M}(\delta) \end{bmatrix} \begin{bmatrix} y_1(x) \\ y_2(x) \\ \vdots \\ y_M(x) \end{bmatrix} = 0. \tag{7.165}$$

The elimination for any of the dependent variables $y_r(x)$ would lead to a single linear unforced ordinary differential equation with homogeneous coefficients (1.291a) whose solution (1.291b) is a power of the independent variable x. Thus, the solutions of the simultaneous system (7.164a, b) $\equiv$ (7.165) are powers of the independent variable (7.166a) with the same exponent and distinct coefficients:

$$y_r(r) = E_r\, x^a: \qquad 0 = \sum_{r=1}^{M} Q_{m,r}(\delta) E_r\, x^a = x^a \sum_{r=1}^{M} Q_{m,r}(a) E_r, \tag{7.166a–c}$$

which substituted in (7.164b) lead to (7.166b), with the use of (7.158d) yielding to (7.166c). The coefficients in (7.166a) cannot be all zero (7.167a), otherwise a trivial solution would result, and also (7.167b) implies (7.167c):

$$\{E_1, \cdots, E_M\} \neq \{0, \cdots, 0\}, \qquad x^a \neq 0: \qquad \sum_{r=1}^{M} Q_{m,r}(a) E_r = 0, \tag{7.167a–c}$$

that the determinant is zero (7.168a):

$$0 = Det\{Q_{m,r}(a)\} = Q_N(a). \tag{7.168a, b}$$

Thus, *the simultaneous system of unforced (7.164a) linear ordinary differential equations with homogeneous coefficients (7.164b) ≡ (7.165) has characteristic polynomial (7.168b), which is the determinant of the matrix of polynomials of homogeneous derivatives (7.152a, b) ≡ (7.153). The degree of the characteristic polynomial is the order of the differential system, and specifies (standard CXLVI) the number of: (i) linearly independent normal integrals; (ii) arbitrary constants of integration; (iii) independent and compatible boundary conditions that ensure unicity of solution. The differential system (7.152b) is non-degenerate (7.59c) [degenerate (7.59b)] if the order equals (is less than) the maximum (7.59a).* For example, the highest order derivative is 2 in (7.162a) and 1 in (7.162b), so the highest possible order is $1 + 2 = 3$, which is the degree of the characteristic polynomial (7.169a, b) as follows from (7.163c):

$$Q_3(\delta) = (\delta - 1)^2 \, \delta - 2(\delta - 1)^2 = (\delta - 1)^2 (\delta - 2), \qquad \text{(7.169a, b)}$$

showing that the system (7.162a, b) is non-degenerate. Next, the natural integrals corresponding to single or multiple roots of the characteristic polynomial (subsection 7.6.4) are considered.

7.6.4 Distinct and Multiple Roots of the Characteristic Polynomial

Each distinct (7.170a, b) root (7.170c) of the characteristic polynomial specifies the exponent of a power of the independent variable (7.170d), which is a **natural integral** of the differential system:

$$Q_N(a_n) = 0 \neq Q'_N(a_n): \qquad Q_N(a) = A \prod_{n=1}^{N} (a - a_n), \qquad q_n(x) = x^{a_n}. \qquad \text{(7.170a–d)}$$

In the case (7.171a, b) of a root a_0 of multiplicity α the method (1.296a, b) of parametric differentiation leads to α linearly independent natural integrals (7.171c–e):

$$Q_N(a) = (a - a_0)^\alpha \, R_{N-\alpha}(a), \quad R_{N-\alpha}(a_0) \neq 0: \quad \beta = 1, ..., \alpha:$$

$$q_\beta(x) = \frac{\partial^{\beta-1}}{\partial a_0^{\beta-1}} \left(x^{a_0} \right) = x^{a_0} \log^{\beta-1} x. \qquad \text{(7.171a–e)}$$

Thus, *the simultaneous linear unforced system of differential equations with homogeneous coefficients, (7.164a, b) ≡ (7.165), has N linearly independent natural integrals, where N is the degree of the characteristic polynomial (7.168b). If (standard CXLVII) all roots (7.170c) are distinct (7.170a, b) they determine the exponent of the powers of the independent variable that specify the natural integrals (7.170d). If (standard CXLVIII) the characteristic polynomial (7.172b) has S roots of multiplicity*

α_s the (7.172a) natural integrals (7.172d) are similar to (7.170d) multiplied by powers of logarithms (7.171e) up to (7.172c) the degree $\alpha_s - 1$:

$$\sum_{s=1}^{S}\alpha_s = N; \quad Q_N(a) = A\prod_{s=1}^{S}(a-a_s)^{\alpha_s}: \quad \beta_s = 1,\cdots,\alpha_s: \quad q_{s,\beta_s}(x) = x^{a_s}\log^{\beta_s-1}x.$$
$$(7.172\text{a–d})$$

For example, the coupled unforced linear system of ordinary differential equations with homogeneous coefficients, (7.162a, b) ≡ (7.163c), has characteristic polynomial (7.169a) ≡ (7.169b) with roots (7.173a):

$$a_{1-3} = 1,1,2: \qquad q_1(x) = x, \qquad q_2(x) = x\log x, \qquad q_3(x) = x^2, \qquad (7.173\text{a–d})$$

and the single (double) root 2 (1) leads to the linearly independent natural integrals (7.173d) [7.173b, c)]. The linearly independent natural integrals (subsection 7.6.5) are used in linear combinations to obtain the general integral of the unforced differential system for all dependent variables (subsection 7.6.5).

7.6.5 Natural Integrals and the General Integral

The simultaneous linear unforced system of ordinary differential equations with homogeneous coefficients (7.164a, b) ≡ (7.165) has the general integral that is a linear combination of normal integrals, namely: (a) if (standard CXLIX) all roots of the characteristic polynomial (7.170c) are distinct (7.170a, b) the general integral (7.174a) ≡ (7.174b) is a linear combination of the normal integrals (7.170a, b):

$$y_m(x) = \sum_{n=1}^{N}C_n F_{m,n}q_n(x) = \sum_{n=1}^{N}C_n F_{m,n}x^{a_n}; \qquad (7.174\text{a, b})$$

(b) if (standard CL) the characteristic polynomial (7.172a, b) has multiple roots the normal integrals in (7.174a) are replaced by (7.172c, d) leading to (7.175):

$$y_m(x) = \sum_{s=1}^{S}x^{a_s}\sum_{\beta_s=1}^{\alpha_s}C_{s,\beta_s}F_{m,s,\beta_s}\log^{\beta_s-1}x. \qquad (7.175)$$

*In both (a) [(b)] cases (7.174b) [(7.175)]: (i) the M dependent variables y_m are linear combinations of the N normal integrals forming an $M \times N$ matrix system; (ii) the N arbitrary constant of integration $C_n\left(C_{s,\beta_s}\right)$ are determined by (standard CLI) N independent and compatible **boundary conditions**; (iii) in the $M \times N$ matrix of coefficients $F_{1,s}\left(F_{1,s,\beta_s}\right)$ any line (standard CLII) can be chosen at will, for example, (7.176a) [(7.176b)]:*

$$F_{m,1} = 1, \qquad\qquad F_{m,\beta_s} = 1, \qquad (7.176\text{a, b})$$

and all others are determined by **compatibility conditions** *resulting from sub-stitution in the system (7.164a, b) ≡ (7.165).* The aspects of (iii) compatibility [(ii) boundary] conditions are illustrated next [subsection 7.6.6 (7.6.7)] using as an example the coupled differential system (7.162a, b) ≡ (7.163c).

7.6.6 Compatibility Conditions for the Dependent Variables

In the case of the coupled linear unforced system of ordinary differential equations with homogeneous coefficients (7.162a, b) both dependent variables (7.177a, b) are linear combinations of the natural integrals (7.173b–d):

$$y(x) = x(C_1 + C_2 \log x) + C_3 x^2, \quad z(x) = x(C_4 + C_5 \log x) + C_6 x^2, \qquad \text{(7.177a, b)}$$

and: (i) of the six constants C_{1-6} only three are arbitrary; (ii) the remaining three are determined by three compatibility conditions resulting from sub-stitution in (7.162a) or (7.162b); (iii) the result is the same regardless of which of (7.162a) or (7.162b) is used. For example, taking C_{1-3} in (7.177a) as the arbitrary constants: (i) substitution of (7.177b) in [(7.177a)] the middle (first and last) term(s) of (7.162b) leads to two sets of terms (7.178) [(7.179)]:

$$x z' = x\left[C_4 + C_5(1 + \log x) + 2C_6 x \right], \qquad \text{(7.178)}$$

$$2y - 2xy' = 2x(C_1 + C_2 \log x) + 2C_3 x^2 - 2x\left[C_1 + C_2(1 + \log x) + 2C_3 x \right]$$
$$= -2C_2 x - 2C_3 x^2; \qquad \text{(7.179)}$$

(ii) from (7.162b) follows (7.178) ≡ (7.179) and equating the coefficients of the natural integrals (7.173b–d) specifies (7.180a–c) the constants C_{4-6} in terms of C_{1-3}:

$$C_4 = -2C_2, \quad C_5 = 0, \quad C_6 = -C_3; \qquad z(x) = -2C_2 x - C_3 x^2, \quad \text{(7.180a–d)}$$

(iii) substituting (7.180a–c) in (7.177b) gives (7.180d). Thus, the general integral of the coupled linear system of ordinary differential equations with constant coefficients (7.162a, b) is (7.177a; 7.180d), where C_{1-3} are arbitrary constants of integration, determined by three independent and compatible boundary conditions (subsection 7.6.7).

7.6.7 Arbitrary Constants and Boundary Conditions

From (7.180d) follows (7.181):

$$z'(x) = -2C_2 - 2C_3 x. \qquad \text{(7.181)}$$

Choosing the three independent and compatible boundary conditions (7.182a):

$$\{3,1,0\}=\{y(1),z(1),z'(1)\}=\{C_1+C_2,-2C_2-C_3,-2C_2-2C_3\}, \quad (7.182a, b)$$

leads to (7.182b) by substitution in (7.177a; 7.180d; 7.181); solving (7.182b) specifies the arbitrary constants (7.183a–c):

$$C_3 = 1, \; C_2 = -C_3 = -1, \; C_1 = 3 - C_3 = 2:$$

$$y(x) = x(2 - \log x) + x^2, \quad z(x) = x(2-x), \quad (7.183a-e)$$

which lead to (7.183d, e) on substitution in (7.177a; 7.180d). Thus, (7.183d, e) is the unique solution of the coupled unforced linear system of ordinary differential equations with homogeneous coefficients (7.162a, b) that satisfies the boundary conditions (7.182a). The dependent variables appear as linear combinations (7.177a; 7.180d) and (7.183d, e) of the natural integrals (7.173b–d) that provide an alternative description of the differential system with either no coupling or minimal coupling (subsection 7.6.8).

7.6.8 Decoupled or Minimally-Coupled Natural Differential System

*Changing from the M dependent variables y_m in the general integral to the N natural integrals leads to a **natural differential system**, which in the case of the characteristic polynomial with: (i) distinct roots (7.170a–c) leads (7.170d) ≡ (7.184a) to (7.184b) ≡ (7.184c):*

$$q_n(x) = x^{a_n}: \qquad \{\delta\}q_n = x \frac{dq_n}{dx} = a_n x^{a_n} = a_n q_n(x), \qquad (7.184a-c)$$

which is a (standard CLIII) diagonal or decoupled system as (7.96c) with homogeneous (7.152a; 7.184a–c) instead of ordinary (7.151a; 7.96a, b) derivatives; (ii) a root a_0 of multiplicity α in (7.171a–c) ≡ (7.185a, b) leads (standard CLIV) to (7.185c) ≡ (7.185d):

$$\beta = 1,...,\alpha: \quad q_\beta(x) = x^{a_0} \log^{\beta-1} x: \qquad (7.185a, b)$$

$$\{\delta\}q_\beta(x) = x\frac{dq_\beta}{dx} = a_0 x^{a_0} \log^{\beta-1} x + x^{a_0}(\beta-1)\log^{\beta-2} x \qquad (7.185d)$$

$$= a_0 q_\beta(x) + (\beta-1)q_{\beta-1}(x), \qquad (7.185d)$$

*which is a two-banded diagonal system like (7.97d) using homogeneous (7.152a) instead of ordinary (7.151a) derivatives and correspondents to **minimal coupling**;*

(iii) for several multiple and/or single roots (7.172a–c) the normal integrals (7.172d) lead (standard CLV) to a diagonal block-banded system.

For example, (7.100) with homogeneous (7.152a) instead of ordinary (7.151a) derivatives, for the characteristic polynomial like (7.98a, b) with one each of single a_1, double a_2 and triple a_3 roots corresponds to: (i) the characteristic polynomial (7.151a; 7.152a, b; 7.153; 7.154a, b) of homogeneous derivatives:

$$\sum_{n=1}^{6} A_n x^n \frac{d^n}{dx^n} = \sum_{n=1}^{6} A_n \delta(\delta-1)...(\delta-n+1) = A_6 (\delta-a_1)(\delta-a_1)^2 (\delta-a_3)^2 \, ;$$

(7.186a, b)

(ii) the natural integrals (7.187a)/(7.187b, c)/(7.187d–f), corresponding, respectively, to the single/double/triple roots of the characteristic polynomial:

$$q_1(x) = x^{a_1}, \qquad q_{2-3}(x) = x^{a_2} \{1, \log x\}, \qquad q_{4-6}(x) = x^{a_3} \{1, \log x, \log^2 x\}.$$

(7.187a–f)

The representation via natural integrals (subsection 7.6.8) is applied next (subsection 7.6.9) to the coupled differential system (7.162a, b).

7.6.9 Block Diagonal-Banded System

The natural integrals (7.173b–d) of the coupled unforced linear system of ordinary differential equations with homogeneous coefficients (7.162a, b) satisfy (7.188a–c):

$$x\frac{dq_1}{dx} = x = q_1(x), \quad x\frac{dq_2}{dx} = x(1+\log x) = q_1(x) + q_2(x), \quad x\frac{dq_3}{dx} = 2x = 2q_3(x),$$

(7.188a–c)

which can be written in matrix form (7.189):

$$\begin{bmatrix} x\dfrac{dq_1}{dx} \\[2mm] x\dfrac{dq_2}{dx} \\[2mm] x\dfrac{dq_3}{dx} \end{bmatrix} = \begin{bmatrix} 1 & 0 & 0 \\ 1 & 1 & 0 \\ 0 & 0 & 2 \end{bmatrix} \begin{bmatrix} q_1(x) \\ q_2(x) \\ q_3(x) \end{bmatrix}, \qquad (7.189)$$

as a block-banded diagonal system with: (i) an upper 2×2 banded matrix for the natural integrals (7.173b, c; 7.188a, b) associated with the double root 1 of the characteristic polynomial (7.169b); (ii) the single root 2 and the natural integral (7.173d; 7.188c) leads to the lower corner as 1×1 "matrix"; (iii) the rest of the matrix is zero because the natural integrals for distinct roots of the characteristic polynomial (7.169b) are decoupled.

The general integral (7.177a; 7.180d) of the coupled unforced linear system of ordinary differential equations with homogeneous coefficients (7.162a, b) can be written as 2×3 matrix (7.190), relating linearly the dependent variables to the natural integrals (7.173b, d):

$$
\begin{bmatrix} y(x) \\ z(x) \end{bmatrix} = \begin{bmatrix} C_1 & C_2 & C_3 \\ -2C_2 & 0 & -C_3 \end{bmatrix} \begin{bmatrix} x \\ \log x \\ x^2 \end{bmatrix} ,
\tag{7.190}
$$

where C_{1-3} are arbitrary constants. The boundary conditions (7.182a) specify the constants (7.183a–c) in (7.190), leading to (7.191):

$$
\begin{bmatrix} y(x) \\ z(x) \end{bmatrix} = \begin{bmatrix} 2 & -1 & 1 \\ 2 & 0 & -1 \end{bmatrix} \begin{bmatrix} x \\ x \log x \\ x^2 \end{bmatrix} ,
\tag{7.191}
$$

in agreement with (7.191) $\equiv$ (7.183d, e).

7.7 Forced and Unforced Homogeneous Systems

The simultaneous linear systems of linear ordinary differential equations with constant (homogeneous) coefficients [(sections 7.4–7.5 (7.6–7.7)] are similar replacing (subsection 7.7.1): (i) ordinary (by homogeneous) derivatives; (ii) exponentials (by powers) of the independent variable; (iii) powers (by logarithms). This leads to the particular integral of a simultaneous linear system of ordinary differential equations with homogeneous derivatives forced by: (i) a power (subsection 7.7.2) in non-resonant (singly/doubly resonant cases) [subsections 7.7.2–7.7.3 (7.7.4/7.7.5)]; (ii) the product of a power by a circular or hyperbolic cosine or sine of a multiple of a logarithm (subsections 7.7.6–7.7.7); (iii) a polynomial of logarithms (subsection 7.7.9) using the inverse matrix of polynomials of homogeneous derivatives (subsection 7.7.8). As for all single (simultaneous systems) of linear differential equation(s) with constant [sections 1.3–1.5 (7.4–7.5)], homogeneous [sections 1.6–1.7 (7.6–7.7)] or variable coefficients the complete integral in the forced case (subsection 7.7.10) consists of a particular integral of the forced case plus the general integral of the unforced case.

7.7.1 Analogy of Constant and Homogeneous Coefficients

Comparing (standard CLVI) the simultaneous linear system of ordinary differential equations (7.45a, b; 7.46a, b) with constant (7.47) ≡ (7.49a–c) ≡ (7.50) ≡ (7.151a, b) ≡ (7.192a)] [homogeneous (7.48) ≡ (7.152a, b; 7.153) ≡ (7.192b)] coefficients:

$$\sum_{r=1}^{M} P_{m,r}(D)y_r(x) = B_m(x) = \sum_{r=1}^{M} Q_{m,r}(\delta)y_r(x), \qquad (7.192a, b)$$

there is a replacement of: (i) ordinary by homogeneous derivatives (7.193a); (ii) exponentials by powers (7.193b); (ii) powers by logarithms (7.193c):

$$D \equiv \frac{d}{dx} \leftrightarrow \delta = x\frac{d}{dx}, \qquad e^{ax} \leftrightarrow x^a, \qquad x^\alpha \leftrightarrow \log^\alpha x. \qquad (7.193a–c)$$

The substitution (7.193a) agrees with (7.194a, b), which is generalized to (7.195a, b):

$$De^{ax} \equiv \frac{d}{dx}(e^{ax}) = a\,e^{ax}, \qquad \delta(x^a) \equiv x\frac{d}{dx}(x^a) = ax^a, \qquad (7.194a, b)$$

$$D^k e^{ax} \equiv \frac{d^k}{dx^k}(e^{ax}) \equiv a^k e^{ax}, \qquad \delta^n(x^a) \equiv \left(x\frac{d}{dx}\right)^k x^a \equiv a^k x^a, \qquad (7.195a, b)$$

$$\{P_N(D)\}e^{ax} = e^{ax}P_N(a), \qquad \{Q_N(\delta)\}x^a = x^a Q_N(a), \qquad (7.196a, b)$$

and extends to polynomials of ordinary (7.196a) [homogeneous (7.196b)] derivatives.

The substitution (7.193b) also agrees with a set of relations similar to (7.194a, b; 7.195a, b; 7.196a, b), namely: (i–ii) for single (multiple) derivatives (7.197a, b) [(7.198a, b)]:

$$D(x^\alpha) = \frac{d}{dx}(x^\alpha) = \alpha x^{\alpha-1}, \qquad \delta(\log^\alpha x) = x\frac{d}{dx}(\log^\alpha x) = \alpha\log^{\alpha-1}x, \qquad (7.197a, b)$$

$$D^n(x^\alpha) = x^{\alpha-n}\alpha(\alpha-1)...(\alpha-n+1), \qquad \delta^n(\log^\alpha x) = \alpha(\alpha-1)...(\alpha-n+1)\log^{\alpha-n}x; \qquad (7.198a, b)$$

(iii) for a polynomial (7.199a) [(7.200a)] of ordinary (homogeneous) derivatives (7.198a) [(7.198b)] lead to (7.199b) [(7.200b)]:

$$P_N(D) \equiv \sum_{n=0}^{N} A_n \frac{d^n}{dx^n}: \quad \{P_N(D)\}x^\alpha = \sum_{n=0}^{N} A_n x^{\alpha-n}\alpha(\alpha-1)...(\alpha-n+1), \qquad (7.199a, b)$$

$$Q_N\left(\delta\right)\equiv\sum_{n=0}^{N}A_n\left(x\frac{d^n}{dx^n}\right):\quad\left\{Q_N\left(\delta\right)\right\}\log^{\alpha}x=\sum_{n=0}^{N}A_n\log^{\alpha-n}x\,\alpha(\alpha-1)...(\alpha-n+1).$$

(7.200a, b)

The substitutions (7.193b, c) suggest the consideration of the particular integral of a simultaneous linear system of ordinary differential equations with constant (7.192a) [homogeneous (7.192b)] coefficients forced by: (i) an exponential (power) in non-resonant and singly and doubly resonant cases [subsections 7.5.2–7.5.3 (7.7.2–7.7.5)]; (ii) the product of an exponential (power) by [subsections 7.5.4–7.5.5 (7.7.6–7.7.7)] the circular or hyperbolic cosine or sine of the (of a multiple of the logarithm of the) independent variable; (iii) a polynomial (polynomial of logarithms) using [subsection 7.5.7 (7.7.9)] the inverse matrix of polynomials of ordinary (homogeneous) derivatives [subsection 7.5.6 (7.7.8)].

7.7.2 Forcing of a Homogeneous System by a Power

Consider a simultaneous linear system of ordinary differential equations with homogeneous derivatives (7.192b) forced by a power (7.201a):

$$\sum_{r=1}^{M}Q_{m,r}\left(\delta\right)y_r\left(x\right)=G_m\,x^b;\qquad y_r\left(x\right)=H_r\,x^b,$$

(7.201a, b)

the particular integral is sought as a similar power (7.201b) and substitution in (7.201a) leads (7.196b) to (7.202a) $\equiv$ (7.202b):

$$G_m\,x^b=\sum_{r=1}^{M}Q_{m,r}\left(\delta\right)H_r\,x^b=x^b\sum_{r=1}^{M}Q_{m,r}\left(b\right)H_r.$$

(7.202a, b)

The condition (7.202c) implies (7.202d):

$$x^b\ne0:\qquad G_m=\sum_{r=1}^{m}Q_{m,r}\left(b\right)H_r,\qquad Q_N\left(b\right)H_r=\sum_{m=1}^{m}\bar{Q}_{m,r}\left(b\right)G_m,$$

(7.202c–e)

which leads as in (7.118a, b; 7.119a–c; 7.120) to (7.202e), involving:

$$m,r,\ell=1,...,M:\qquad\sum_{m=1}^{M}\bar{Q}_{\ell,m}\left(b\right)Q_{m,r}\left(b\right)=\delta_{\ell r}\,Det\left[Q_{m,r}\left(b\right)\right]=\delta_{\ell r}\,Q_N\left(b\right),$$

(7.203a–c)

the matrix of co-factors (7.203a–c) and characteristic polynomial (7.168b).

The inversion of (7.203c) and substitution in (7.201b) in the non-resonant case when b is not a root of the characteristic polynomial (7.204a):

$$Q_N(b) \neq 0: \qquad\qquad y_r(x) = \frac{x^a}{Q_N(a)} \sum_{m=1}^{M} \overline{Q}_{r,m}(b) G_m , \qquad\qquad (7.204a, b)$$

specifies the particular integral (7.204b).

If b is a root of multiplicity α of the characteristic polynomial (7.205a) $\equiv$ (7.122a), then the application of the L'Hospital rule, as in (7.122b), leads to (7.205b):

$$Q_N(b) = Q'_N(b) = \ldots = Q_N^{(\alpha-1)}(b) = 0 \neq Q_N^{(\alpha)}(b):$$

$$y_r(x) = \left[Q_N^{(\alpha)}(b) \right]^{-1} \sum_{m=1}^{M} G_m \frac{\partial^\alpha}{\partial b^\alpha} \left[x^b \, \overline{Q}_{r,m}(b) \right]. \qquad (7.205a, b)$$

The Leibnitz rule $(I.13.31) \equiv (7.123) \equiv (7.206)$:

$$\frac{\partial^\alpha}{\partial b^\alpha} \left[x^b \overline{Q}_{r,m}(b) \right] = \sum_{\gamma=0}^{\alpha} \binom{\alpha}{\gamma} \overline{Q}_{r,m}^{(\alpha-\gamma)}(b) \frac{\partial^\gamma}{\partial b^\gamma} \left(x^b \right), \qquad (7.206)$$

substituted in (7.205b) leads to (7.207):

$$y_r(x) = \frac{x^b}{Q_N(b)} \sum_{\gamma=0}^{\alpha} \frac{\alpha! \log^\gamma x}{\gamma!(\alpha-\gamma)!} \sum_{m=1}^{M} G_m \overline{Q}_{r,m}^{(\alpha-\gamma)}(b). \qquad (7.207)$$

The α-times resonant solution (7.207) involves: (i) in the denominator, the lowest-order derivative of the characteristic polynomial (7.168b) that is not zero (7.205a): (ii) in the numerator, a linear combination of terms of the form $x^b \log^\gamma x$, as for the unforced solution (7.171a–e) with $\gamma = 0, \ldots, \alpha - 1$ plus $x^b \log^\alpha x$ that is not an unforced solution. Thus, *a particular integral of the simultaneous linear system of ordinary differential equations with homogeneous coefficients (7.192b) forced by a power (7.201a) is (standard CLVII) (7.204b) [(7.205b) $\equiv$ (7.207)] in the non-resonant (resonant) case when the exponent is not a root (7.204a) [is a root (7.205a) of multiplicity α] of the characteristic polynomial (7.168b)*. The coupled differential system (7.162a, b) with single and double roots of the characteristic polynomial (7.169b) serves as example of non-resonant/singly/doubly resonant particular integrals (subsections 7.7.3/7.7.4/7.7.5).

7.7.3 Non-Resonant and Multiply Resonant Particular Integrals

Consider the coupled linear system of ordinary differential equations with homogeneous coefficients (7.162a, b) with forcing by powers (7.208a, b):

$$x^2 y'' - xy' + xz' + y - z = -x^b, \qquad 2xy' + xz' - 2y = 2x^b, \qquad (7.208a, b)$$

which can be written (7.163a–c) in the matrix form (7.209):

$$\begin{bmatrix} \delta^2 - 2\delta + 1 & \delta - 1 \\ 2\delta - 2 & \delta \end{bmatrix} \begin{bmatrix} y(x) \\ z(x) \end{bmatrix} = x^b \begin{bmatrix} -1 \\ 2 \end{bmatrix}. \qquad (7.209)$$

The matrix of polynomials of homogeneous derivatives (7.210a) has matrix of co-factors (7.210b):

$$Q_{m,r}(\delta) = \begin{bmatrix} \delta^2 - 2\delta + 1 & \delta - 1 \\ 2\delta - 2 & \delta \end{bmatrix}, \quad \bar{Q}_{m,r}(\delta) = \begin{bmatrix} \delta & 1 - \delta \\ 2 - 2\delta & \delta^2 - 2\delta + 1 \end{bmatrix},$$

$$(7.210a, b)$$

and determinant specifying the characteristic polynomial (7.169b). The particular integral (7.211c) of (7.209) is non-resonant (7.211d):

$$b \neq 1, 2: \qquad \begin{bmatrix} y(x) \\ z(x) \end{bmatrix} = \frac{x^b}{(b-1)^2 (b-2)} \begin{bmatrix} b & 1-b \\ 2-2b & b^2 - 2b + 1 \end{bmatrix} \begin{bmatrix} -1 \\ 2 \end{bmatrix}$$

$$= \frac{x^b}{(b-1)^2 (b-2)} \begin{bmatrix} 2 - 3b \\ -2b + 2b^2 \end{bmatrix}, \qquad (7.211a–d)$$

provided that the exponent is not a root (7.211a, b) of the characteristic polynomial (7.169b). The case of the simple (double) root leads to single (double) resonance [subsection 7.7.4 (7.7.5)].

7.7.4 Power Forcing and Single Resonance

The first-order (7.212c) [second-order (7.212d)] derivative of the characteristic polynomial (7.169b) ≡ (7.212a) ≡ (7.212b):

$$Q_3(b) = (b-2)(b^2 - 2b + 1) = b^3 - 4b^2 + 5b - 2:$$
$$Q_3'(b) = 3b^2 - 8b + 5, \quad Q_3''(b) = 6b - 8, \qquad (7.212a–d)$$

is the lowest-order derivative that does not vanish (7.213b, c) [(7.213e–g)] for the single root (7.213a) [double root (7.213d)]:

$$b = 2: \quad Q_3(2) = 0 \neq 1 = Q_3'(2); \quad b = 1: \quad Q_3(1) = Q_3'(1) = 0 \neq -2 = Q_3''(1),$$

$$(7.213a\text{–}g)$$

implying a **single (double) resonance**. The particular integral (7.205a, b) with $\alpha = 1$ is (7.214b) in the case (7.214a) of single resonance:

$$b = 2: \quad \begin{bmatrix} y(x) \\ z(x) \end{bmatrix} = \frac{1}{Q_3'(2)} \lim_{b \to 2} \frac{\partial}{\partial b} \left\{ x^b \begin{bmatrix} 2 - 3b \\ 2b^2 - 2b \end{bmatrix} \right\}$$

$$= \lim_{b \to 2} x^b \left\{ \begin{bmatrix} -3 \\ 4b - 2 \end{bmatrix} + \begin{bmatrix} 2 - 3b \\ 2b^2 - 2b \end{bmatrix} \log x \right\}$$

$$= x^2 \left\{ \begin{bmatrix} -3 \\ 6 \end{bmatrix} + \begin{bmatrix} -4 \\ 4 \end{bmatrix} \log x \right\},$$

$$(7.214a, b)$$

which correspond to the particular integrals (7.215b, c):

$$b = 2: \quad y(x) = -x^2(3 + 4\log x), \quad z(x) = 2x^2(3 + 2\log x), \quad (7.215a\text{–}c)$$

that involve at least one logarithmic factor because the exponent (7.215a) is a simple root of the characteristic polynomial (7.169b). A double (multiple) resonance involves a square (a higher power) of the logarithm, as shown next (subsection 7.7.5).

7.7.5 Double Root and Double Resonance

The double root (7.213d–g) of the characteristic polynomial (7.169b) ≡ (7.212a–d) leads in (7.205a, b) with $\alpha = 2$, as in (7.130b) to (7.216b), a double resonance (7.216a):

$$b = 1: \quad \begin{bmatrix} y(x) \\ z(x) \end{bmatrix} = \frac{1}{Q_3''(1)} \lim_{b \to 1} \frac{\partial^2}{\partial b^2} \left\{ x^b \begin{bmatrix} 2 - 3b \\ 2b^2 - 2b \end{bmatrix} \right\}, \quad (7.216a, b)$$

which simplifies to (7.217a, b):

$$
\begin{bmatrix} y(x) \\ z(x) \end{bmatrix} = -\frac{1}{2} \lim_{b \to 1} x^b \left\{ \begin{bmatrix} 0 \\ 4 \end{bmatrix} + 2\log x \begin{bmatrix} -3 \\ 4b-2 \end{bmatrix} + \log^2 x \begin{bmatrix} 2-3b \\ 2b^2-2b \end{bmatrix} \right\}
$$

$$
= -\frac{x}{2} \left\{ \begin{bmatrix} 0 \\ 4 \end{bmatrix} + 2\log x \begin{bmatrix} -3 \\ 2 \end{bmatrix} + \log^2 x \begin{bmatrix} -1 \\ 0 \end{bmatrix} \right\};
$$

$$(7.217a, b)$$

the particular integrals (7.218b, c):

$$
b=1: \qquad y(x) = x\log x\left(3 + \frac{1}{2}\log x\right), \qquad z(x) = -2x\left(1 + \log x\right), \qquad (7.218a\text{-c})
$$

involve as factors polynomials of degree 2 of the logarithm because the exponent (7.218a) is a double root of the characteristic polynomial (7.169b). The circular and hyperbolic cosines of a multiple of a logarithm are a sum of powers (subsections 7.7.6–7.7.7) leading to an extension of the forcing by powers (subsections 7.7.2–7.7.5).

7.7.6 Cosine and Sine of Multiples of Logarithms

The hyperbolic (circular) cosine and sine of a multiple of a logarithm are a sum of powers with real (7.219a, b) [imaginary (7.220a, b)] exponents:

$$
\cosh, \sinh\left(c\log x\right) = \frac{1}{2}\left[\exp\left(c\log x\right) \pm \exp\left(-c\log x\right)\right] = \frac{x^c \pm x^{-c}}{2}, \qquad (7.219a, b)
$$

$$
\cos, \sin\left(g\log x\right) = \frac{\exp\left(ig\log x\right) \pm \exp\left(-ig\log x\right)}{2,2i} = \frac{x^{ig} \pm x^{-ig}}{2,2i}. \qquad (7.220a, b)
$$

Applying (7.219a, b; 7.220a, b) to the forcing by a power (7.204a, b) leads to the following results: *the simultaneous linear system of ordinary differential equations (7.192b) with homogeneous coefficients and forcing by the product of a power by: (i) the hyperbolic cosine or sine of the multiple of a logarithm (7.221a, b) has (standard CLVIII) particular integral (7.221c):*

$$
B_m(x) = G_m x^b \cosh, \sinh\left(c\log x\right) = \frac{1}{2}G_m\left(x^{b+c} \pm x^{b-c}\right), \qquad (7.221a, b)
$$

$$
y_r(x) = \frac{x^b}{2}\sum_{m=1}^{M} G_m\left[\frac{x^c}{Q_N(b+c)}\bar{Q}_{r,m}(b+c) \pm \frac{x^{-c}}{Q_N(b-c)}\bar{Q}_{r,m}(b-c)\right]; \qquad (7.221c)
$$

(ii) circular cosine or sine of a multiple of a logarithm (7.222a, b) has (standard CLIX) particular integral (7.222c):

$$B_m(x) = G_m\, x^b \cos, \sin(g \log x) = G_m \frac{x^{b+ig} \pm x^{b-ig}}{\{2, 2i\}}; \qquad (7.222a, b)$$

$$y_r(x) = x^b \sum_{m=1}^{M} \frac{G_m}{\{2, 2i\}} \left[\frac{x^{ig}}{Q_N(b+ig)} \bar{Q}_{r,m}(b+ig) \pm \frac{x^{-ig}}{Q_N(b-ig)} \bar{Q}_{r,m}(b-ig) \right];$$

$$(7.222c)$$

(iii) the case of real b, g and real matrix of polynomials of homogeneous derivatives (7.223a–c) simplifies the forcing (7.223d) and particular integrals (7.223e):

$$b, c, g, Q_{m,r} \in |R: \qquad\qquad B_m(x) = G_m\, x^b \operatorname{Re}, \operatorname{Im}(x^{ig}), \qquad (7.223a\text{–}d)$$

$$y_r(x) = x^b \sum_{m=1}^{M} G_m \operatorname{Re}, \operatorname{Im}\left\{ \frac{x^{ig}}{Q_N(b+ig)} \bar{Q}_{r,m}(b+ig) \right\}; \qquad (7.223e)$$

(ii) circular and hyperbolic cosine and sine of a multiple of logarithm (7.224e) with real b, c, g and real matrix of polynomials of homogeneous derivatives (7.224a–d) has (standard CLX) particular integral (7.224f):

$$b, c, g, Q_{m,r} \in |R: \qquad B_m(x) = G_m\, x^b \cosh, \sinh(c \log x) \cos, \sin(g \log x)$$

$$(7.224a\text{–}e)$$

$$= \frac{1}{2} G_m \operatorname{Re}, \operatorname{Im}\left(x^{b+c+ig} \pm x^{b-c+ig} \right),$$

$$y_r(x) = \frac{x^b}{2} \sum_{m=1}^{M} G_m \operatorname{Re}, \operatorname{Im}\left\{ \left[\frac{x^{ig+c}}{Q_N(b+c+ig)} \bar{Q}_{r,m}(b+c+ig) - \right.\right.$$

$$(7.224f)$$

$$\left.\left. \frac{x^{ig-c}}{Q_N(b-c+ig)} \bar{Q}_{r,m}(b-c+ig) \right] \right\},$$

In (7.221c)/(7.222c)/(7.223e)/(7.224f), it is assumed that, respectively, $b \pm c/b \pm ig/b + ig/b \pm c + ig$ is not a root of the characteristic polynomial, otherwise the particular integrals have to be modified as in the passage from (7.204a, b) to (7.205a, b). The case (7.224a–f) of a power multiplied by the hyperbolic cosine and the circular sine of multiples of a logarithm is chosen as an example (subsection 7.7.7).

7.7.7 Forcing by a Power Multiplied by a Double Product

Consider the coupled linear system of ordinary differential equations with homogeneous coefficients (7.162a, b) forced by the product of a power by the hyperbolic cosine and circular sine of multiples of the logarithm of the independent variable:

$$x^2 y'' - xy' + xz' + y - z = 4x\cosh(\log x)\sin(2\log x) = 2\operatorname{Im}\left(x^{2+2i} + x^{2i}\right),$$
(7.225a)

$$2xy' - xz' - 2y = -2 \, x\cosh(\log x)\sin(2\log x) = -\operatorname{Im}\left(x^{2+2i} + x^{2i}\right). \quad (7.225b)$$

Since $2i$ and $2+2i$ are not roots of the characteristic polynomial (7.169b), the particular integral (7.224a–f) of (7.225a, b) is obtained in four steps: (i) multiply the matrix of co-factors (7.210b) of the matrix of polynomials of inhomogeneous derivatives (7.210a) by the coefficients of the forcing vector in (7.225a, b):

$$\begin{bmatrix} b & 1-b \\ 2-2b & b^2-2b+1 \end{bmatrix} \begin{bmatrix} 2 \\ -1 \end{bmatrix} = \begin{bmatrix} 3b-1 \\ 3-2b-b^2 \end{bmatrix}; \qquad (7.226)$$

(ii) substitute (7.226) together with the characteristic polynomial (7.169b) in:

$$\begin{bmatrix} y(x) \\ z(x) \end{bmatrix} = \operatorname{Im}\left\{ \frac{x^{2+2i}}{Q_3(2+2i)} \lim_{b\to 2+2i} \begin{bmatrix} 3b-1 \\ 3-2b-b^2 \end{bmatrix} + \frac{x^{2i}}{Q_3(2i)} \lim_{b\to 2i} \begin{bmatrix} 3b-1 \\ 3-2b-b^2 \end{bmatrix} \right\}$$

$$= x^2 \operatorname{Im}\left\{ \frac{x^{2i}}{(1+2i)^2 \, 2i} \begin{bmatrix} 3(2+2i)-1 \\ 3-2(2+2i)-(2+2i)^2 \end{bmatrix} \right\}$$

$$+ \operatorname{Im}\left\{ \frac{x^{2i}}{(2i-1)^2(2i-2)} \begin{bmatrix} 6i-1 \\ 3-4i-(2i)^2 \end{bmatrix} \right\}$$
(7.227a–e)

$$= x^2 \operatorname{Im}\left\{ -\frac{x^{2i}}{8+6i} \begin{bmatrix} 5+6i \\ -1-12i \end{bmatrix} \right\} + \operatorname{Im}\left\{ \frac{x^{2i}}{14+2i} \begin{bmatrix} 6i-1 \\ 7-4i \end{bmatrix} \right\}$$

$$= \frac{x^2}{2} \operatorname{Im}\left\{ \frac{3i-4}{25} x^{2i} \begin{bmatrix} 5+6i \\ -1-12i \end{bmatrix} \right\} + \operatorname{Im}\left\{ \frac{7-i}{100} x^{2i} \begin{bmatrix} 6i-1 \\ 7-4i \end{bmatrix} \right\}$$

$$= \frac{x^2}{50} \operatorname{Im}\left\{ x^{2i} \begin{bmatrix} -38-9i \\ 40+45i \end{bmatrix} \right\} + \operatorname{Im}\left\{ \frac{x^{2i}}{100} \begin{bmatrix} 43i-1 \\ 45-35i \end{bmatrix} \right\};$$

(iii) the corresponding (7.227e) ≡ (7.228a, b) particular integrals of (7.225a, b) are:

$$y(x) = -\frac{x^2}{50}\left[9\cos(2\log x) + 38\sin(2\log x)\right] + \frac{1}{100}\left[43\cos(2\log x) - \sin(2\log x)\right],$$

(7.228a)

$$z(x) = \frac{x^2}{10}\left[9\cos(2\log x) + 8\sin(2\log x)\right] + \frac{1}{20}\left[-7\cos(2\log x) + 9\sin(2\log x)\right].$$

(7.228b)

An alternative method of obtaining particular integrals is (subsection 7.7.8) to "invert" (7.192b), in particular in the case of forcing by polynomials of logarithms (subsection 7.7.9).

7.7.8 Inverse Matrix of Polynomials of Homogeneous Derivatives

The coupled forced linear system (7.192b) of linear ordinary differential equations with homogeneous coefficients may be (standard CLXI) formally inverted:

$$y_r(x) = \frac{1}{Q_N(\delta)}\sum_{m=1}^{M}\bar{Q}_{rm}(\delta)B_m(x),$$

(7.229)

where appear: (i) the matrix of co-factors (7.203a–c) of the matrix of polynomials of homogeneous derivatives; (ii) the inverse (7.230a) of the characteristic polynomial (7.168b) that can be expanded (section 1.5) as a series of homogeneous derivatives, which applies to (7.229) and must converge (chapter I.21):

$$\frac{1}{Q_N(\delta)} = \sum_{k=0}^{\infty}q_k\,\delta^k\,; \qquad B_m(x) = \sum_{\ell=0}^{L_m}B_{m,\ell}\log^\ell x,$$

(7.230a, b)

(iv) if the forcing vector is a polynomial of logarithms (7.230b), there is no convergence issue because the derivatives of order $k > L_m$ vanish:

$$\delta^k\left(\log^\ell x\right) = \begin{cases} \ell(\ell-1)...(\ell-k+1)\log^{\ell-k}x & \text{if} \quad \ell \le k, \\ \ell! = k! & \text{if} \quad \ell = k, \\ 0 & \text{if} \quad \ell > k. \end{cases}$$

(7.231a–c)

The relation, (7.231a) ≡ (7.198b), was obtained before, the case $\ell = k$ leads to a constant (7.231b), and hence, further homogeneous differentiation $\ell > k$ gives zero (7.231c).

7.7.9 Homogeneous Forcing by a Polynomial of Logarithms

Consider the coupled linear system of ordinary differential equations (7.162a, b) forced by (7.232a, b) powers of the logarithm:

$$x^2 y'' - xy' + xz' + y - z = -\log^2 x, \qquad 2xy' + xz' - 2y = 3\log x. \qquad (7.232a, b)$$

The particular integral (7.229) is obtained in four steps, starting with (7.233):

$$\begin{bmatrix} y(x) \\ z(x) \end{bmatrix} = \frac{1}{-2 + 5\delta - 4\delta^2 + \delta^3} \begin{bmatrix} \delta & 1 - \delta \\ 2 - 2\delta & \delta^2 - 2\delta + 1 \end{bmatrix} \begin{bmatrix} -\log^2 x \\ 3\log x \end{bmatrix}. \qquad (7.233)$$

where appears: (i) the matrix of co-factors (7.210b) of the matrix of polynomials of homogeneous derivatives; (ii) the inverse of the characteristic polynomial (7.169a) ≡ (7.169b) ≡ (7.212b). Step 2 uses (7.231a–c) in (7.233) leading to (7.234a):

$$\begin{bmatrix} y(x) \\ z(x) \end{bmatrix} = -\frac{1}{2} \frac{1}{1 - \frac{5}{2}\delta + 2\delta^2 - \frac{1}{2}\delta^3} \begin{bmatrix} -2\log x + 3\log x - 3 \\ -2\log^2 x + 4\log x - 6 + 3\log x \end{bmatrix}$$

$$(7.234a, b)$$

$$= -\frac{1}{2} \frac{1}{1 - \frac{5}{2}\delta + 2\delta^2 + O(\delta^3)} \begin{bmatrix} \log x - 3 \\ -2\log^2 x + 7\log x - 6 \end{bmatrix}.$$

which simplifies to (7.234b).

In (7.234b) the homogeneous derivatives of an order higher than order 2 can be omitted by (7.231c), and the geometric series (I.21.62c) ≡ (7.235a) in step 3 leads to (7.235b):

$$\frac{1}{1 - \frac{5}{2}\delta + 2\delta^2 + O(\delta^3)} = 1 + \left(\frac{5}{2}\delta - 2\delta^2 \right) + \left(\frac{5}{2}\delta - 2\delta^2 \right)^2 + O(\delta^3)$$

$$(7.235a, b)$$

$$= 1 + \frac{5}{2}\delta + \frac{17}{4}\delta^2 + O(\delta^3).$$

Step 4 substitutes (7.235b) in (7.234b) and uses (7.231a–c) again (7.236a, b):

$$
\begin{bmatrix} y(x) \\ z(x) \end{bmatrix} = \left(-\frac{1}{2} - \frac{5}{4}\delta - \frac{17}{8}\delta^2 \right) \begin{bmatrix} \log x - 3 \\ -2\log^2 x + 7\log x - 6 \end{bmatrix}
$$

$$
= \begin{bmatrix} -\dfrac{1}{2}\log x + \dfrac{3}{2} - \dfrac{5}{4} \\[2mm] \log^2 x - \dfrac{7}{2}\log x + 3 + 5\log x - \dfrac{35}{4} + \dfrac{17}{2} \end{bmatrix},
$$

(7.236a, b)

leading to:

$$
y(x) = \frac{1}{4} - \frac{1}{2}\log x, \qquad z(x) = \frac{11}{4} + \frac{3}{2}\log x + \log^2 x, \tag{7.237a, b}
$$

as the particular integrals (7.237a, b) of (7.232a, b).

7.7.10 Complete Integral of the Forced Homogeneous Derivatives

Using the principle of superposition (section 1.2) the preceding examples (sections 7.6–7.7) can be combined in a single statement: the coupled system of ordinary differential equations with homogeneous coefficients if unforced (7.162a, b) ≡ (7.222a, b):

$$
x^2 y'' - xy' + xz' + y - z = -x^3 - x^2 - x - \log^2 x + 4x\cosh(\log x)\sin(2\log x), \tag{7.238a}
$$

$$
2xy' + xz' - 2y = 2x^3 + 2x^2 + 2x + 3\log x - 2x\cosh(\log x)\sin(2\log x), \tag{7.238b}
$$

has the general integral (7.177a; 7.180d) ≡ (7.239a, b):

$$
\bar{y}(x) = x(A + B\log x) + Cx^2 - \frac{7}{4}x^3 - x^2(3 + 4\log x) + x\log x\left(3 + \frac{1}{2}\log x\right)
$$

$$
+ \frac{1}{4} - \frac{1}{2}\log x - \left(\frac{9x^2}{50} - \frac{43}{100}\right)\cos(2\log x) - \left(\frac{19x^2}{25} + \frac{1}{100}\right)\sin(2\log x), \tag{7.239a}
$$

$$\bar{z}(x) = -2Bx - Cx^2 + 3x^3 + 2x^2(3 + 2\log x) - 2x(1 + \log x)$$

$$+ \frac{11}{4} + \frac{3}{2}\log x + \log^2 x + \left(\frac{9x^2}{10} - \frac{7}{20}\right)\cos(2\log x) + \left(\frac{4x^2}{5} + \frac{9}{20}\right)\sin(2\log x),$$

(7.239b)

to which may be added forcing (7.238a, b) by a: (i) the non-resonant power (7.208a, b; 7.211a–d) with exponent $b = 3$; (ii–iii) singly (doubly) resonant power (7.215a–c) [(7.218a–c)]; (iv) the power of logarithms (7.232a, b; 7.237a, b); (v) the product of a power by a hyperbolic cosine and a circular sine of multiples of logarithms (7.225a, b; 7.228a, b).

Thus, *the coupled linear system of ordinary differential equations with homogeneous coefficients in the unforced (7.162a, b) [forced (7.238a, b)] case has (standard CLXII) general (complete) integral (7.177a; 7.180d) [(7.239a, b)], involving three arbitrary constants C_1, C_2, C_3 (A, B, C). The three independent and compatible boundary conditions (7.182a) [≡(7.240a)] lead to (7.182b) [(7.240b)]:*

$$\{\bar{y}(1), \bar{z}(1), \bar{z}'(1)\} = \{3, 1, 0\} = \left\{ A + C - \frac{17}{4}, -2B - C + \frac{103}{10}, -2B - 2C + \frac{154}{5} \right\},$$

(7.240a, b)

the constants (7.183a–c) [(7.241a–c)]:

$$C = \frac{43}{2}, \qquad B = -\frac{61}{10}, \qquad A = -\frac{57}{4},$$

(7.241a–c)

specifying to a unique solution (7.183d, e) [(7.239a, b; 7.241a–c)]. In (7.241c) the derivative (7.242) of (7.239b) was used:

$$\bar{z}'(x) = -2B - 2Cx + 9x^2 + 16x - 4 + \frac{3}{2x} - 2\log x + 8x\log x + \frac{2}{x}\log x$$

(7.242)

$$+ \left(\frac{17x}{5} + \frac{9}{10x}\right)\cos(2\log x) - \left(\frac{x}{5} - \frac{7}{10x}\right)\sin(2\log x).$$

In (7.239a, b) the particular integrals of the forced differential system that coincide with normal integrals, such as x ($x \log x$) should not be included in the arbitrary constants of integration $A(B)$, because this could be inconsistent with the compatibility relations between the dependent variables y and z.

7.8 Simultaneous Finite Difference Equations

A characteristic polynomial (as the determinant of a matrix of polynomials) exists for a single (a simultaneous system of): (i) linear ordinary differential equations with constant coefficients involving ordinary derivatives [sections 1.3–1.5 (7.4–7.5)]; (ii) linear ordinary differential equations with power coefficients involving homogeneous derivatives [sections 1.6–1.7 (7.6–7.7)]; (iii) linear finite difference equations with constants coefficients involving finite forward differences [sections(s) 1.9 (7.8–7.9)]. In the latter case (iii), a simultaneous system of finite difference equations relates the values of several dependent variables at several points (subsection 7.8.1). In the linear case with constant coefficients (subsection 7.8.2), there is a matrix of polynomials of finite differences whose determinant is the characteristic polynomial (subsection 7.8.3). The single (multiple) roots of the characteristic polynomial specify the natural sequences (subsection 7.8.4), which are integral powers (multiplied by powers of the exponent). The general solution of the simultaneous unforced system of finite difference equations is a linear combination of natural sequences (subsection 7.8.5), with arbitrary constants determined by starting conditions (subsection 7.8.6) and the dependent variables related by compatibility conditions (subsection 7.8.7). Whereas the dependent variables satisfy a square system, the natural sequences lead (subsection 7.8.8) for distinct (multiple) roots to a diagonal (lower triangular) system [subsection 7.8.9 (7.8.10)].

7.8.1 Non-Linear and Linear Finite Difference Equations

Consider a set of M dependent variables (7.243a, b) of a single independent variable and let (7.243c) be their values at particular points:

$$r = 1, \ldots, M: \qquad y_r = y_r(x); \qquad y_{r,\ell} = y_r(x_\ell). \qquad (7.243\text{a–c})$$

A simultaneous system of finite difference equations is a set of M relations (7.244a, b) among all values (7.243c) of the variables (7.243a, b):

$$m = 1, \ldots, M: \qquad 0 = F_m\left(y_{r,\ell}\right). \qquad (7.244\text{a, b})$$

The absence of powers or products of any of the values (7.243c) leads to a linear simultaneous system of finite difference equations (7.245a, b):

$$N_{m,r} \in |N: \qquad B_{m,\ell} = \sum_{r=1}^{m} \sum_{k=0}^{N_{m,r}} A_{m,r,k,\ell}\, y_{r,\ell+k}. \qquad (7.245\text{a, b})$$

The case of coefficients that do not depend on the particular point:

$$B_{m,\ell} = \sum_{r=1}^{m} \sum_{k=0}^{N_{m,r}} A_{m,r,k}\, y_{r,\ell+k} \,, \qquad (7.246)$$

corresponds to a linear simultaneous system of finite difference equations with constant coefficients. The relation (7.246), for example (7.247a, b):

$$y_{\ell+2} + z_{\ell+1} - y_{\ell} + z_{\ell} = 0 = 2\, y_{\ell+1} + z_{\ell+1} - 2\, y_{\ell} \,. \qquad (7.247a,\ b)$$

can be written as polynomials of forward finite differences (subsection 7.8.2).

7.8.2 Operator Forward Finite Difference

The forward finite difference operator (7.248a) steps from one value to the next of each dependent variable and may be applied iteratively (7.248b):

$$\Delta y_{r,\ell} = y_{r,\ell+1} \,, \qquad \Delta^k y_{r,\ell} = y_{r,\ell+k} \,. \qquad (7.248a,\ b)$$

Substituting (7.248b) in (7.246) leads to:

$$B_{m,\ell} = \sum_{r=1}^{m} \sum_{k=0}^{N_{m,r}} A_{m,r,k}\, \Delta^k\, y_{r,\ell} \,. \qquad (7.249)$$

Introducing the matrix of polynomials of finite differences:

$$R_{m,r}(\Delta) = \sum_{k=0}^{N_{m,r}} A_{m,r,k}\, \Delta^k \,, \qquad (7.250)$$

leads to the system:

$$B_{m,\ell} = \sum_{r=1}^{m} R_{m,r}(\Delta)\, y_{r,\ell} \,, \qquad (7.251)$$

showing *that a simultaneous system of finite difference equations (7.243a–c; 7.244a, b) that (standard CLXIII) is linear (7.245a, b) with constant coefficients (7.246) ≡ (7.249) ≡ (7.251) corresponds to a matrix of polynomials of forward differences (7.250) applied to the matrix of values of the dependent variables (7.243c) equated to a forcing matrix:*

$$
\begin{bmatrix}
R_{1,1}(\Delta) & R_{1,2}(\Delta) & \cdots & R_{1,M}(\Delta) \\
R_{2,1}(\Delta) & R_{2,2}(\Delta) & \cdots & R_{1,M}(\Delta) \\
\vdots & \vdots & \ddots & \vdots \\
R_{M-1}(\Delta) & R_{M,2}(\Delta) & \cdots & R_{M,M}(\Delta)
\end{bmatrix}
\begin{bmatrix}
y_{1,\ell} \\
y_{2,\ell} \\
\vdots \\
y_{M,\ell}
\end{bmatrix}
=
\begin{bmatrix}
B_{1,\ell} \\
B_{2,\ell} \\
\vdots \\
B_{M,\ell}
\end{bmatrix}.
\tag{7.252}
$$

For example, the coupled linear system of finite difference equations with constant coefficients constant coefficients (7.247a, b) can be written in matrix form:

$$
\begin{bmatrix}
\Delta^2 - 1 & \Delta + 1 \\
2\Delta - 2 & \Delta
\end{bmatrix}
\begin{bmatrix}
y_\ell \\
z_\ell
\end{bmatrix}
= 0.
\tag{7.253}
$$

The method of the matrix of polynomials applies with ordinary/homogeneous derivatives (finite differences) to simultaneous systems of ordinary differential (finite difference) equations, with constant/homogeneous (constant) coefficients [sections 7.4–7.5/7.6–7.7 (7.8–7.9)].

7.8.3 Matrix of Polynomials of Finite Differences

The simultaneous linear unforced (7.254a) system of finite difference equations with constant coefficients (7.254b):

$$
B_{m,\ell} = 0: \qquad\qquad \sum_{r=1}^{M} R_{m,r}(\Delta) y_{r,\ell} = 0,
\tag{7.254a, b}
$$

is equivalent to the matrix system:

$$
\begin{bmatrix}
R_{1,1}(\Delta) & R_{1,2}(\Delta) & \cdots & R_{1,M}(\Delta) \\
R_{2,1}(\Delta) & R_{2,2}(\Delta) & \cdots & R_{1,M}(\Delta) \\
\vdots & \vdots & \ddots & \vdots \\
R_{M-1}(\Delta) & R_{M,2}(\Delta) & \cdots & R_{M,M}(\Delta)
\end{bmatrix}
\begin{bmatrix}
y_{1,\ell} \\
y_{2,\ell} \\
\vdots \\
y_{M,\ell}
\end{bmatrix}
= 0.
\tag{7.255}
$$

Elimination for any of the dependent variables $y_{m,\ell}$ would lead to a single linear finite difference equation with constant coefficients (1.447a–d) whose solution is power with integer exponent (7.256a) with a distinct constant coefficient for each dependent variable:

$$y_{m,\ell} = E_m\, a^\ell; \qquad\qquad \Delta^k y_{m,\ell} = E_m\, \Delta^k a^\ell = E_m\, a^{\ell+k}, \qquad (7.256a, b)$$

the application of forward finite differences (7.248a, b) to (7.256a) leads to (7.256b), that:

$$\left\{R_{m,r}(\Delta)\right\}a^\ell = \sum_{k=0}^{N_{m,r}} A_{m,r,k}\, \Delta^k a^\ell = a^\ell \sum_{k=0}^{N_{m,r}} A_{m,r,k}\, a^k = a^\ell\, R_{m,r}(a), \qquad (7.257a\text{--}c)$$

extends to a polynomial of finite differences (7.257a–c).
  Substituting (7.256a) in (7.254b) and using (7.257c) leads to:

$$0 = \sum_{r=0}^{M} R_{m,r}(\Delta) E_r\, a^\ell = a^\ell \sum_{r=0}^{M} R_{m,r}(a) E_r. \qquad (7.258)$$

The coefficients in (7.256a) cannot be all zero (7.259b), otherwise a trivial solution would result; using also (7.259a) from (7.258) follows (7.259c):

$$a^\ell \neq 0; \qquad \left\{E_1....E_M\right\} \neq \left\{0,...,0\right\}: \qquad 0 = \sum_{r=1}^{M} R_{m,r}(a) E_m, \qquad (7.259a\text{--}c)$$

implying that the *characteristic polynomial (7.260a), which is the determinant of the matrix of polynomials of finite differences (standard CLXIV), must be zero (7.260b):*

$$R_N(a) \equiv Det\left[R_{m,r}(a)\right] = 0. \qquad (7.260a, b)$$

For example, in the case of the coupled linear system of finite difference equations with constant coefficients (7.247a, b) the matrix of polynomials of finite differences (7.253) leads to:

$$R_3(\Delta) = \left(\Delta^2 - 1\right)\Delta - 2(\Delta+1)(\Delta-1) = \left(\Delta^2 - 1\right)(\Delta - 2), \qquad (7.261a, b)$$

as the characteristic polynomial.

7.8.4 Simple and Multiple Roots of the Characteristic Polynomial

*If the characteristic polynomial (7.260a, b) has (standard CLXV) all roots (7.262c) distinct (7.262a, b) the corresponding **natural sequences** (7.256a) are (7.262d):*

$$R_N(a_n) = 0 \neq R'_N(a_n): \qquad R_N(a_n) = A \prod_{n=1}^{N}(a - a_n) \Rightarrow q_{n,\ell} = (a_n)^{\ell}. \qquad (7.262\text{a–d})$$

To a root (7.263a) of multiplicity α of the characteristic polynomial (7.263b) correspond (standard CLXVI) α natural sequences (7.263c, d):

$$S_{N-\alpha}(a_0) \neq 0: \quad R_N(a) = (a - a_0)^{\alpha} S_{N-\alpha}(a), \quad \beta = 1,...,\alpha: \quad q_{n,\ell,\beta} = \ell^{\beta-1}(a_0)^{\ell},$$
$$(7.263\text{a–d})$$

similar to (7.262d) and multiplied by powers with integer base $1, \ell, \ell^2, ..., \ell^{\alpha-1}$. For example, the coupled linear system of finite difference equations with constant coefficients, (7.247a, b) $\equiv$ (7.253), has characteristic polynomial, (7.261a, b) $\equiv$ (7.264a), with three simple roots (7.264b):

$$R_3(\Delta) = (\Delta - 1)(\Delta + 1)(\Delta - 2); \quad a_{1-3} = 1, -1, 2: \quad q_{1,\ell} = 1, \ q_{2,\ell} = (-)^{\ell}, \quad q_{3,\ell} = 2^{\ell},$$
$$(7.264\text{a–e})$$

leading to the normal sequences (7.264c–e).

7.8.5 General Solution of an Unforced System

The general solution of a simultaneous linear unforced system of finite difference equations (7.254a, b) $\equiv$ (7.255) is a linear combination of normal sequences leading to two cases: (i) if (standard CLXVII) the characteristic polynomial has distinct roots (7.262a–c) every solution is a linear combination (7.265a, b) of natural sequences (7.262d):

$$y_{m,\ell} = \sum_{N=1}^{N} C_n F_{n,m} q_{m,\ell} = \sum_{N=1}^{N} C_n F_{n,m} (a_n)^{\ell}; \qquad (7.265\text{a, b})$$

(ii) in the case (standard CLXVIII) of a multiple root (7.266a) with multiplicities α_s of the characteristic polynomial (7.266b) the linear combination of natural sequences (7.263a–d) is (7.266c, d):

$$\sum_{s=1}^{S} \alpha_s = M; \qquad R_N(a) = A \prod_{s=1}^{S} (a - a_s)^{\alpha_s}:$$
$$(7.266\text{a–d})$$

$$y_{m,\ell} = \sum_{s=1}^{S} \sum_{\beta_s=1}^{\alpha_S} C_{s\beta_S} F_{n,s,\beta_S} q_{m,\ell,\beta_S} = \sum_{s=1}^{S} (a_s)^{\ell} \sum_{\beta_s=1}^{\alpha_S} \ell^{\beta_S-1} C_{s,\beta_S} F_{n,S,\beta_S}.$$

Both in (7.265a, b) [(7.266c, d)], there are n arbitrary constants $C_s (C_{s,\beta_s})$ determined (standard CLXIX) from N independent and compatible **starting conditions**. In the $N \times M$ matrix of coefficients $F_{n,m} (F_{n,s,\beta_s})$ in (7.265a, b) [(7.266c, d)] one row (standard CLXX) can be chosen at will, for example, (7.267a) [(7.267b)]:

$$F_{1,m} = 1, \qquad\qquad F_{1,s,\beta,s} = 1, \qquad\qquad (7.267a, b)$$

and all others are determined (standard CLXX) by **compatibility conditions** obtained by substituting the solution (7.265a, b) [(7.266a–d)] back into the unforced system of finite differences (7.254a, b) ≡ (7.255). The application of compatibility (starting) conditions is illustrated [subsection 7.8.6 (7.8.7)] by the system (7.247a, b) ≡ (7.253).

7.8.6 Compatibility Conditions for the Dependent Variables

In the case of the coupled linear uniform system of finite difference equations with constant coefficients (7.247a, b) ≡ (7.253) the characteristic polynomial (7.261a) ≡ (7.261b) ≡ (7.264a) has distinct roots (7.264b) leading to the natural sequences (7.264c–e) whose linear combination specifies the dependent variables (7.268a, b):

$$y_\ell = C_1 + C_2 (-)^\ell + C_3 2^\ell, \qquad z_\ell = C_4 + C_5 (-)^\ell + C_6 2^\ell. \qquad (7.268a, b)$$

Of the six constants C_{1-6} only three are independent, and the remaining three are determined by compatibility relations obtained substituting the solutions (7.268a, b) back into the system (7.247a, b). Substituting (7.268a) [(7.268b)] in (7.247b) leads to the two sets of terms (7.269b) [(7.269a)]:

$$z_{\ell+1} = C_4 + C_5 (-)^{\ell+1} + C_6 2^{\ell+1} = C_4 - C_5 (-)^\ell + 2C_6 2^\ell, \qquad (7.269a)$$

$$2y_\ell - 2y_{\ell+1} = 2C_1 + 2C_2 (-)^\ell + 2C_3 2^\ell - 2C_1 - 2C_2 (-)^{\ell+1} - 2C_3 2^{\ell+1}$$
$$= 4C_2 (-)^\ell - 2C_3 2^\ell. \qquad (7.269b)$$

From (7.247b) follows the equality of (7.269a) = (7.269b), and equating the coefficients of the normal sequences (7.264c–e) specifies (7.270a–c) the constants C_{4-6} in terms of C_{1-3}:

$$C_4 = 0, \quad C_5 = -4C_2, \quad C_6 = -C_3; \quad z_\ell = -4C_2 (-)^\ell - C_3 2^\ell, \qquad (7.270a–d)$$

substituting (7.270a–c) in (7.268b) leads to (7.270d). Thus, the coupled linear unforced system of finite difference equations (7.247a, b) ≡ (7.253) has for general solution the sequences of dependent variables (7.268a; 7.270d) where C_{1-3} are arbitrary constants determined by three independent and compatible starting conditions (subsection 7.8.7).

7.8.7 Arbitrary Constants and Starting Conditions

The three independent and compatible starting conditions (7.271a–c) applied to (7.268a; 7.270d) lead to (7.271d–f):

$$\{y_0, z_0, z_1\} = \{0, 1, 1\} = \{C_1 + C_2 + C_3, -4C_2 - C_3, \quad 4C_2 - 2C_3\}. \quad (7.271a-f)$$

The solution of (7.271d–f) is (7.272a–c):

$$C_3 = -\frac{2}{3}, \qquad C_2 = \frac{1}{4} + \frac{C_3}{2} = -\frac{1}{12}, \qquad C_1 = -C_2 - C_3 = \frac{3}{4}. \quad (7.272a-c)$$

Substitution of (7.272a–c) in (7.268a; 7.270d) gives:

$$y_\ell = \frac{3}{4} - \frac{(-)^\ell}{12} - \frac{2^{\ell+1}}{3}, \qquad z_\ell = \frac{(-)^\ell}{3} + \frac{2^{\ell+1}}{3}, \quad (7.273a, b)$$

as the unique solutions of the coupled linear unforced system of finite difference equations with constant coefficients (7.247a, b) $\equiv$ (7.253) that meets the starting conditions (7.271a–c). If the starting condition (7.271a) was replaced by (7.274a):

$$g \equiv z_2 = -4C_2 - 4C_3 \begin{cases} = 3 & redundant, \\ \neq 3 & incompatible, \end{cases} \quad (7.274a-c)$$

there would be three equations (7.271e, f; 7.274a) to determine two constants (C_2, C_3) leading to two possibilities: (i) the case (7.274b) is consistent but redundant, and leaves C_1 undetermined; (ii) the case (7.274c) is inconsistent. Thus, the starting conditions specifying $\{z_0, z_1, z_2\}$ cannot be independent and compatible.

7.8.8 Diagonal or Lower Triangular System

The simultaneous unforced system of finite differences equations with constant coefficients (7.254a, b) $\equiv$ (7.255) has for: (i) distinct roots (standard CLXXI) of the characteristic polynomial (7.262a–c) the natural sequences (7.262d) $\equiv$ (7.275a) that satisfy (7.275b):

$$q_{n,\ell} = (a_n)^\ell: \qquad\qquad \Delta q_{n,\ell} = (a_n)^{\ell+1} = a_n q_{n,\ell}, \quad (7.275a, b)$$

leading to a decoupled or diagonal system (7.276):

$$
\begin{bmatrix} \Delta q_{1,\ell} \\ \Delta q_{1,\ell} \\ \vdots \\ \Delta q_{1,\ell} \end{bmatrix} = \begin{bmatrix} a_1 & 0 & \cdots & 0 \\ 0 & a_2 & \cdots & 0 \\ \vdots & \vdots & \ddots & \vdots \\ 0 & 0 & \cdots & a_N \end{bmatrix} \begin{bmatrix} q_{1,\ell} \\ q_{2,\ell} \\ \vdots \\ q_{N,\ell} \end{bmatrix} ; \qquad (7.276)
$$

(ii) a root of multiplicity α of the characteristic polynomial (7.263a, b) a (standard CLXXII) set of α natural sequences, (7.263c, d) $\equiv$ (7.277a, b), satisfying (7.277c):

$$
\beta = 1,\ldots, \alpha_s; \qquad q_{s,\ell,\beta} = \ell^{\beta-1}(a_s)^{\ell}: \qquad \Delta q_{s,\ell,\beta} = (\ell+1)^{\beta-1}(a_s)^{\ell+1}. \qquad (7.277a\text{–}c)
$$

In the latter case (7.261c) the binomial theorem (I.25.38) $\equiv$ (7.278a) leads to:

$$
\Delta q_{s,\ell,\beta} = (a_s)^{\ell+1}\,\ell^{\beta-1} + (a_s)^{\ell+1} \sum_{\gamma=1}^{\beta-2} \binom{\beta-1}{\gamma} \ell^{\gamma} = a_s\, q_{s,\ell,\beta} + a_s \sum_{\gamma=1}^{\beta-2} \binom{\beta-1}{\gamma} q_{s,\ell,\gamma},
$$

$$(7.278a, b)$$

*a **lower triangular system** (7.278b), which is illustrated next (subsection 7.8.9) for the simplest cases of double or triple roots of the characteristic polynomial.*

7.8.9 Block-Diagonal Lower Triangular System

Consider a characteristic polynomial with one single a_1 root, one double a_2 root, and one triple a_3 root:

$$
R_6(\Delta) = \sum_{n=1}^{6} A_n \Delta^n = A_6(\Delta - a_1)(\Delta - a_2)^2(\Delta - a_3)^3. \qquad (7.279)
$$

The single root leads to a natural sequence (7.280a) satisfying (7.280b):

$$
q_{1,\ell} = (a_1)^{\ell}: \qquad \Delta q_{1,\ell} = (a_1)^{\ell+1} = a_1(a_1)^{\ell} = a_1\, q_{\ell,1}; \qquad (7.280a, b)
$$

(ii) the double root gives, in addition to (7.280a, b) $\equiv$ (7.281a, b):

$$
q_{2,\ell,1} = (a_2)^{\ell}: \qquad \Delta q_{2,\ell,1} = (a_2)^{\ell+1} = a_2\, q_{2,\ell,1}; \qquad (7.281a, b)
$$

also (7.282a, b):

$$
q_{2,\ell,2} = \ell(a_2)^{\ell}: \quad \Delta q_{2,\ell,2} = (\ell+1)(a_2)^{\ell+1} = (a_2)^{\ell+1} + \ell(a_2)^{\ell+1} = a_2\, q_{2,\ell,1} + a_2\, q_{2,\ell,2},
$$

$$(7.282a, b)$$

(ii) the triple root adds to (7.283a, b) ≡ (7.281a, b) ≡ (7.280a, b) and (7.284a, b) ≡ (7.282a, b):

$$q_{3,\ell,1} = (a_3)^\ell: \qquad\qquad \Delta q_{3,\ell,1} = a_3\, q_{3,\ell,1}, \qquad\qquad (7.283a, b)$$

$$q_{3,\ell,2} = \ell(a_3)^\ell: \quad \Delta q_{3,\ell,2} = (\ell+1)(a_3)^{\ell+1} = (a_3)^{\ell+1} + \ell(a_3)^{\ell+1} = a_3\, q_{3,\ell,1} + a_3\, q_{3,\ell,2},$$
$$(7.284a, b)$$

also (7.285a, b).

$$q_{3,\ell,3} = \ell^2 (a_3)^\ell: \qquad \Delta q_{3,\ell,3} = (\ell+1)^2 (a_3)^{\ell+1}$$
$$= (a_3)^{\ell+1} + 2a_3\,\ell(a_3)^\ell + a_3\,\ell^2(a_3)^\ell \qquad (7.285a, b)$$
$$= a_3\, q_{3,\ell,1} + 2\, a_3\, q_{3,\ell,2} + a_3\, q_{3,\ell,3}.$$

Thus, the set of six natural sequences (7.280a; 7.281a, 7.282a; 7.283a, 7.284a, 7.285a) satisfies (7.280b; 7.281b, 7.282b; 7.283b, 7.284b, 7.285b):

$$
\begin{bmatrix}
\Delta q_{1,\ell} \\
\Delta q_{2,\ell,1} \\
\Delta q_{2,\ell,2} \\
\Delta q_{3,\ell,1} \\
\Delta q_{3,\ell,2} \\
\Delta q_{3,\ell,3}
\end{bmatrix}
=
\begin{bmatrix}
a_1 & 0 & 0 & 0 & 0 & 0 \\
0 & a_2 & 0 & 0 & 0 & 0 \\
0 & a_2 & a_2 & 0 & 0 & 0 \\
0 & 0 & 0 & a_3 & 0 & 0 \\
0 & 0 & 0 & a_3 & a_3 & a_3 \\
0 & 0 & 0 & a_3 & 2a_3 & a_3
\end{bmatrix}
\begin{bmatrix}
q_{1,\ell} \\
q_{2,\ell,1} \\
q_{2,\ell,2} \\
q_{3,\ell,1} \\
q_{3,\ell,2} \\
q_{3,\ell,3}
\end{bmatrix},
\qquad (7.286)
$$

which is a block diagonal system consisting of lower triangular submatrices. In general, *an unforced linear simultaneous system of finite difference equations with constant coefficients, (7.254a) ≡ (7.255), whose characteristic polynomial, (7.257a–c; 7.260a, b), has distinct multiple roots (7.266a–d) leads (standard CLXXIII) to natural sequences forming a block lower triangular system, for example (7.279; 7.286).*

7.8.10 Diagonalization of a Finite Difference System

In the case of the coupled linear unforced system of finite difference equations with constant coefficients (7.247a, b) ≡ (7.253), the natural sequences (7.264c–e) satisfy (7.287a–c):

$$\Delta q_{1,\ell} = \Delta(1^\ell) = 1^{\ell+1} = 1 = q_{1,\ell}, \qquad (7.287a)$$

$$\Delta q_{2,\ell} = \Delta\left[(-)^\ell\right] = (-)^{\ell+1} = -(-)^\ell = -q_{2,\ell}, \qquad (7.287b)$$

$$\Delta q_{3,\ell} = \Delta(2)^\ell = 2^{\ell+1} = 2^\ell = 2\, q_{3,\ell}, \qquad (7.287c)$$

and leads to a diagonal system:

$$
\begin{bmatrix} \Delta q_{1,\ell} \\ \Delta q_{2,\ell} \\ \Delta q_{3,\ell} \end{bmatrix} = \begin{bmatrix} 1 & 0 & 0 \\ 0 & -1 & 0 \\ 0 & 0 & 2 \end{bmatrix} \begin{bmatrix} q_{1,\ell} \\ q_{2,\ell} \\ q_{3,\ell} \end{bmatrix},
\tag{7.288}
$$

because the roots (7.264b) of the characteristic polynomial (7.264a) are distinct as shown by the diagonal in (7.288).

The dependent variables are a linear combination of the natural sequences (7.264c–e) leading to the 2×3 rectangular system for: (i) the general integral (7.268a; 7.270d) of the unforced system:

$$
\begin{bmatrix} y_\ell \\ z_e \end{bmatrix} = \begin{bmatrix} C_1 & C_2 & C_3 \\ 0 & -4\,C_2 & -C_3 \end{bmatrix} \begin{bmatrix} q_{1,\ell} \\ q_{2,\ell} \\ q_{3,\ell} \end{bmatrix};
\tag{7.289}
$$

(ii) the unique solution (7.290) satisfying the starting conditions (7.271a–c):

$$
\begin{bmatrix} y_\ell \\ z_e \end{bmatrix} = \begin{bmatrix} \dfrac{3}{4} & -\dfrac{1}{12} & -\dfrac{2}{3} \\ 0 & \dfrac{1}{3} & \dfrac{2}{3} \end{bmatrix} \begin{bmatrix} q_{1,\ell} \\ q_{2,\ell} \\ q_{3,\ell} \end{bmatrix};
\tag{7.290}
$$

using the constants (7.272a–c) in (7.273a, b).

7.9 Unforced and Forced Finite Difference

The simultaneous linear system of ordinary differential (finite difference) equations with constant/homogeneous (constant) coefficients: (i) involve ordinary/homogeneous derivatives (finite differences) in the unforced case [section 7.4/7.6 (7.8)]; (ii) in the forced case [section 7.5/7.7 (7.9)] with (subsection 7.9.2) the forcing vector similar to the natural integral (sequence) there are non-resonant (resonant) solutions [subsection 7.9.3 (7.9.4)] when there is not (there is) coincidence with the roots of the characteristic polynomial; this may be extended (subsection 7.9.5) to the products of powers by circular or hyperbolic sines and cosines of multiple angles (subsection 7.9.6). For all two differential (one finite difference) linear systems (subsection 7.9.8) the complete integral (solution) (subsection 7.9.7) is the sum of the general integral (solution) of the unforced system and a particular integral (solution) of the forced system. The finite difference equations and systems may use (subsection 7.9.1) either forward or backward differences, or also their arithmetic mean as central differences.

7.9.1 Forward, Backward, and Central Differences

A simultaneous system of linear finite difference equations with constant coefficients (7.245a, b) can be considered for **forward** (7.248a) ≡ (7.291a), **backward** (7.291b), or **central** (7.291c) differences:

$$\Delta y_{r,\ell} = y_{r,\ell+1}, \quad \nabla y_{r,\ell} = y_{r,\ell-1}, \quad \delta y_{r,\ell} = \frac{1}{2}\left(y_{r,\ell+1} + y_{r,\ell-1}\right) = \frac{1}{2}\left(\Delta y_{r,\ell} + \nabla y_{r,\ell}\right),$$

$$(7.291\text{a--c})$$

with the central difference equating (7.291d) to the arithmetic mean of the forward and backward differences. The forward differences (7.248a) ≡ (7.291a) are used in the comparison with a simultaneous system of linear ordinary differential equations with constant (homogeneous) coefficients that: (i) uses ordinary (homogeneous) (7.49a, b) [(7.152a)] derivatives (7.292a) [(7.293a)]: (ii) has exponential (power) natural integrals (7.292b) [(7.293b)] for single roots a_n of the characteristic polynomial; and (iii) inserts power (logarithmic) factors (7.292c) [(7.293c)] for multiple roots a of the characteristic polynomial:

$$Dy_m = \frac{dy_m}{dx}: \qquad q_n(x) = e^{a_s x}, \qquad q_{s,\beta}(x) = e^{a_s x} x^{\beta-1}, \qquad (7.292\text{a--c})$$

$$\delta y_m = x\frac{dy_m}{dx}: \qquad q_{s,\beta}(x) = x^{a_n}, \qquad q_{s,\beta}(x) = x^{a_s} \log^{\beta-1} x, \qquad (7.293\text{a--c})$$

$$\Delta y_{m,\ell} = y_{m,\ell+1}: \qquad y_{n,\ell} = (a_n)^\ell, \qquad y_{s,\ell,\beta} = (a_n)^\ell \ell^{\beta-1}. \qquad (7.294\text{a--c})$$

In the case of a simultaneous linear system of finite difference equations with constant coefficients: (i) ordinary (7.292a) [homogeneous (7.293a)] derivatives are replaced by (7.294a)] finite differences; (ii) for single roots of the characteristic polynomial the exponential (7.292b) [power (7.293b)] natural integrals are replaced (7.294b) by natural sequences consisting of powers with integer exponents; (iii) for multiple roots of the characteristic polynomial the powers (7.292c) [powers of logarithms (7.293c)] as factors are replaced (7.294c) by powers of integers. The corresponding forced systems of simultaneous equations have two important cases: (i) forcing similar to (7.292b; 7.293b) [(7.294b)] the natural integral (sequences) leads to non-resonant (resonant) solutions [subsection 7.9.3–(7.9.4)] in the case of non-coincidence (coincidence) with roots of the characteristic polynomial; this can be extended to include as factor circular or hyperbolic cosines and sines of multiple angles (subsections 7.9.5–7.9.6). The preceding examples (sections 7.8–7.9) lead to the complete solution of a coupled linear system of finite difference equations with constant coefficients (subsection 7.9.7), for which the arbitrary constants can be determined from starting conditions (subsection 7.9.8) in analogy with simultaneous linear systems of ordinary differential equations with constant or homogeneous coefficients (Table 7.1, p. 76).

7.9.2 Forcing by a Power with Integer Exponent

Consider the simultaneous linear system of finite difference equations with constant coefficients (7.250; 7.251) forced by powers with integral exponents (7.295a):

$$\sum_{r=1}^{M} R_{m,r}(\Delta) y_{r,\ell} = G_r b^\ell ; \qquad\qquad y_{r,\ell} = H_r b^\ell ; \qquad (7.295a, b)$$

the solution is sought in a similar form (7.295b) to the forcing (7.295a) with unknown coefficients H_r related to the known forcing coefficients G_r by substitution of (7.295b) in (7.295a) leading to (7.296a):

$$G_r b^\ell = \sum_{r=1}^{M} R_{m,r}(\Delta) H_r b^\ell = b^\ell \sum_{r=1}^{M} R_{m,r}(b) H_r , \qquad (7.296a, b)$$

where (7.257c) was substituted to obtain (7.296b). As in (7.119a–c; 7.203a–c) the system (7.296b) can be inverted to specify the unknown response coefficients G_r in terms of the known forcing coefficients F_r:

$$\sum_{m=1}^{M} \bar{R}_{m,r}(b) G_r = H_r Det\left[R_{m,r}(b)\right] = H_r R_N(b), \qquad (7.297a, b)$$

where appears the matrix of co-factors $\bar{R}_{r,m}$ of the matrix of polynomials of finite differences that satisfies:

$$\sum_{q=1}^{M} \bar{R}_{m,q}(b) \bar{R}_{q,r}(b) = \delta_{mr} R_N(b), \qquad (7.298)$$

involving the characteristic polynomial (7.260a).

TABLE 7.1

Simultaneous Systems of Linear Equations

Type	Ordinary Differential	Ordinary Differential	Finite Difference
Coefficients	Constant	Homogeneous	Constant
Equation	(7.49a–c)	(7.159)	(7.249)
Matrix form	(7.50)	(7.161)	(7.252)
Characteristic Polynomial	(7.58c)	(7.168a, b)	(7.260a, b)
Matrix of Co-factors	(7.119a–c)	(7.203a–c)	(7.298)
Unforced	section 7.4	section 7.6	section 7.8
Equation	(7.54)	(7.165)	(7.255)
Single Roots	(7.64a–c)	(7.170a–c)	(7.262a–c)
Natural Integrals	(7.64d)	(7.170d)	(7.262d)
General Integral	(7.79a–c)	(7.174a, b)	(7.265a, b)
Diagonalization	(7.96a–c)	(7.184a–c)	(7.276)
Multiple Roots	(7.70a–d)	(7.172a–c)	(7.263a–c)
Natural Integral	(7.71a–d)	(7.172d)	(7.263d)
General Integral	(7.80)	(7.175)	(7.266a–d)
Diagonalization	(7.97a–d)	(7.185a–d)	(7.278a, b)
Forcing	section 7.5	section 7.7	section 7.9
General	(7.50)	(7.161)	(7.252)
Non-Resonant	(7.116a, b; 7.121a, b)	(7.201a; 7.204a, b)	(7.295a; 7.299a, b)
Resonant	(7.116a, b; 7.122a, b)	(7.201a; 7.205a, b)	(7.295a; 7.300a, b)
Extension	subsections 7.5.3–7.5.7	subsections 7.7.3–7.7.9	subsections 7.9.3–7.9.6
Inverse Matrix of Polynomials	(7.141)	(7.229)	–
Example with Forcing	(7.148a, b)	(7.238a, b)	(7.322a, b)
Complete Integral	(7.149a, b)	(7.239a, b)	(7.323a, b)
Initial Conditions General Integral	(7.93a; 7.94a, b)	(7.182a; 7.183d, e)	(7.271a; 7.273a, b)
Initial Conditions Complete integral	(7.150a–c)	(7.240a; 7.241a–c)	(7.324a; 7.325a–c)

Note: Comparison of linear systems of simultaneous equations with matrix of polynomials of: (i)(ii) ordinary (homogeneous) derivatives for ordinary differential equations with constant (homogeneous) coefficients; (iii) forward finite difference equations with constant coefficients.

Thus, *the simultaneous linear system of finite difference equations with constant coefficients (7.250; 7.251) ≡ (7.252) forced by powers with integer exponents (7.295a) has (standard CLXXIV) particular solutions: (i) given by (7.299b) in the non-resonant case when b is not a root of the characteristic polynomial (7.299a):*

$$R_N(b) \neq 0: \qquad y_{r,\ell} = \left[R_N(b)\right]^{-1} b^\ell \sum_{m=1}^{M} \bar{R}_{r,m}(b) G_m ; \qquad (7.299a, b)$$

(ii) in the resonant case when b is a root of multiplicity α of the characteristic polynomial (7.300a) the solution is given by (7.300b):

$$R_N(b) = R_N'(b) = \ldots R_N^{(\alpha-1)}(b) = 0 \neq R_N^{(\alpha)}(b):$$

$$y_{r,\ell} = \left[R_N^{(\alpha)}(b)\right]^{-1} \frac{\partial^\alpha}{\partial b^\alpha} \left\{ b^\ell \sum_{m=1}^{M} \bar{R}_{r,m}(b) G_m \right\},$$

$$(7.300a, b)$$

where L'Hôspital rule was used, as in (7.121a, b; 7.122a, b) and (7.204a, b; 7.205a, b). Next are given non-resonant (resonant) examples [subsection 7.9.3 (7.9.4)] for the system (7.247a, b).

7.9.3 Non-Resonant Forcing by Integral Powers

Consider the coupled linear system of finite difference equations with constant coefficients (7.247a, b) forced by powers with integral exponents (7.301a, b):

$$y_{\ell+2} + z_{\ell'+1} - y_\ell + z_\ell = b^\ell, \qquad 2y_{\ell+1} + z_{\ell+1} - 2y_\ell = -b^\ell, \qquad (7.301a, b)$$

which can be written using forward finite differences:

$$\begin{bmatrix} \Delta^2 - 1 & \Delta + 1 \\ 2\Delta - 2 & \Delta \end{bmatrix} \begin{bmatrix} y_\ell \\ z_\ell \end{bmatrix} = b^\ell \begin{bmatrix} 1 \\ -1 \end{bmatrix}, \qquad (7.302)$$

where the matrix of polynomials (7.253) ≡ (7.303a) has co-factors (7.303b):

$$R_{m,r}(\Delta) = \begin{bmatrix} \Delta^2 - 1 & \Delta + 1 \\ 2(\Delta - 1) & \Delta \end{bmatrix}, \qquad \bar{R}_{m,r} = \begin{bmatrix} \Delta & -\Delta - 1 \\ 2(1 - \Delta) & \Delta^2 - 1 \end{bmatrix}.$$

$$(7.303a, b)$$

The solution (7.299b) of (7.301a, b) is (7.304b) ≡ (7.304c):

$$b \neq \pm 1, 2: \qquad \begin{bmatrix} y_\ell \\ z_\ell \end{bmatrix} = \frac{b^\ell}{(b^2-1)(b-2)} \begin{bmatrix} b & -b-1 \\ 2-2b & b^2-1 \end{bmatrix} \begin{bmatrix} 1 \\ -1 \end{bmatrix}$$

$$= \frac{b^\ell}{(b^2-1)(b-2)} \begin{bmatrix} 1+2b \\ 3-2b-b^2 \end{bmatrix},$$

(7.304a–c)

provided that b is not (7.304a–c) one of the three roots (7.264b) of the characteristic polynomial (7.264a). The three single roots (7.264b) lead to three simple resonances (subsection 7.9.4).

7.9.4 Three Cases of Simple Resonance

The characteristic polynomial (7.261a) ≡ (7.305a) has derivative (7.305b):

$$R_3(b) = b^3 - 2b^2 - b + 2; \qquad R_3'(b) = 3b^2 - 4b - 1, \qquad \text{(7.305a, b)}$$

which does not vanish for any of the three single roots (7.269b) leading to three simply resonant solutions (7.300b) of the system (7.301a, b), namely: (i) for the root (7.306a):

$$b = 1: \qquad \begin{bmatrix} y_\ell \\ z_\ell \end{bmatrix} = \frac{1}{R_3'(1)} \lim_{b \to 1} \frac{\partial}{\partial b} \left\{ b^\ell \begin{bmatrix} 1+2b \\ 3-2b-b^2 \end{bmatrix} \right\}$$

$$= -\frac{1}{2} \lim_{b \to 1} \left\{ b^\ell \begin{bmatrix} 2 \\ -2-2b \end{bmatrix} + \ell \begin{bmatrix} 1+2b \\ 3-2b-b^2 \end{bmatrix} b^{\ell-1} \right\} \qquad \text{(7.306a–d)}$$

$$= -\frac{1}{2} \left\{ \begin{bmatrix} 2 \\ -4 \end{bmatrix} + \ell \begin{bmatrix} 3 \\ 0 \end{bmatrix} \right\},$$

the resonant solution is (7.306b) ≡ (7.306c) ≡ (7.306d); (ii) for the root (7.307a), the resonant solution is (7.307b) ≡ (7.307c):

$$b = -1: \qquad \begin{bmatrix} y_\ell \\ z_\ell \end{bmatrix} = \frac{1}{R_3'(-1)} \lim_{b \to -1} \frac{\partial}{\partial b} \left\{ b^\ell \begin{bmatrix} 2 \\ -2-2b \end{bmatrix} + \ell \begin{bmatrix} 1+2b \\ 3-2b-b^2 \end{bmatrix} b^{\ell-1} \right\}$$

$$= \frac{1}{6} \left\{ (-)^\ell \begin{bmatrix} 2 \\ 0 \end{bmatrix} + \ell \begin{bmatrix} -1 \\ 4 \end{bmatrix} (-)^{\ell-1} \right\};$$

(7.307a–c)

(iii) for the third root (7.308a), the resonant solution (7.308b) ≡ (7.308c):

$$b=2: \quad \begin{bmatrix} y_\ell \\ z_\ell \end{bmatrix} = \frac{1}{R_3'(2)} \lim_{b\to 2} \left\{ b^\ell \begin{bmatrix} 2 \\ -2-2b \end{bmatrix} + \ell \begin{bmatrix} 1+2b \\ 3-2b-b^2 \end{bmatrix} b^{\ell-1} \right\}$$

$$= \frac{1}{3} \left\{ 2^\ell \begin{bmatrix} 2 \\ -6 \end{bmatrix} + \ell \begin{bmatrix} 5 \\ -5 \end{bmatrix} 2^{\ell-1} \right\},$$

$$(7.308a\text{--}c)$$

follows as in (7.306b, c).

Thus, the coupled linear system of finite difference equations with constant coefficients (7.301a, b) forced by powers with integral exponents has resonant solutions for the three single roots (7.264b) of the characteristic polynomial (7.264a), namely: (i) for the root (7.306a), the system (7.309a, b) has the solution (7.306d) ≡ (7.309c, d):

$$y_{\ell+2} + z_{\ell+1} - y_\ell + z_\ell = 1, \quad 2y_{\ell+1} + z_{\ell+1} - 2y_\ell = -1: \quad y_\ell = -1-\frac{3}{2}\ell, \quad z_\ell = 2;$$

$$(7.309a\text{--}d)$$

(ii) for the root (7.307a), the system (7.310a, b) has solution (7.307c) ≡ (7.310c, d):

$$y_{\ell+2} + z_{\ell+1} - y_\ell + z_\ell = (-)^\ell, \quad 2y_{\ell+1} + z_{\ell+1} - 2y_\ell = (-)^{\ell+1}:$$

$$y_\ell = \frac{(-)^\ell}{3}\left(1+\frac{\ell}{2}\right), \quad z_\ell = \frac{2\ell}{3}(-)^{\ell-1};$$

$$(7.310a\text{--}d)$$

(iii) for the root (7.308a), the system (7.311a, b) has solution (7.308c) ≡ (7.311c, d):

$$y_{\ell+2} + z_{\ell+1} - y_\ell + z_\ell = 2^\ell, \quad 2y_{\ell+1} + z_{\ell+1} - y_\ell = -2^\ell:$$

$$y_\ell = \frac{2^{\ell+1}}{3}\left(1+\frac{15\ell}{4}\right), \quad z_\ell = -2^{\ell+1}\left(1+\frac{5\ell}{12}\right).$$

$$(7.311a\text{--}d)$$

The forcing by powers (subsection 7.9.4) can be extended via a complex base (subsection 7.9.5) to include the product by circular and/or hyperbolic cosine and sines of multiple angles (subsection 7.9.6).

7.9.5 Product of Power by Circular and Hyperbolic Functions

The forcing term corresponding to the product of a power by a circular (7.312a) [hyperbolic (7.313a)] cosine or sine of a multiple angle:

$$b^\ell \cosh, \sinh(c\ell\phi) = \frac{b^\ell}{2}\left(e^{c\ell\phi} \pm e^{-c\ell\phi}\right) = \frac{\left(be^{c\phi}\right)^\ell \pm \left(be^{-c\phi}\right)^\ell}{2}, \qquad (7.312\text{a, b})$$

$$b^\ell \sin, \cos(g\ell\phi) = b^\ell \frac{e^{ig\ell\phi} \pm e^{-ig\ell\phi}}{\{2, 2i\}} = \frac{\left(be^{ig\phi}\right)^\ell \pm \left(be^{-ig\phi}\right)^\ell}{\{2, 2i\}} = \mathrm{Re}, \mathrm{Im}\left\{\left(be^{ig\phi}\right)^\ell\right\},$$

$$(7.313\text{a–c})$$

can be written as a sum of powers (7.312b) [(7.313b)] or the real and imaginary part of a power with a complex base (7.133c). The latter can also be extended to products of circular and hyperbolic cosines and sines (7.314a–c):

$$b^\ell \cosh, \sinh(c\,\ell\phi)\cos, \sin(g\ell\phi) = \mathrm{Re}, \mathrm{Im}\left\{b^\ell e^{ig\ell\phi}\frac{e^{c\ell\phi} \pm e^{-c\ell\phi}}{2}\right\}$$

$$= \frac{1}{2}\mathrm{Re}, \mathrm{Im}\left\{\left[be^{(ig+c)\phi}\right]^\ell \pm \left[be^{(ig-c)\phi}\right]^\ell\right\}.$$

$$(7.314\text{a–c})$$

Using (7.299a, b; 7.300a, b) leads to the solution of the system (7.295a) with the forcings (7.312a, b; 7.313a–c; 7.314a–c).

Thus, *the simultaneous linear system of finite difference equations with constant coefficients (7.250; 7.251) ≡ (7.252) forced by the product of a power (7.295a) times: (i) an hyperbolic cosine or sine (7.312a, b) of the same multiple of an angle (7.315a) has (standard CLXXV) solution (7.315b):*

$$\sum_{r=1}^{M} R_{m,r}(\Delta)y_{r,\ell} = G_m b^\ell \cosh, \sinh(c, \ell, \phi):$$

$$(7.315\text{a, b})$$

$$y_{r,\ell} = \frac{b^\ell}{2}\sum_{m=1}^{M} G_m\left[e^{c\ell\phi}\frac{\bar{R}_{r,m}\left(be^{c\phi}\right)}{R_N\left(be^{c\phi}\right)} \pm e^{-c\ell\phi}\frac{\bar{R}_{r,m}\left(be^{-c\phi}\right)}{R_N\left(be^{-c\phi}\right)}\right];$$

(ii) a circular cosine or sine (7.313a, b) of the same multiple of an angle (7.316a) has (standard CLXXVI) solution (7.316b):

$$\sum_{r=1}^{M} R_{m,r}(\Delta) y_{r,\ell} = F_m b^{\ell} \cos, \sin(c, \ell, \phi):$$

$$y_{r,\ell} = \frac{b^{\ell}}{\{2, 2i\}} \sum_{m=1}^{M} G_m \left[e^{ig\ell\phi} \frac{\bar{R}_{r,m}\left(be^{ig\phi}\right)}{R_N\left(be^{ig\phi}\right)} \pm e^{-ig\ell\phi} \frac{\bar{R}_{r,m}\left(be^{-ig\phi}\right)}{R_N\left(be^{-ig\phi}\right)} \right],$$

(7.316a, b)

which in the case of real parameters (7.317a, b) and matrix of polynomials of finite differences (7.317c) simplifies the forcing term (7.316a) to (7.317d) with solution (7.317e):

$$b, g, R_{m,r} \in | R: \qquad \sum_{r=1}^{M} R_{m,r}(\Delta) y_{r,\ell} = G_m \operatorname{Re}, \operatorname{Im}\left(be^{ig\ell\phi}\right)$$

$$y_{r,\ell} = b^{\ell} \sum_{r=1}^{M} G_m \operatorname{Re}, \operatorname{Im}\left\{ e^{ig\ell\phi} \frac{\bar{R}_{r,m}\left(be^{ig\phi}\right)}{R_N\left(be^{ig\phi}\right)} \right\};$$

(7.317a–e)

(iii) the product of an hyperbolic by a circular cosine or sine (7.314a, b) in the same case (7.314c) of real parameters (7.318a–c) and matrix of polynomials of finite differences (7.318d) leads (standard CLXXVII) to (7.318e, f):

$$b, c, g, R_{m,r} \in | R: \qquad \sum_{r=1}^{M} R_{m,r}(\Delta) y_{r,\ell} = F_m b^{\ell} \cosh, \sinh(c\ell\phi) \cos, \sin(g\ell\phi);$$

$$y_{r,\ell} = \frac{b^{\ell}}{2} \sum_{r=1}^{M} G_m \operatorname{Re}, \operatorname{Im}\left\{ \left[e^{(ig+c)\ell\phi} \frac{\bar{R}_{r,m}\left(be^{(ig+c)\phi}\right)}{R_N\left(be^{(ig+c)\phi}\right)} \pm e^{(ig-c)\ell\phi} \frac{\bar{R}_{r,m}\left(be^{(ig-c)\phi}\right)}{R_N\left(be^{(ig-c)\phi}\right)} \right] \right\}.$$

(7.318a–f)

The solution (7.315a, b; 7.316a, b; 7.317a–e; 7.318a–f) are non-resonant cases (7.299a, b) that need to be modified as (7.300a, b) in the cases of resonance. The forcing by the product of a power by a hyperbolic cosine (7.315a, b) [circular sine (7.317a–e)] are chosen as illustrations in subsection 7.9.6 (example 10.18).

7.9.6 Products of Powers by Cosines of Multiple Angles

The coupled linear system of finite difference equations with constant coefficients (7.247a, b) ≡ (7.253) is considered with forcing (7.319a, b) by the product of a power by a hyperbolic cosine:

$$y_{\ell+2} + z_{\ell+1} - y_\ell + z_\ell = 4b^\ell \cosh(\ell\phi) = 2\left[\left(be^\phi\right)^\ell + \left(be^{-\phi}\right)^\ell\right], \qquad (7.319a)$$

$$2y_{\ell+1} + z_{\ell+1} - 2y_\ell = -2b^\ell \cosh(\ell\phi) = -\left[\left(be^\phi\right)^\ell + \left(be^{-\phi}\right)^\ell\right]. \qquad (7.319b)$$

Provided that $be^{\pm\phi}$ is not a root of the characteristic polynomial for (7.320a) the solution (7.299a, b) is similar to (7.304a–c) replacing b by $be^{\pm\phi}$ thus, leading to (7.320b):

$$be^{\pm c\phi} \neq \pm 1, 2: \qquad \begin{bmatrix} y_\ell \\ z_\ell \end{bmatrix} = \begin{bmatrix} 2 \\ -1 \end{bmatrix} \left(\lim_{\Delta \to be^\phi} + \lim_{\Delta \to be^{-\phi}} \right) \frac{\Delta^\ell}{(\Delta^2 - 1)(\Delta - 2)} \begin{bmatrix} 1 + 2\Delta \\ 3 - 2\Delta - \Delta^2 \end{bmatrix}.$$

$$(7.320a, b)$$

Thus, the solution of the system (7.319a, b) is (7.320b) ≡ (7.321a, b):

$$\left\{ \frac{1}{2} y_\ell, -z_\ell \right\} = b^\ell e^{\ell\phi} \frac{\left\{ 1 + 2be^\phi, 3 - 2be^\phi - b^2 e^{2\phi} \right\}}{\left(b^2 e^{2\phi} - 1 \right)\left(be^\phi - 2 \right)}$$

$$+ b^\ell e^{-\ell\phi} \frac{\left\{ 1 + 2be^{-\phi}, 3 - 2be^{-\phi} - b^2 e^{-2\phi} \right\}}{\left(b^2 e^{-2\phi} - 1 \right)\left(be^{-\phi} - 2 \right)},$$

$$(7.321a, b)$$

excluding the cases (7.320a) that have been considered before (7.309a–d; 7.310a–d; 7.311a–d).

7.9.7 Complete Integral of Forced Finite Differences

Using the principle of superposition (section 1.2), the preceding examples (sections 7.8–7.9) can be combined in a single statement: the coupled linear system of finite difference equations with constant coefficients if unforced (7.247a, b) ≡ (7.322a, b):

$$y_{\ell+2} + z_{\ell+1} - y_\ell + z_\ell = 3^\ell + 1 + (-)^\ell + 2^\ell, \quad 2y_{\ell+1} + z_{\ell+1} - 2y_\ell = -3^\ell - 1 - (-)^\ell - 2^\ell,$$

$$(7.322a, b)$$

has the general solution (7.268a; 7.270d) ≡ (7.323a, b):

$$y_\ell = A + (-)^\ell B + 2^\ell C + \frac{7}{8} 3^\ell - 1 - \frac{3}{2}\ell + \frac{(-)^\ell}{3}\left(1+\frac{\ell}{2}\right) + \frac{2^{\ell+1}}{3}\left(1+\frac{15\ell}{4}\right), \quad (7.323a)$$

$$z_\ell = -4(-)^\ell B - 2^\ell C - \frac{3^{\ell+1}}{2} + 2 + \frac{2\ell}{3}(-)^{\ell-1} - 2^{\ell+1}\left(1+\frac{5\ell}{12}\right), \quad (7.323b)$$

to which may be added by forcing: (i) a power of $b = 3$ with integer exponent (7.301a, b) leading to the non-resonant solution (7.304e); (ii–iv) three resonant solutions (7.309a–d; 7.310a–d; 7.311a–d).

7.9.8 Comparison of Three Matrix Polynomial Systems

Thus, *the coupled linear system of finite difference equations with constant coefficients in the unforced (7.247a, b) [forced (7.322a, b)] case has (standard CLXXVIII) a general (7.268a; 7.270d) [complete (7.323a, b)] solution involving three arbitrary constants. The starting conditions (7.271a) [≡(7.324a)] lead to (7.271b) [(7.324b)]:*

$$\{y_0, z_0, z_1\} = \{0,1,1\} = \left\{A+B+C+\frac{7}{8}, -4B-C-\frac{3}{2}, 4B-2C-\frac{15}{2}\right\},$$

$$(7.324a, b)$$

which determine the constants, (7.272a–c) [(7.325a–c)]:

$$C = -\frac{11}{3}, \qquad B = \frac{7}{24}, \qquad A = \frac{5}{2}, \qquad (7.325a–c)$$

in the unique general, (7.273a, b) [complete (7.323a, b; 7.325a, b)] solution.

This example is included in Table 7.1, which compares three simultaneous systems of equations with matrix of polynomials namely: (i/ii) ordinary differential equations with constant (homogeneous) coefficients [sections 7.4–7.5 (7.6–7.7)]; (iii) finite difference equations with constant coefficients (sections 7.8–7.9). Table 7.1 includes: (a) the matrix of polynomials, its co-factors, inverse and the characteristic polynomial; (b) for the unforced system, the simple and multiple roots of the characteristic polynomial, the natural solutions, the general integral, and the diagonal or block-diagonal forms; (d) for the forced system, the non-resonant and resonant solutions and extensions, and the use of the inverse matrix of polynomials; (d) an example of the use of initial and compatibility conditions to determine the arbitrary constants of integration in the general (complete) solution of a coupled linear system of equations.

NOTE 7.1: **Classification of Differential Equations**

The simplest equations (Diagram 7.1) are **algebraic** of two types: (i) **rational,** if they reduce to the ratio of polynomials (chapter I.31); (ii) **transcendental,** if they involve infinite sequences, such as series of powers (chapters I.21, 23, 25, 27, 29) or fractions (sections II.1.2–II.1.3), infinite products (sections II.1.4–II.1.5) or continued fractions (sections II.1.6–II.1.9). The next level above algebraic equations are those that involve analytical methods like differentiation (chapter I.11) and/or integration (chapters I.13, 15, 17, 19). The differential equations can be classified (Table 7.2) by four criteria (Diagram 7.2): (i/ii) number of independent (dependent) variables; (iii) order; (iv) type. An **ordinary (partial) differential equation** [o.d.e (p.d.e)] has (i) one (several) independent variable(s). A **single** or separate (**simultaneous system** of) **differential equations** [s.d.e. (s.s.d.e)] has (ii) one (several) dependent variable(s). The (iii) order of a single differential equation is that of the highest derivative present; in the case of a simultaneous system of differential equations the order is the highest of all single differential equations obtained by elimination for each dependent variable (section 7.3). The most common are first-order and second-order differential equations (chapters 2, 3, 4, 5, and 9); besides higher-order equations and systems (chapters 1, 6, 7, 8,

TYPES OF EQUATIONS

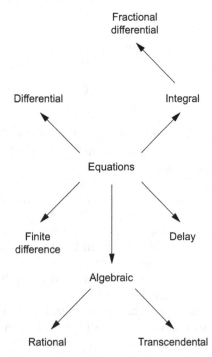

DIAGRAM 7.1
Types of equations, (a) algebraic, (b) finite difference, (c) differential, (d) integral, (e) fractional differential and (f) delay with some combinations in the Diagram 7.3.

TABLE 7.2

Classification of Differential Equations

	Differential Equation	
Variables	**One**	**Several**
Independent	ordinary	partial
Dependent	single equation	simultaneous system

Note: Basic classification of differential equations, more detailed in the Diagram 7.2.

and 9) also have many applications. The most general (iv) are (chapters 3–9) non-linear differential equations; an important class is linear differential equations, excluding (chapters 1–9) powers and products of the dependent variable(s) and their derivative(s). The coefficients of a linear differential equation may be functions of the independent variable; two sub-classes are the cases of homogeneous (constant) coefficients [sections (1.7–1.8 and 7.6–7.7 (1.3–1.6 and 7.4–7.5)]. There are also other types related to differential equations (note 7.2).

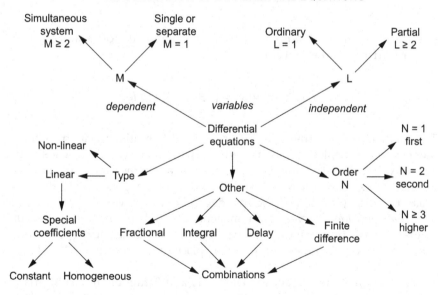

CLASSIFICATION OF DIFFERENTIAL EQUATIONS

DIAGRAM 7.2
Classification of differential equations according to: (i)(ii) the number of independent and dependent variables; (iii) the order; (iv) the non-linear and linear, the latter with special types of coefficients. The ordinary and partial differential equations may be combined with up to four other types of equations from Diagram 7.1.

NOTE 7.2: **Difference, Fractional, Delay, and Integral Equations**

Diagram 7.1 also indicates other equations with some properties related to differential equations namely: (a) finite difference equations; (b) fractional differential equations; (c) integral equations; (d) delay differential equations. The single or separate (simultaneous systems of) (a) finite difference equations [section(s) 1.9 (7.8–7.9)] can be solved by methods similar to differential equations in the linear case with constant [sections 1.3–1.6 (7.4–7.5)] or homogeneous [sections 1.7–1.8 (7.6–7.7)] coefficients. The fractional differential equations involve derivatives of non-integer order, that is, the order may be a rational, real, or complex number. They are a particular case of (c) linear **integral equations**, of which an example is:

$$y(x) = \int_a^x K(x;\xi)\, y(\xi)\, d\xi;\qquad(7.326)$$

the integral equation (7.326) is linear because the **kernel** or nucleus $K(x;\xi)$ does not involve the dependent variable y, though it may involve the independent variable. A **delay differential equation** involves (d) the dependent variable and its derivatives for different values of the independent variable, for example:

$$0 = F\big(y(x), y(x-x_1), y'(x-x_2), y''(x-x_3)\big).\qquad(7.327)$$

The various types of equations may be combined, for example, as an **integro-differential equation**:

$$y''(x) + e^x\, y(x) = \int_a^x K(x;\xi) y(\xi) d\xi.\qquad(7.328)$$

Two methods are illustrated for linear partial differential equations with two independent variables: (i) the method of separation of variables, leads to two ordinary differential equations, and applies always in the case of constant coefficients, for example, one-dimensional waves in homogeneous steady media (notes 6.1–6.22); (ii) if the coefficients depend only one variable, for example, for one-dimensional waves in inhomogeneous steady media (notes 7.6–7.50), a single ordinary differential equation is obtained using the Fourier series (notes 1.9–1.10) or integrals (notes 1.11–1.14) or Laplace transforms (notes 1.15–1.28).

NOTE 7.3: **Non-Linear Waves in Unsteady and Inhomogeneous Media**

An single (simultaneous system of) ordinary differential equation(s) has one independent variable, for example, (chapters 2 and 4) time t or (chapter 6) position x. A single (coupled system of) partial differential equation(s) has several independent variables, for example, time and one position coordinate

x for **one-dimensional waves**. The dependent variable(s) may be designated wave variable(s) of which several examples are given in the sequel (notes 7.8–7.17). For example, (problem 366) *a one-dimensional non-linear wave in an inhomogeneous and unsteady medium satisfies:*

$$0 = F\left(x, t; \Phi, \frac{\partial \Phi}{\partial x}, \frac{\partial \Phi}{\partial t}, \frac{\partial^2 \Phi}{\partial x^2}, \frac{\partial^2 \Phi}{\partial x^2}, \frac{\partial^2 \Phi}{\partial t^2}, \frac{\partial^2 \Phi}{\partial x \partial t}, \ldots, \frac{\partial^{N+M} \Phi}{\partial x^M \partial t^N} \right), \qquad (7.329)$$

which involves partial derivatives with regard to position x (time t) up to order M (N). For **linear waves** (problem 367), usually of small amplitude, there are no products or powers of the wave variable and its derivatives:

$$\sum_{m=0}^{M} \sum_{n=0}^{N} A_{m,n}(x,t) \frac{\partial^{m+n} \Phi}{\partial x^m \partial t^n} = B(x,t), \qquad (7.330)$$

and: (i) there may be a forcing or **source** term depending on position and time on the r.h.s. of (7.330); (ii) in its absence may exist **free waves**, and the coefficients $A_{m,n}$ may depend on position x (time t) for an **inhomogeneous (unsteady) medium**. The coefficients are constant (7.331b) in the case of an homogeneous and steady medium:

$$P_{M,N}\left(\frac{\partial}{\partial x}, \frac{\partial}{\partial t} \right) \equiv \sum_{m=0}^{M} \sum_{n=0}^{N} A_{m,n} \frac{\partial^{m+n}}{\partial x^m \partial t^n}: \qquad \left\{ P_{M,N}\left(\frac{\partial}{\partial x}, \frac{\partial}{\partial t} \right) \right\} \Phi(x,t) = B(x,t),$$

$$(7.331a, b)$$

when the differential operator is a polynomial of derivatives (7.331a). The linear waves in a steady homogeneous medium (7.331a, b) are considered next (note 7.4) followed by an intermediate case to (7.330), namely a steady inhomogeneous medium.

NOTE 7.4: **Linear Waves in Steady Homogeneous Media**

A linear partial differential equation with constant coefficients in unlimited space time (7.332a) suggests (notes 1.11–1.14) the use of a double direct (1.549a–c) [inverse (1.549d)] Fourier transform for the wave variable (7.332b) [forcing (7.332c)]:

$$-\infty < x, t < +\infty: \qquad \Phi(x,t) = \int_{-\infty}^{+\infty} dx \int_{-\infty}^{+\infty} dt\, \tilde{\Phi}(k,\omega)\, e^{i(kx - \omega t)}, \qquad (7.332a, b)$$

$$\tilde{B}(k,\omega) = \frac{1}{4\pi^2} \int_{-\infty}^{+\infty} dk \int_{-\infty}^{+\infty} d\omega\, e^{-i(kx - \omega t)} B(x,t); \qquad (7.332c)$$

the implication is that linear waves in homogeneous (steady) media have sinusoidal waveforms in space (time) with wavenumber k (frequency ω) defined by (7.333a) [(7.333c)] where $\lambda(\tau)$ is the wavelength (period) because (7.333b) [(7.333d)]:

$$\lambda \equiv \frac{2\pi}{\lambda}: \quad \exp(ikx) = \exp\left(\frac{i2\pi x}{\lambda}\right) = \exp\left(\frac{i2\pi x}{\lambda} + i2\pi\right) = \exp\left[\frac{i2\pi}{\lambda}(x+\lambda)\right]$$

(7.333a, b)

$$\tau \equiv \frac{2\pi}{\omega}: \quad \exp(-i\omega t) = \exp\left(-\frac{i2\pi t}{\tau}\right) = \exp\left(-\frac{i2\pi t}{\lambda} - i2\pi\right)$$

$$= \exp\left[-\frac{i2\pi}{\tau}(t+\tau)\right],$$

(7.333c, d)

the wave field repeats itself after a wavelength λ (period τ) or a multiple of it. Bearing in mind that the spatial (7.334a) [temporal (7.334b)] derivatives of a wave variable are equivalent to multiplying by i ($-i$) times the wavenumber (frequency):

$$\left\{\frac{\partial}{\partial x}, \frac{\partial}{\partial t}\right\} \exp\left[i(kx - \omega t)\right] = \{ik, -i\omega\} \exp\left[i(kx - \omega t)\right], \quad (7.334a, b)$$

the double Fourier transform of (7.331a, b) leads to an algebraic relation (7.335):

$$P_{M,N}(ik, -i\omega)\tilde{\tilde{\Phi}}(k, \omega) = \tilde{\tilde{B}}(k, \omega),$$

(7.335)

between the wave $\tilde{\tilde{\Phi}}$ (forcing $\tilde{\tilde{B}}$) double spectrum, having as factor:

$$P_{M,N}(ik, -i\omega) = \sum_{m=0}^{M}\sum_{n=0}^{N} A_{m,n}(ik)^m(-i\omega)^n,$$

(7.336)

the characteristic polynomial (7.336) in two variables.

Solving (7.335) for the wave double spectrum and substituting in (7.332b) leads to the wave field as a function of position and time (7.337):

$$\Phi(x, t) = \int_{-\infty}^{+\infty} dk \int_{-\infty}^{+\infty} d\omega \frac{\tilde{\tilde{B}}(k, \omega)}{P_{M,N}(ik, -i\omega)} e^{i(kx - \omega t)}.$$

(7.337)

Thus, *for linear waves in a homogeneous steady media (problem 368), specified by a forced linear partial differential equation with constant coefficients (7.331a, b) and characteristic polynomial (7.336) the wave field is determined by the double Fourier integral (7.337), where (7.332c) is the double spectrum of the forcing and thus, the sequence of solution is:*

$$B(x,t) \quad \rightarrow \quad \tilde{\tilde{B}}(K,\omega) \quad \rightarrow \quad \tilde{\tilde{\Phi}}(K,\omega) \quad \rightarrow \quad \Phi(x,t). \qquad (7.338a\text{--}c)$$

The integral (7.337) may be evaluated by residues (section I.17.5; notes III.3.11–III.3.19; notes 1.11–1.14). The result (7.337): (i) cannot be extended to non-linear waves (7.329) because the application of Fourier transforms (7.331a, b) does not allow suppression of the dependence on position x and time t; (ii) cannot be extended to linear waves (7.330) in inhomogeneous and unsteady media because the coefficients depend on position and time; (iii) (iv) can be extended to linear waves in inhomogeneous steady (homogeneous unsteady) media, when the coefficients in (7.330) depend only on position x (time t), using a single Fourier transform in the other variable $t(x)$, implying that there exists a frequency ω (wavenumber k) but no (wavenumber k) (frequency ω), that is, the waveforms are sinusoidal in time (space) but not in space (time). The case (iii) of linear waves in a inhomogeneous steady medium is detailed next (note 7.5).

NOTE 7.5: **Linear Waves in an Inhomogeneous Steady Medium**

Consider the case (iii) of linear waves in a inhomogeneous steady medium, specified by a linear partial differential equation whose coefficients depend only on position x, but not on time t:

$$\sum_{n=0}^{N}\sum_{m=0}^{M} A_{nm}(x)\frac{\partial^{n+m}\Phi}{\partial x^{n}\,\partial t^{m}} = B(x,t); \qquad (7.339)$$

taking the direct (inverse) Fourier transform (7.340a) [(7.340b)] only in frequency (time) leads to the spectra with frequency ω at position x for the wave variable (7.340a) [forcing (7.340b)]:

$$\Phi(x,t) = \int_{-\infty}^{+\infty} d\omega\, e^{i\omega t}\, \tilde{\Phi}(x;\omega), \qquad \tilde{B}(x;\omega) = \frac{1}{2\pi}\int_{-\infty}^{+\infty} dt\, e^{-i\omega t}\, B(x,t); \qquad (7.340a, b)$$

Substitution of (7.340a, b) leads from (7.339) to (7.341b):

$$P_{M}\!\left(\frac{d}{dx};-i\omega\right) \equiv \sum_{n=0}^{N}\sum_{m}^{m}(-i\omega)^{m} A_{nm}(x): \quad \left\{P_{M}\!\left(\frac{d}{dx};-i\omega\right)\right\}\tilde{\Phi}(x;\omega) = \tilde{B}(x;\omega),$$

$$(7.341a, b)$$

where (7.341a) is: (i) an algebraic polynomial of degree M in the frequency ω; (ii) a polynomial of degree N of spatial derivatives, implying that (7.341b) is a linear ordinary differential equation with constant coefficients of order N, whose solution specifies the wave field. Thus, *linear waves in an inhomogeneous steady medium (problem 369) are specified by a linear partial differential equation with forcing (7.339) whose coefficients depend only on position and not on time. The Fourier direct (7.340a) and inverse (7.340b) transforms in time relate the wave field and forcing for a wave of frequency ω at position x leading to an ordinary differential equation (7.341b) with coefficients dependent on position. The reduction of a partial (7.339) to an ordinary (7.341a, b) differential equation corresponds to the sequence of calculations:*

$$B(x,t) \quad \rightarrow \quad \tilde{B}(x;\omega) \quad \rightarrow \quad \tilde{\Phi}(x;\omega) \quad \rightarrow \quad \Phi(x,t), \qquad (7.342\text{a–c})$$

which is similar to (7.338a–c) with Fourier transforms in one instead of two independent variables. Comparing linear waves in steady homogeneous (inhomogeneous) media [note 7.4 (7.5)]: (i) the wave equation (7.331a, b) [(7.339)] is linear with coefficients that are constant (functions of position); (ii) the Fourier transforms (7.332b, c) [(7.340a, b)] are taken over time and position (time only); (iii) the characteristic polynomial (7.336) [(7.341a)] is algebraic on frequency and wavenumber (algebraic on frequency and a linear differential operator of position); (iv) the double (single) wave spectrum satisfies an algebraic (7.335) [linear ordinary differential (7.341b)] equation. The sequence of steps of the solution is similar for linear waves in steady homogeneous (7.338a–c) [inhomogeneous (7.342a–c)] media, showing the reduction of a linear partial differential equation to an algebraic system (linear ordinary differential equation). Several examples of linear second-order waves in steady inhomogeneous media are considered next (notes 7.6–7.19).

NOTE 7.6: Second-Order One-Dimensional Waves in Spatially Varying Media

The partial differential equation (7.339) applies to linear one-dimensional waves in steady inhomogeneous media and six second-order cases (Table 7.3) will be considered: (i) transverse vibrations with small slope of an elastic string with steady non-uniform mass density and tangential tension (notes 7.8–7.9); (ii) (iii) linear torsional (longitudinal) vibrations of a straight elastic rod with [note 7.10 (7.11)] steady non-uniform mass density and torsional stiffness (Young modulus); (iv) longitudinal water waves in a channel with depth and/or width varying slowly along its length (notes 7.12–7.13); (v) electromagnetic waves in a medium with dielectric permittivity and magnetic permeably depending on position (notes 7.14–7.15); (vi) sound waves in a horn, that is, duct with cross-section varying along its

TABLE 7.3

Quasi-One-Dimensional Propagation

Medium	Physical Properties	Dual Variables	Wave	Notes
elastic string	mass density axial tension	displacement slope	transversal	7.8–7.9
elastic rod	mass density Young modulus	displacement strain	longitudinal	7.11
elastic rod	moment of inertia torsional stiffness	rotation torsion	torsional	7.10
water channel	cross-section gravity	transverse displacement longitudinal velocity	longitudinal	7.12–7.13
electromagnetic waveguide	dielectric permittivity magnetic permeability	electric field magnetic field	transversal	7.14–7.15
sound in horn	cross-sectional area sound speed	pressure velocity	longitudinal	7.16–7.17

Note: A set of six cases of quasi-one-dimensional wave propagation in inhomogeneous media, including transverse vibrations of strings, torsional and longitudinal oscillations of rods, water waves in a non-uniform channel, electromagnetic waves in an inhomogeneous waveguide, and acoustic waves in a horn.

length (notes 7.16–7.17). The quasi-one-dimensional propagation (note 7.18) assumes in all cases (i–vi) that the wavelength is larger than the transverse dimensions; otherwise transverse modes have to be considered. All six wave equations (i–vi) involve a propagation speed and a lengthscale of inhomogeneity. The waves (i, ii, iv, v) [(iii) (vi)] are transversal (longitudinal), that is, the perturbations are orthogonal to (along) the direction of propagation.

The wave equation in homogeneous media is the same for all variables, whereas in inhomogeneous media it is generally different for distinct variables. Two variables are used (Table 7.3), leading to distinct wave equations, namely: (i) the transverse displacement and slope for transversal elastic waves along a non-uniform string (notes 7.8–7.9); (ii/iii) the torsion and rate-of-torsion (displacement and strain) for transversal torsional (longitudinal) waves along a non-uniform straight rod [note 7.10 (7.11)]; (iv) vertical surface displacement and slope for water waves in a non-uniform channel (notes 7.12–7.13); (v) electric and magnetic fields for transversal electromagnetic waves in a non-uniform waveguide (notes 7.14–7.15); (vi) fluid pressure and bulk velocity (that is, the velocity multiplied by cross-sectional area) for longitudinal sound waves in a horn or duct of varying cross-sections (notes 7.16–7.17). All these six analogous waves (i–vi) lead to the same pair of dual-wave equation (note 7.18) that have similar properties (note 7.19), including duality principles relating a pair of wave variables (notes 7.20–7.21). The linear quasi-one-dimensional propagation in a steady inhomogeneous medium leads to properties illustrated for sound in a **horn** (note 7.7), that is, a duct of varying cross-section containing a fluid at rest.

NOTE 7.7: **Filtering/Transparency and Reflection/Transmission/ Absorption**

Two opposite limits of wave diffraction (notes 7.27 and 7.55) are using the terminology for quasi-one-dimensional acoustic waves (notes 7.22–7.24), the ray (scattering) approximation for wavelength short (large) compared with the lengthscale of changes in cross-section [notes 7.25–7.26 (7.47–7.54)]; in the ray (compactness) approximation of gradual (abrupt) changes of cross-section on a wavelength scale excludes (causes) reflection and/or absorptions and allows total (partial or no) transmission. For intermediate wavelengths, comparable to the lengthscale of variation of the cross-section, exact solutions of the horn wave equation are necessary, and can be obtained in terms of elementary functions only (note 7.35) for five shapes: (i) the exponential horn (note 7.28) that has, both for the acoustic pressure and acoustic velocity perturbations (note 7.30), a filtering function excluding propagation below a cut-off frequency (note 7.29); (ii) (iii) the catenoidal (inverse catenoidal) horn that has a filtering function for the acoustic pressure (velocity) perturbation [note 7.31 (7.32)]; (iv) (v) the sinusoidal (inverse sinusoidal) duct that leads to a transparency function allowing propagation of all frequencies for the acoustic pressure (velocity) perturbation [note 7.33 (7.34)].

The exact solutions of the horn wave equations for all shapes (note 7.35) other than (i–v) involve special functions, for example, (vi) [(vii)] Hermite polynomials (Bessel functions) for the Gaussian (power law) horns [notes 7.36–7.38 (7.39–7.46)]. The latter (vii) power law horns (notes 7.39–7.41) include, for particular choices of the exponent, the (viii) cylindrical [(ix) spherical] waves in a wedge-shaped (conical) horn [notes 7.42–7.43 (7.44)], which can also be obtained from the solution of the classical wave equation (note 7.45) in cylindrical (spherical) coordinates (note 7.46). The second-order waves (note 7.55) can: (a) propagate in opposite directions in an infinite horn (notes 7.25–7.46) with choice of direction of propagation by a radiation conditions; (b) be reflected in a semi-infinite horn with a rigid or impedance wall boundary condition, specifying the reflection and adsorption coefficients (notes 7.47–7.48); (c) form standing modes in a finite horn with two rigid or impedance boundaries (notes 7.49–7.50); (d) partial reflection, transmission, and absorption can occur for the acoustic matching of two horns with different cross-sections and fluid mass density and sound speed (notes 7.52–7.53), leading to the scattering matrix (note 7.54).

NOTE 7.8: **Transverse Vibrations of a Non-Uniform String**

The transverse displacement in the vibrations (Figure 7.8a) of an elastic string (6.755) lead to (7.343d) in: (i) the absence of forcing (7.343a); (ii) for mass

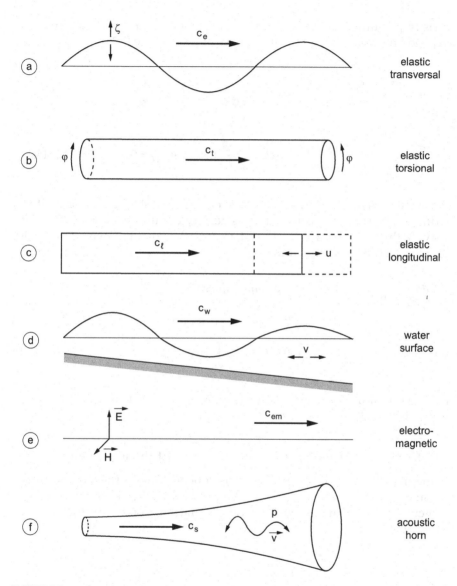

FIGURE 7.8
Six analogous cases of quasi-one-dimensional wave propagation in inhomogeneous media
(Tables 7.3 and 7.4) are: (a) transverse vibrations of an elastic string with variable mass per unit
length and/or tangential tension; (b)(c) torsional (longitudinal) waves along an elastic rod with
non-uniform moment of inertia and torsional stiffness of the cross-section (mass density per
unit length and Young modulus); (d) waves on the surface of a water channel with variable
depth and width (Figures 7.9a–c); (e) electromagnetic waves (Figure 7.10) in a waveguide with
non-uniform dielectric permittivity and/or magnetic permeability; (f) sound waves in a horn
whose shape depends on the variation of the cross-sectional area along its length, for example,
in Figures 7.11, 7.12a–f, 7.14a, and 7.15a–c.

density per unit length (7.343b) that does not depend on time t, but may depend on position x; (iii) the linear case of small slope (7.343c):

$$f_a = 0 = \frac{\partial \sigma}{\partial t}, \left(\frac{\partial \zeta}{\partial x}\right)^2 \ll 1: \qquad \frac{\partial^2 \zeta}{\partial t^2} - \frac{1}{\sigma(x)} \frac{\partial}{\partial x}\left[T(x,t)\frac{\partial \zeta}{\partial x}\right] = 0; \qquad (7.343\text{a--d})$$

$$\zeta' \equiv \frac{\partial \zeta}{\partial x}: \qquad \frac{\partial^2 \zeta'}{\partial t^2} - \frac{\partial}{\partial x}\left\{\frac{1}{\sigma(x)} \frac{\partial}{\partial x}\left[T(x,t)\zeta'\right]\right\} = 0, \qquad (7.344\text{a, b})$$

the slope (7.344a) satisfies a dual-wave equation (7.344b) for a non-uniform string, such as: (i) with constant mass density per unit volume (7.345a) with varying thickness or cross-sectional area $A(x)$ so that the mass density per unit length (7.345b) is non-uniform:

$$\rho = \frac{dm}{dV} = const: \qquad \sigma(x) = \frac{dm}{dx} = \frac{dm}{dV}\frac{dV}{dx} = \rho A(x); \qquad (7.345\text{a, b})$$

$$g = const: \qquad T(x) = T(0) + g \int_0^x \sigma(\xi)d\xi, \qquad (7.346\text{a, b})$$

(ii) under non-uniform tension due to the weight (7.346b) in a uniform gravity field (7.346a).

NOTE 7.9: **Propagation Speed and Lengthscale of Inhomogeneity**

If the mass density (tension) does not depend [7.347a) (7.347b)] on time t (position x), only the **elastic wave speed** (7.347c) appears in the one-dimensional **modified classical wave equation**, for the transverse displacement (7.347d):

$$\frac{\partial \sigma}{\partial t} = 0 = \frac{\partial T}{\partial x}: \qquad c_e(x,t) = \sqrt{\frac{T(t)}{\sigma(x)}}, \qquad \left\{\frac{\partial^2}{\partial t^2} - \left[c_e(x,t)\right]^2 \frac{\partial^2}{\partial x^2}\right\}\zeta(x,t) = 0.$$

$$(7.347\text{a--e})$$

The elastic wave speed (7.347c) is the square of the ratio of the tension to the mass density per unit length (7.345b) and, in particular, the classical wave equation (7.347d) applies with a constant wave speed (7.347c) also to the slope (7.344b). In the case of a non-uniform string, that is, with tension (7.348a) and mass density per unit length (7.348b) depending on position x but not time t, the displacement (7.343d) [slope (7.344b)] satisfy distinct dual-wave equations (7.348c) [(7.348e)]:

$$\frac{\partial T}{\partial t} = 0 = \frac{\partial \sigma}{\partial t}: \qquad \left\{ \frac{\partial^2}{\partial t^2} - \left[c_e(x) \right]^2 \left[\frac{\partial^2}{\partial x^2} + \frac{1}{L_T(x)} \frac{\partial}{\partial x} \right] \right\} \zeta(x,t) = 0, \qquad (7.348a\text{–}c)$$

$$L_T(x) = \frac{T(x)}{T'(x)}: \qquad \left\{ \frac{\partial^2}{\partial t^2} - \frac{\partial}{\partial x} \left\{ \left[c_e(x) \right]^2 \left[\frac{\partial}{\partial x} + \frac{1}{L_T(x)} \frac{\partial}{\partial x} \right] \right\} \right\} \zeta'(x,t) = 0,$$

$$(7.348d, e)$$

involving the **lengthscale** (7.348d) of variation of the tension that is large (small) if the tension varies slowly (fast) with distance. It has been shown that *the transverse displacement [slope (7.334a)] of the free linear vibrations with small slope (7.343c) of an elastic string satisfy (problem 370) different wave equations (7.343d) [(7.344b)] involving the mass density (tangential tension) of the elastic string that may depend on position (and on time). It follows that if the tension (mass density per unit length) does not (7.347b) [(7.347a)] depend on time (position) the transverse displacement (7.347d) satisfies the modified classical wave equation with elastic wave speed (7.347c) that also applies to the scope for constant wave speed. If instead the tension (7.348a) and mass density per unit length (7.348b) do not depend on time, but depend on position for a non-uniform string, the displacement (slope) satisfy distinct primal (7.348c) [dual (7.348e)] **dual-wave equations**, involving the lengthscale of variation of the tension (7.348d). The classical wave equation applies (dual-wave equations apply) to other waves in homogeneous (inhomogeneous) media (notes 7.10–7.17)* with suitable choice of wave variables, wave speed, and lengthscale of non-uniformity.

NOTE 7.10: Torsional Vibrations of an Elastic Rod

The linear torsional vibrations (Figure 7.8b) of a straight elastic rod are given by (6.768b) that simplifies to the primal wave equation (7.349e) in: (i) the absence of forcing torque (7.349a); (ii) for moment of inertia (7.349b) and torsional stiffness (7.349c) of the cross-section that do not depend on time t but may depend on position x; (iii) using as variable the torsion, that is, the rate of change of the angle of rotation along the axis (7.349d):

$$M_a = 0 = \frac{\partial I}{\partial t} = \frac{\partial C}{\partial t}, \quad \tau \equiv \frac{\partial \phi}{\partial x}: \qquad \frac{\partial^2 \tau}{\partial t^2} - \frac{1}{I(x)} \frac{d}{dx} \left[C(x) \frac{\partial \tau}{\partial x} \right] = 0; \qquad (7.349a\text{–}e)$$

$$\tau' \equiv \frac{d^2 \phi}{dx^2}: \qquad \frac{\partial^2 \tau'}{\partial t^2} - \frac{\partial}{\partial x} \left\{ \frac{1}{I(x)} \frac{\partial}{\partial x} \left[C(x) \tau' \right] \right\} = 0, \qquad (7.350a, b)$$

the rate of torsion (7.350a) satisfies a dual-wave equation (7.350b). Comparing (7.343a–d) ≡ (7.349a–e) and (7.344a, b) ≡ (7.350a, b) leads to the following analogies between transverse (torsional) vibrations of an elastic string (rod): (i) the mass density per unit length corresponds to moment of inertia the cross-section (7.351a); (ii) the tangential tension corresponds to the torsional stiffness (7.351b):

$$\sigma(x) \leftrightarrow I(x), \qquad T(x) \leftrightarrow C(x); \qquad \zeta(x,t) \leftrightarrow \tau(x,t), \qquad \frac{\partial \zeta}{\partial x} \leftrightarrow \frac{\partial \tau}{\partial x},$$

$$(7.351a\text{–}d)$$

(iii) the transverse displacement corresponds to the torsion (7.351c) in the main-wave equation (7.343d) ≡ (7.349e); (iv) the slope corresponds to the rate of torsion (7.351d) in the dual-wave equation (7.344b) ≡ (7.350b); (v) the speed of propagation of elastic waves (7.347c) ≡ (7.352a) is replaced by the **torsional wave speed** (7.352b), which equals the square root of the ratio of the bending stiffness to the moment of inertia of the cross-section:

$$c_e(x) = \sqrt{\frac{T(x)}{\sigma(x)}} \leftrightarrow c_t(x) = \sqrt{\frac{C(x)}{I(x)}}; \qquad L_T(x) = \frac{T(x)}{T'(x)} \leftrightarrow L_C(x) = \frac{C(x)}{C'(x)},$$

$$(7.352a\text{–}d)$$

(iv) the lengthscale of inhomogeneity (7.352d) applies to the torsional stiffness instead of the tangential tension (7.348d) ≡ (7.352c); (vii) with the preceding substitution, the torsion (rate of torsion) of an elastic rod satisfies the same wave equations as the displacement (slope) of an elastic string. Thus, *the free torsional vibrations, in the absence of applied moment (7.349a) of a straight non-uniform elastic rod, whose moment of inertia (torsional stiffness) of the cross-section may depend on position x but not time t, (7.349b) [(7.349c)] are specified (problem 371) by distinct primal (dual) wave equations for the torsion (7.349e) [rate-of-torsion (7.350b) that: (i) reduce to the same classical-wave equation (7.353c, d) with constant elastic-wave speed (7.352b) for a homogeneous rod (7.353a, b):*

$$I, C = const: \qquad \left\{ \frac{\partial^2}{\partial t^2} - c_t^2 \frac{\partial^2}{\partial x^2} \right\} \tau, \tau'(x,t) = 0; \qquad (7.353a\text{–}d)$$

(ii) for an inhomogeneous rod, the torsion (rate of torsion) satisfies distinct primal (7.354a) [dual (7.354b)] wave equations involving also the lengthscale of variation of the torsional stiffness (7.352d):

$$\frac{\partial^2 \tau}{\partial t^2} - \left[c_t(x) \right]^2 \left\{ \frac{\partial^2 \tau}{\partial t^2} + \frac{1}{L_C(x)} \frac{\partial \tau}{\partial x} \right\} = 0, \qquad (7.354a)$$

$$\frac{\partial^2 \tau'}{\partial t^2} - \frac{\partial}{\partial x} \left[c_t(x) \right]^2 \left\{ \left[\frac{\partial^2 \tau'}{\partial x} + \frac{1}{L_C(x)} \tau' \right] \right\} = 0, \qquad (7.354b)$$

Similar results apply to the longitudinal oscillations of a straight elastic rod (note 7.11).

NOTE 7.11: **Longitudinal Oscillations of an Elastic Rod**

The linear longitudinal vibrations (Figure 7.8c) of a straight elastic rod (6.772b) lead to the primal wave equation (7.355d) for the longitudinal displacement (6.772a): (i) in the absence of forcing (7.355a); (ii) for mass density per unit length (7.355b) and Young modulus (7.355c), which do not depend on time t but may depend on position x:

$$F_a = 0 = \frac{\partial \sigma}{\partial t} = \frac{\partial E}{\partial t}: \qquad \frac{\partial^2 u}{\partial t^2} - \frac{1}{\sigma(x)} \frac{\partial}{\partial x} \left[E(x) \frac{\partial u}{\partial x} \right] = 0; \qquad (7.355a\text{–}d)$$

$$S \equiv \frac{\partial u}{\partial x}: \qquad \frac{\partial^2 S}{\partial t^2} - \frac{\partial}{\partial x} \left\{ \frac{1}{\sigma(x)} \frac{\partial}{\partial x} [E(x)S] \right\} = 0, \qquad (7.356a, b)$$

the strain (7.356a) satisfies the dual-wave equation (7.356b). Comparing (7.349a–e) ≡ (7.355a–d) and (7.350a, b) ≡ (7.356a, b) leads to the following analogies between the torsional (longitudinal) vibrations of a straight elastic rod: (i) the mass density per unit length (7.357a) is unchanged; (ii) the torsional stiffness corresponds to the Young modulus (7.357b):

$$\sigma(x) \leftrightarrow \sigma(x), \quad C(x) \leftrightarrow E(x); \quad \tau(x,t) \leftrightarrow u(x,t), \quad \tau'(x,t) \leftrightarrow S(x,t), \qquad (7.357a\text{–}d)$$

(iii) the torsion is replaced by the longitudinal displacement (7.357c) in the primal wave equation (7.349e) ≡ (7.355d); (iv) the rate of torsion corresponds to the strain (7.355d) ≡ (7.356d) in the dual-wave equation (7.350b) ≡ (7.356b); (v) the torsional wave speed (7.352b) ≡ (7.358a) is replaced (7.358b) by the **longitudinal wave speed,** which is equal to the square root of the Young modulus divided by the mass density:

$$c_t(x) = \sqrt{\frac{C(x)}{I(x)}} \leftrightarrow c_\ell(x) = \sqrt{\frac{E(x)}{\sigma(x)}}; \quad L_C(x) = \frac{C(x)}{C'(x)} \leftrightarrow L_E(x) = \frac{E(x)}{E'(x)}, \qquad (7.358a\text{–}d)$$

(vi) the lengthscale for the torsional stiffness (7.352d) ≡ (7.358c) is replaced by the lengthscale for the Young modulus (7.358d); (vii) with the preceding substitutions the longitudinal displacement (strain) satisfy the same equations as the torsion (rate of torsion). Thus, *the free longitudinal vibrations, in the absence of forces (7.355a), of a straight non-uniform elastic rod, whose mass density*

*per unit length (Young modulus) may depend on position x but not on time t (7.355b)
[(7.355c)] satisfy (problem 372) distinct primal (7.355d) [dual (7.356b)] wave equations for the longitudinal displacement [strain (7.356a)] that: (i) coincide with the classical wave equation (7.359c, d) with constant longitudinal wave speed for a homogeneous rod (7.359a, b):*

$$\sigma, E = const: \qquad \left\{ \frac{\partial^2}{\partial t^2} - c_\ell^2 \frac{\partial^2}{\partial x^2} \right\} u, S(x,t) = 0; \qquad (7.359a–d)$$

(ii) for an inhomogeneous rod, the longitudinal displacements (strains) satisfy distinct primal (7.360a) [dual (7.360b)] wave equations also involving the lengthscale of variation of the Young modulus (7.358d):

$$\frac{\partial^2 u}{\partial t^2} - \left[c_\ell^2(x) \right]^2 \left\{ \frac{\partial^2 u}{\partial x^2} + \frac{1}{L_E(x)} \frac{\partial u}{\partial x} \right\} = 0, \qquad (7.360a)$$

$$\frac{\partial^2 S}{\partial t^2} - \frac{\partial}{\partial x} \left\{ \left[c_\ell(x) \right]^2 \left[\frac{\partial S}{\partial x} + \frac{1}{L_E(x)} S \right] \right\} = 0. \qquad (7.360b)$$

Similar results apply to longitudinal surface waves in a water channel with varying cross-section (notes 7.12–7.13).

NOTE 7.12: **Water Waves in a Variable Channel**

Consider water waves at the surface of a channel (Figure 7.8d) with variable depth h and width b, leading to the cross-sectional area (7.361b) when the elevation of the water surface is ζ; the mass density per unit length (7.361c) equals the mass density per unit volume (7.345a) $\equiv$ (7.361a) times the cross-sectional area (7.361b), where the vertical surface displacement adds to the depth:

$$\rho \equiv \frac{dm}{dV}, \qquad A = b(h+\zeta): \qquad \sigma = \frac{dm}{dx} = \frac{dm}{dV} \frac{dV}{dx} = \rho A = \rho b(h+\zeta). \qquad (7.361a–c)$$

The equation of continuity or mass conservation (section I.14.1) in the one-dimensional form (7.362a) balances: (i) the rate of change in time of the mass density per unit length (7.361c) against (ii) the rate of change with position of the mass flux, obtained by multiplication by the velocity along the x-axis:

$$0 = \frac{\partial \sigma}{\partial t} + \frac{\partial}{\partial x}(\sigma v) = \frac{\partial}{\partial t} \left[\rho b(h+\zeta) \right] + \frac{\partial}{\partial x} \left[\rho b(h+\zeta) v \right], \qquad (7.362a, b)$$

leading to (7.362b). The inviscid momentum or Euler equation, (I.14.9) ≡ (6.539b), in the absence of external forces (7.363a) when the stresses reduce to an inward pressure (7.363b), simplifies in one dimension to (7.363c):

$$F = 0, \quad T = -p: \qquad -\frac{\partial p}{\partial x} = \rho \frac{dv}{dt} = \rho \left(\frac{\partial v}{dt} + v \frac{\partial v}{\partial x} \right), \qquad \text{(7.363a–d)}$$

leading to (7.363d) where were used: (i) the mass density per unit volume (7.361a); (ii) the acceleration in one dimension (7.364b):

$$\frac{d}{dt} \equiv \frac{\partial}{\partial t} + v \frac{\partial}{\partial x}: \qquad a = \frac{dv}{dt} = \frac{\partial v}{\partial t} + \frac{\partial v}{\partial x}\frac{dx}{dt} = \frac{\partial v}{\partial t} + v \frac{\partial v}{\partial x}, \qquad \text{(7.364a, b)}$$

which equals the material derivative (7.364a) of the velocity.

The variables for water waves (Figure 7.8d) are: (i) the vertical displacement of the surface $\zeta(x,t)$; (ii) the longitudinal velocity $v(x,t)$ along the axis of the channel. For one-dimensional waves, the wavelength must be larger than the transverse dimensions of the channel, which is larger than the width (7.365a) and the depth (7.365b), otherwise transverse modes could exist. Also, for linear waves, the surface elevation must be small compared with the depth (7.365c), and the product or powers of wave variables (ζ, v) and their derivatives are negligible, so that the continuity (7.362b) [momentum (7.363d)] equations are linearized to (7.365d) [(7.365e)]:

$$b < \lambda > h, \quad \zeta^2 \ll h^2: \qquad \frac{\partial}{\partial t}(\rho b \zeta) + \frac{\partial}{\partial x}(\rho b h v) = 0 = \frac{\partial p}{\partial x} + \rho \frac{\partial v}{\partial t}. \qquad \text{(7.365a–e)}$$

It is assumed that the water is incompressible (7.366a) and that the breadth and width of the channel may vary along the length (Figures 7.9a–c), but not with time (7.366b, c), so that the continuity (7.365d) [momentum (7.365e)] equations simplify further to (7.366d) [(7.366e)]:

$$\rho = const, \quad \frac{\partial b}{\partial t} = 0 = \frac{\partial h}{\partial t}: \qquad \frac{\partial \zeta}{\partial t} + \frac{1}{b(x)}\frac{\partial}{\partial x}\left[b(x)h(x)v \right] = 0 = \frac{\partial p}{\partial x} + \rho \frac{\partial v}{\partial t}.$$

$$\text{(7.366a–e)}$$

For the mean state of hydrostatic equilibrium with constant mass density (7.366a) the pressure difference from the atmospheric value p_0 is proportional

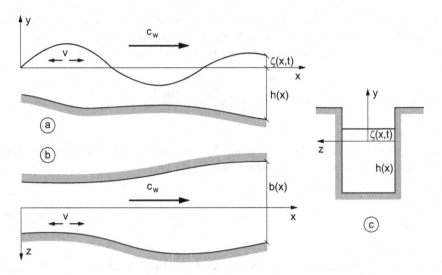

FIGURE 7.9
The quasi-one-dimensional propagation of hydraulic waves (Figure 7.8d) at the surface of a water channel (a) allows (Figure 7.9) for variations of width (b) and depth (c) along the channel with the restrictions (I) that: (I-i) the wavelength must be larger than the width $b < \lambda$ (depth $h < \lambda$); (I-ii)) thus, transverse horizontal (vertical) modes cannot exist; (I-iii) only a fundamental longitudinal mode can exist; (I-iv) all wave variables are uniform over the cross-section and can vary only with the longitudinal coordinate and time. In addition, (II) for linear waves, the surface elevation $\zeta(x,t)$ must at all times be small $\zeta^2 \ll h^2$ compared with the local depth h. It is also assumed that: (III) the mass density is constant because water is nearly incompressible; (IV) the acceleration of gravity is uniform because the water depth is small compared with the radius of the earth.

(7.367b) to the weight of a column of fluid of height $h + \zeta$ in the uniform gravity field with downward acceleration (7.367a):

$$g = const: \qquad p = p_0 + \rho g (h + \zeta); \qquad p_0 + \rho g\, h = p_a = const. \qquad (7.367a\text{--}c)$$

At the mean height of the surface, the pressure equals the atmospheric pressure (7.367c), which is constant, implying (7.368a):

$$p = \rho g \zeta + const: \qquad g\frac{\partial \zeta}{\partial x} = \frac{1}{\rho}\frac{\partial p}{\partial x} = -\frac{\partial v}{\partial t}, \qquad (7.368a\text{--}c)$$

for uniform gravity (7.367a); from (7.368a) follows (7.368b) where (7.366e) may be substituted leading to (7.368c). Thus, the continuity (momentum) equations simplify to (7.366d) [(7.368c)], which lead to the wave equations by eliminating either of the two variables (notes 7.13).

NOTE 7.13: Channel with Non-Uniform Depth and Width

Elimination between the equations of continuity (7.366d) and momentum (7.368c) for the surface elevation (7.369a) [longitudinal velocity (7.369b)] in the case (7.367a) of uniform gravity:

$$\frac{\partial^2 \zeta}{\partial t^2} = -\frac{1}{b(x)}\frac{\partial}{\partial x}\left[h(x)b(x)\frac{\partial v}{\partial t}\right] = \frac{g}{b(x)}\frac{\partial}{\partial x}\left[h(x)b(x)\frac{\partial \zeta}{\partial x}\right], \qquad (7.369a)$$

$$\frac{\partial^2 v}{\partial t^2} = -g\frac{\partial^2 \zeta}{\partial x \partial t} = g\frac{\partial}{\partial x}\left\{\frac{1}{b(x)}\frac{\partial}{\partial x}\left[h(x)b(x)v\right]\right\}, \qquad (7.369b)$$

shows that *the vertical surface displacement (longitudinal velocity) of linear (7.365c) one-dimensional (7.365a, b) water waves (Figure 7.8d) satisfy (problem 373) the primal (7.369a) ≡ (7.370a) [dual (7.369b) ≡ (7.370b)] wave equations in a channel whose width (7.366b) and depth (7.366c) may vary with position x but not time t:*

$$\frac{\partial^2 \zeta}{\partial t^2} - \frac{1}{b(x)}\frac{\partial}{\partial x}\left[g\,h(x)b(x)\frac{\partial \zeta}{\partial x}\right] = 0, \qquad (7.370a)$$

$$\frac{\partial^2 v}{\partial t^2} - \frac{\partial}{\partial x}\left\{\frac{1}{b(x)}\frac{\partial}{\partial x}\left[g\,h(x)b(x)v\right]\right\} = 0, \qquad (7.370b)$$

*assuming constant mass density (7.366a) and a uniform gravity field (7.367a). The **water wave speed** (7.371a), which equals the square root of the depth multiplied by the acceleration of gravity and the lengthscale of variation (7.371d) of the cross-sectional area (7.371c):*

$$c_w(x) \equiv \sqrt{g\,h(x)}: \qquad \frac{\partial^2 \zeta}{\partial t^2} - \left[c_w(x)\right]^2\left\{\frac{\partial^2 \zeta}{\partial x^2} + \frac{1}{L_A(x)}\frac{\partial \zeta}{\partial x}\right\} = 0, \qquad (7.371a, b)$$

$$A(x) = b(x)h(x); \quad L_A = \frac{A(x)}{A'(x)}: \qquad \frac{\partial^2 v}{\partial t^2} - \frac{\partial}{\partial x}\left\{\left[c_w(x)\right]\left[\frac{\partial v}{\partial x} + \frac{1}{L_A(x)}v\right]\right\} = 0,$$

$$(7.371c\text{–}e)$$

appears in the primal (7.371b) [dual (7.371e)] wave equations for the surface elevation (longitudinal velocity), which simplify to the classical wave equation (7.372c) [≡ (7.372d)] for a water channel with uniform cross-section (7.372a, b):

$$h, b = const: \qquad \left\{\frac{\partial^2}{\partial t^2} - c_w^2\frac{\partial^2}{\partial x^2}\right\}\zeta, v(x,t) = 0. \qquad (7.372a\text{–}d)$$

These wave equations are similar (7.370a, b) ≡ (7.355d; 7.356b) to linear longitudinal vibrations of an inhomogeneous elastic rod replacing: (i) the moment of inertia of the cross-section by the width of the channel (7.373a); (ii) the Young modulus of the material by the depth of the channel multiplied by the acceleration of gravity (7.373b); (iii) the longitudinal by the vertical displacement (7.373c); (iv) the elastic strain by the longitudinal velocity (7.373d):

$$I(x) \leftrightarrow b(x), \quad E(x) \leftrightarrow g\,h(x), \quad u(x,t) \leftrightarrow \zeta(x,t), \quad S(x,t) \leftrightarrow v(x,t).$$

$$(7.373\text{a–d})$$

As a consequence: (v) the longitudinal elastic wave speed (7.358a) ≡ (7.374a) is replaced by the water wave speed (7.374b), which is equal to the square root of the product of the depth by the acceleration of gravity:

$$c_\ell(x) = \sqrt{\frac{E(x)}{\sigma(x)}} \leftrightarrow c_w(x) = \sqrt{g\,h(x)}; \quad L_E(x) = \frac{E(x)}{E'(x)} \leftrightarrow L_A(x) = \frac{A(x)}{A'(x)}.$$

$$(7.374\text{a–d})$$

(vi) the lengthscale for the variation of the Young modulus (7.358d) ≡ (7.374d) by that for the cross-sectional area of the channel (7.374d). From (7.374b) it follows that the speed of propagation of water waves in a channel increases with the square root of the depth, but the result does not apply to: (i) shallow water, when the surface displacement is no longer small compared with the depth (7.365c) and the waves become non-linear; (ii) deep waters, when the depth exceeds the wavelength violating (7.365b) so that vertical wave modes may exist. In addition to water waves and the preceding analogues, another concerns electromagnetic waves (notes 7.14–7.15).

NOTE 7.14: **Electromagnetic Waves in an Inhomogeneous Waveguide**

The electromagnetic waves are described by the two pairs of Maxwell equations, (2.25a, b) [(2.26a, b)], that are considered, (7.375b, c) [(7.376b, c)], in the absence of electric charges, (7.375a) [currents (7.376a)], for a medium with dielectric permittivity (2.28a) [magnetic permeability (2.28b)]:

$$q = 0: \qquad \nabla \cdot (\varepsilon \vec{E}) = 0, \qquad \nabla \wedge \vec{E} = -\frac{1}{c_0} \frac{\partial}{\partial t}(\mu H), \qquad (7.375\text{a–c})$$

$$\vec{J} = 0: \qquad \nabla \cdot (\mu \vec{H}) = 0, \qquad \nabla \wedge \vec{H} = \frac{1}{c_0} \frac{\partial}{\partial t}(\varepsilon \vec{E}), \qquad (7.376\text{a–c})$$

where c_0 is the speed of light *in vacuo*. Considering one-dimensional waves (Figure 7.8e), the electric (magnetic) field depends only on time and longitudinal coordinate (7.377a) [(7.377b)]:

$$\vec{E} = \vec{E}(x,t),\ \vec{H} = \vec{H}(x,t): \qquad \frac{\partial}{\partial x}(\varepsilon E_x) = 0 = \frac{\partial}{\partial x}(\mu H_x),\ E_x = 0 = H_x, \qquad (7.377\text{a–f})$$

from (7.375b) [(7.376b)] follow (7.377c) [(7.377d)] showing that $\varepsilon E_x\ (\mu H_x)$ do not depend on position. Thus propagation, which must depend on position and time is not possible, and both must vanish (7.377e) [(7.377f)]. Thus, electromagnetic waves are transverse, that is, the electric and magnetic field are transverse to the direction of propagation.

Choosing (Figure 7.10) the y-axis in the direction of the electric field (7.378a) the equation (7.375c) becomes (7.378b):

$$\vec{E} = \vec{e}_y\, E(x,t): \qquad \vec{e}_z\frac{\partial E}{\partial x} = \nabla \wedge \vec{E} = -\frac{1}{c_0}\frac{\partial}{\partial t}(\mu\vec{H}), \qquad (7.378\text{a, b})$$

showing that the magnetic field lies in the z-direction, which is (7.379a) perpendicular to the electric field and to the direction of propagation:

$$\vec{H} = \vec{e}_z\, H(x,t); \qquad -\vec{e}_y\frac{\partial H}{\partial x} = \nabla \wedge \vec{H} = \frac{1}{c_0}\frac{\partial}{\partial t}(\varepsilon\,\vec{E}), \qquad (7.379\text{a, b})$$

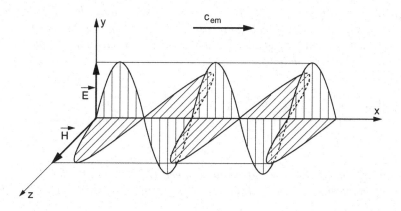

FIGURE 7.10
The quasi-one-dimensional (Figure 7.9e) propagation of an electromagnetic wave in an inhomogeneous waveguide with dielectric permittivity and magnetic permeability varying along its length (Figure 7.10) has electric $\vec{E}$ and magnetic $\vec{H}$ field orthogonal to each other and transverse to the direction of propagation $\vec{e}_x$, so that $(e_x, \vec{E}, \vec{H})$ from an orthogonal right-handed triad.

substituting (7.379a) in (7.376c) leads to (7.379b), which confirms that the electric field lies in the y-direction (7.378a). Thus the Maxwell equations for one-dimensional waves, (7.378a) [(7.379a)], simplify to (7.380c) [(7.380d)] in the case of dielectric permittivity, (7.380a) [magnetic permeability (7.380b)], independent of time, which may depend on position:

$$\frac{\partial \varepsilon}{\partial t} = 0 = \frac{\partial \mu}{\partial t}: \qquad \frac{\partial E}{\partial x} = -\frac{\mu(x)}{c_0}\frac{\partial H}{\partial t}, \qquad \frac{\partial H}{\partial x} = -\frac{\varepsilon(x)}{c_0}\frac{\partial E}{\partial t}. \qquad \text{(7.380a–d)}$$

Elimination between (7.380c, d) leads to:

$$\frac{\partial^2 E}{\partial t^2} = -\frac{c_0}{\varepsilon(x)}\frac{\partial^2 H}{\partial x \partial t} = \frac{c_0^2}{\varepsilon(x)}\frac{\partial}{\partial x}\left[\frac{1}{\mu(x)}\frac{\partial E}{\partial x}\right], \qquad \text{(7.381a)}$$

$$\frac{\partial^2 H}{\partial t^2} = -\frac{c_0}{\mu(x)}\frac{\partial^2 E}{\partial x \partial t} = \frac{c_0^2}{\mu(x)}\frac{\partial}{\partial x}\left[\frac{1}{\varepsilon(x)}\frac{\partial H}{\partial x}\right], \qquad \text{(7.381b)}$$

as the wave equation for the electric (7.381a) [magnetic (7.381b)] field.

NOTE 7.15: **Non-Uniform Dielectric Permittivity and Magnetic Permeability**

It has been shown that *the electric (magnetic) field of a one-dimensional electromagnetic wave (Figure 7.8e) propagating in a medium with dielectric permittivity (magnetic permeability), depending on position x but not on time t (7.380a; 7.380b), form (problem 374) an orthogonal triad (Figure 7.10) and satisfy the primal (7.382a) [dual (7.382b)] wave equations:*

$$\frac{\partial^2 E}{\partial t^2} - \frac{c_0^2}{\mu(x)}\frac{\partial}{\partial x}\left[\frac{1}{\varepsilon(x)}\frac{\partial E}{\partial x}\right] = 0, \qquad \frac{\partial^2 H}{\partial t^2} - \frac{c_0^2}{\varepsilon(x)}\frac{\partial}{\partial x}\left[\frac{1}{\mu(x)}\frac{\partial H}{\partial x}\right] = 0.$$

$$\text{(7.382a, b)}$$

*Introducing the **electromagnetic wave speed** (7.383a) and the lengthscales for variation of the dielectric permittivity (7.383b) [magnetic permeability (7.383c)]:*

$$c_{em}(x) = \frac{c_0}{\sqrt{\varepsilon(x)\mu(x)}}, \qquad L_\varepsilon(x) = \frac{\varepsilon(x)}{\varepsilon'(x)}, \qquad L_\mu(x) = \frac{\mu(x)}{\mu'(x)}, \qquad \text{(7.383a–c)}$$

the dual-wave equations for the electric (7.382a) [magnetic (7.382b)] field become (7.384a) [(7.384b)]:

$$\frac{\partial^2 E}{\partial t^2} - \left[c_{em}(x)\right]^2 \left\{\frac{\partial^2 E}{\partial x^2} - \frac{1}{L_\varepsilon(x)}\frac{\partial E}{\partial x}\right\} = 0, \tag{7.384a}$$

$$\frac{\partial^2 H}{\partial t^2} - \left[c_{em}(x)\right]^2 \left\{\frac{\partial^2 H}{\partial x^2} - \frac{1}{L_\mu(x)}\frac{\partial H}{\partial x}\right\} = 0. \tag{7.384b}$$

In the case of a homogeneous medium (7.385a, b) the electric (magnetic) field satisfy the same classical wave equation (7.385c) [≡ (7.385d)]:

$$\varepsilon, \mu = const: \qquad \left\{\frac{\partial^2}{\partial t^2} - c_{em}^2 \frac{\partial^2}{\partial x^2}\right\} E, H(x,t) = 0, \tag{7.385a–d}$$

with a constant electromagnetic wave speed (7.383a). The sixth and last wave analogy concerns sound in a duct with varying cross-sections (notes 7.16–7.17).

NOTE 7.16: Sound Waves in an Acoustic Horn

The propagation of sound (water waves) in a duct (channel) of varying cross-sections [Figure 7.8d(f)] is specified [notes 7.12–7.13 (7.16–7.17)] by the equations of continuity and momentum in a different form. The mass density per unit length (7.345b) [(7.386a)], which equals the mass density per unit volume (7.345a) ≡ (7.386b) times the cross-sectional area, appears in the equation of continuity or mass conservation, (7.362a) ≡ (7.386c), where (7.386d) the total mass density $\bar{\rho}$ has been split into (7.386b), a mean state mass density ρ_0 and an acoustic perturbation ρ:

$$\bar{\sigma} \equiv \bar{\rho}A, \quad \bar{\rho}(x,t) = \rho_0 + \rho(x,t): \quad 0 = \frac{\partial\bar{\sigma}}{\partial t} + \frac{\partial}{\partial x}(\bar{\sigma}v) = \frac{\partial}{\partial t}(A\bar{\rho}) + \frac{\partial}{\partial x}(A\bar{\rho}v). \tag{7.386a–d}$$

In the case of water waves (notes 7.12–7.13), the fluid is assumed to be incompressible (7.366a); in the case of sound waves in fluid, including water and air, compressibility must be considered, and thus, the mass density (7.386b) consists of a constant mean state value plus an acoustic perturbation; a similar decomposition is made for the pressure (7.387a):

$$\bar{p}(x,t) = p_0 + p(x,t): \qquad -\frac{\partial\bar{p}}{\partial x} = \bar{\rho}\frac{dv}{dt} = \bar{\rho}\left(\frac{dv}{dt} + v\frac{\partial v}{\partial x}\right), \tag{7.387a–c}$$

in the momentum equation, (7.363c, d) ≡ (7.387b, c). The medium is assumed to be at rest, so the total velocity is due to the acoustic velocity perturbation alone. The perturbations of pressure and density are assumed to be adiabatic (5.105a) ≡ (7.388a) with a **sound speed** (5.107a, b) ≡ (7.388b, c) that simplifies to (5.107c) ≡ (7.388d) for a perfect gas:

$$p = c_s^2 \, \rho: \qquad c_s^2 = \left(\frac{\partial p_0}{\partial \rho_0} \right)_s = \gamma \frac{p_0}{\rho_0} = \gamma R T_0 ; \qquad\qquad (7.388\text{a--d})$$

in (7.388b–d) all quantities are calculated for the mean state of rest, including the adiabatic exponent (5.101a) and the gas constant (5.111a–d).

For linear sound waves (note III.7.14) the mass density (pressure) perturbations are small compared with mean state values (7.389a) [(7.389b)], and the velocity perturbation is small compared with the sound speed (7.389c):

$$\left(\frac{\rho}{\rho_0} \right)^2 \sim \left(\frac{p}{p_0} \right)^2 \sim \left(\frac{v}{c_0} \right)^2 \ll 1: \qquad 0 = \frac{\partial p}{\partial x} + \rho_0 \frac{\partial v}{\partial t}, \qquad\qquad (7.389\text{a--d})$$

$$-\frac{\partial}{\partial x}(\rho_0 \, A v) = \frac{\partial}{\partial t}(\rho A) = \frac{1}{c_s^2} \frac{\partial}{\partial t}(A p), \qquad\qquad (7.389\text{e, f})$$

and the equation of: (i) momentum (7.387c) simplifies to (7.389d); (ii) continuity (7.366d) simplifies to (7.389e), which leads to (7.389f) using the adiabatic condition (7.388a). Assuming that the cross-sectional area does not depend on time t (7.390a) but may depend on position x for a **horn** (Figures 7.11a–c), the elimination of (7.389d, f) leads to:

$$\frac{\partial A}{\partial t} = 0: \qquad \frac{\partial^2 p}{\partial t^2} = -\frac{c_s^2}{A} \frac{\partial}{\partial x}\left(\rho_0 A \frac{\partial v}{\partial t} \right) = \frac{c_s^2}{A} \frac{\partial}{\partial x}\left(A \frac{\partial p}{\partial x} \right), \qquad\qquad (7.390\text{a, b})$$

$$\frac{\partial^2 v}{\partial t^2} = -\frac{1}{\rho_0} \frac{\partial^2 p}{\partial x \partial t} = \frac{c_s^2}{\rho_0} \frac{\partial}{\partial x}\left[\frac{1}{A} \frac{\partial}{\partial x}(\rho_0 A v) \right], \qquad\qquad (7.390\text{c})$$

(7.390b) [(7.390c)] for the acoustic pressure (velocity) perturbations.

NOTE 7.17: **Acoustic Pressure and Velocity Perturbations**

It has been shown that *the acoustic pressure (longitudinal velocity) perturbation of linear (7.389a–c)* **quasi-one-dimensional sound** *(Figure 7.8f) in a horn with cross-section depending on position x (Figures 7.11a–c) but not on time t (7.390a)*

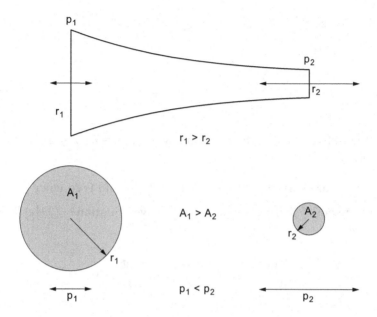

FIGURE 7.11
In the ray limit of wavelength short compared with the lengthscales of variation of the cross-sectional area of an acoustic horn (Figure 7.9f), the amplitude (Figure 7.10) is inversely proportional to: (i) the square-root of the cross-sectional area; (ii) the radius r for an axisymmetric horn. Thus, the amplitude of sound is smaller p_1 (larger $p_2 > p_1$) in larger A_1 (smaller $A_2 < A_1$) cross-sections.

containing and homogeneous steady fluid at rest with adiabatic sound speed (7.388a–d) satisfies (problem 375) the dual pair of wave equations (7.391a) [(7.391b)]:

$$\frac{\partial^2 p}{\partial t^2} - \frac{c_s^2}{A(x)}\frac{\partial}{\partial x}\left[A(x)\frac{\partial p}{\partial x}\right],$$
(7.391a)

$$\frac{\partial^2 v}{\partial t^2} - c_s^2 \frac{\partial}{\partial x}\left\{\frac{1}{A(x)}\frac{\partial}{\partial x}\left[A(x)v\right]\right\}.$$
(7.391b)

Introducing the lengthscale for the variation of the cross-section (7.392a) ≡ (7.371b) the primal (dual) acoustic wave equation for the pressure (7.391a) [velocity (7.391b)] perturbation becomes (7.392b) [(7.392c)]:

$$L_A = \frac{A(x)}{A'(x)}: \qquad \frac{\partial^2 p}{\partial t^2} - c_s^2\left[\frac{\partial^2 p}{\partial x^2} + \frac{1}{L_A(x)}\frac{\partial p}{\partial x}\right] = 0,$$
(7.392a, b)

$$\frac{\partial^2 v}{\partial t^2} - c_s^2 \frac{\partial}{\partial x}\left[\frac{\partial v}{\partial x} + \frac{v}{L_A(x)}\right] = 0.$$
(7.392c)

In the case of a duct of constant cross-section (7.393a), the dual-wave equations for the acoustic pressure (7.392b) [velocity (7.392c)] lead to the classical wave equation (7.393b) [≡ (7.393c)]:

$$A = const: \qquad \left\{ \frac{\partial^2}{\partial t^2} - c_s^2 \frac{\partial^2}{\partial x^2} \right\} p, v(x,t) = 0. \qquad (7.393a\text{–}c)$$

This is the sixth and last of the wave analogies (Tables 7.2–7.3) is summarized next (notes 7.18–7.19).

NOTE 7.18: **Dual Wave Equations in Space Time and Frequency**

It has been shown that the **primal (dual) wave equations** (7.394a) [(7.394b)] *in space-time:*

$$\frac{\partial^2 \Phi}{\partial t^2} - \left[c(x) \right]^2 \left[\frac{\partial^2 \Phi}{\partial x^2} + \frac{1}{L(x)} \frac{\partial \Phi}{\partial x} \right] = 0, \qquad (7.394a)$$

$$\frac{\partial^2 \Psi}{\partial t^2} - \frac{\partial}{\partial x} \left\{ \left[c(x) \right]^2 \left[\frac{\partial \Psi}{\partial x} + \frac{\Psi}{L(x)} \right] \right\} = 0, \qquad (7.394b)$$

*are (problem 376) satisfied (Table 7.2) by linear waves in inhomogeneous steady medium for six pairs of **primary (dual) wave variables** [problem 377 (378)]. The analogy is closest for the following five cases: (i) the displacement (7.395a) [slope (7.396a)] of the transverse vibrations (Figure 7.8a) of a non-uniform elastic string (7.348c) [(7.348e)]: (ii) the torsion (7.395b) [rate or torsion (7.396b)] of the torsional oscillations (Figure 7.8b) of a straight rod of varying cross-section (7.354a) [(7.354b)]; (iii) the longitudinal displacement (7.395c) [strain (7.396c)] of the longitudinal vibrations (Figure 7.8c) of a straight inhomogeneous rod (7.360a) [(7.360b)]; (iv) the surface elevation (7.395d) [longitudinal velocity (7.396d)] of water waves (Figures 7.8d and 7.9a–c) in a channel of variable depth and width (7.371b) [(7.371e)]; (v) the acoustic pressure (7.395e) [longitudinal velocity (7.396e)] perturbation of sound waves (Figures 7.8f and 7.11a–c) in a horn with variable cross-section containing an homogeneous fluid at rest (7.390b) [(7.390c)]:*

$$\zeta(x,t) \ \leftrightarrow \ \tau(x,t) \ \leftrightarrow \ u(x,t) \ \leftrightarrow \ \zeta(x,t) \ \leftrightarrow \ p(x,t) \ \leftrightarrow \ E(x,t), H(x,t),$$
$$(7.395a\text{–}g)$$

$$\frac{\partial \zeta(x,t)}{\partial x} \ \leftrightarrow \ \frac{\partial \tau(x,t)}{\partial x} \ \leftrightarrow \ S(x,t) \ \leftrightarrow \ \frac{\partial \zeta(x,t)}{\partial x} \ \leftrightarrow \ v(x,t). \qquad (7.396a\text{–}e)$$

The sixth somewhat distinct case (vi) is the electric (7.395f) [magnetic (7.395g)] field of electromagnetic waves (Figures 7.8e, and 7.10) in an inhomogeneous waveguide that satisfy the same primal wave equation (7.384a) [(7.384b)], with distinct length-scales (7.383b) [(7.383c)]. The lengthscales of non-uniformity and wave speeds are considered next (note 7.19).

NOTE 7.19: Combination of Inertia and Restoring Effects

*The properties of the inhomogeneous steady medium that depend on position x are [problem 379 (380)] the **inertial (restoring) effects,** that is, respectively, in the six cases: (i) the mass density per unit length (7.397a) [tangential tension (7.398a); (ii) the moment of inertia (7.397b) [torsional stiffness (7.398b)] of the cross-section; (iii) the mass density per unit length (7.397a) [Young modulus of the material (7.398c)]:*

$$\sigma(x) \;\leftrightarrow\; I(x) \;\leftrightarrow\; \sigma(x) \;\leftrightarrow\; h(x) \;\leftrightarrow\; \gamma p_0(x) \;\leftrightarrow\; c_0^2. \qquad (7.397\text{a--f})$$

$$T(x) \;\leftrightarrow\; C(x) \;\leftrightarrow\; E(x) \;\leftrightarrow\; \frac{1}{g} \;\leftrightarrow\; \rho_0(x) \;\leftrightarrow\; \varepsilon(x)\mu(x),$$

$$(7.398\text{a--f})$$

(iv) the depth (7.397d) [inverse of the acceleration of gravity (7.398d)]; (v) the mean-state pressure (7.397e) [mass density (7.398e)] with the former multiplied by the adiabatic exponent; (vi) the square of the speed of light in vacuo (7.397f) [product of the dielectric permittivity by the magnetic permeability (7.398f)].

*The **phase speed** of propagation is (problem 381) the square root of the restoring effect to the inertia in all six cases: (i) (iii) the elastic transversal, (7.347c) ≡ (7.399a) [longitudinal (7.358b) ≡ (7.399c)] wave speed is the square root of the ratio of the tangential tension (Young modulus of the material) by the mass density per unit length; (ii) the torsional wave speed (7.352b) ≡ (7.399b) is the square root of the ratio of the bending stiffness to the moment of inertia of the cross-section:*

$$\left[c(x) \right]^2 = \frac{T(x)}{\sigma(x)}, \frac{C(x)}{I(x)}, \frac{E(x)}{\sigma(x)}, \, g\,h(x), \, \gamma\frac{p_0}{\rho_0}, \, \frac{c_0^2}{\varepsilon(x)\mu(x)}, \qquad (7.399\text{a--f})$$

*(iv) the water-wave speed (7.371a) ≡ (7.399d) is the square root of the depth multiplied by the acceleration of gravity; (v) the sound speed (7.388c) ≡ (7.399e) is the square root of the ratio of the pressure (restoring effect) to the mass density (inertia) in isothermal conditions (5.130c), but since acoustic propagation is adiabatic (5.107b), the adiabatic coefficient appears as a factor; (vi) the electromagnetic wave speed (7.383a) ≡ (7.399f) is the ratio of the speed of light in vacuo to the square root of the product of the dielectric permittivity and magnetic permeability. The **lengthscale** for variations of the properties of the medium (problem 382) is the algebraic inverse of the logarithmic derivative of: (i) the tangential tension (7.348b) ≡ (7.400a); (ii) the torsional stiffness of the cross-section (7.352d) ≡ (7.400b); (iii) the Young modulus of the material (7.358d) ≡ (7.400c); (iv) the cross-sectional area of the water channel (7.374d) ≡ (7.400d);*

(v) the cross-sectional area of the horn (7.392a) ≡ (7.400e); (vi) the dielectric permittivity (7.383b) ≡ (7.400f) and magnetic permeability (7.383c) ≡ (7.400g):

$$\frac{1}{L(x)} = \frac{d}{dx}\left\{\log\left[T(x),C(x),E(x),A(x),A(x),\varepsilon(x),\mu(x)\right]\right\}.$$

$$(7.400\text{a–g})$$

The six analogue cases (Tables 7.2–7.3) of quasi-one dimensional waves in inhomogeneous media (notes 7.1–7.19) lead to duality principles (notes 7.20–7.21).

NOTE 7.20: Acoustic Duality Principle (Pyle, 1967) and Analogues

Bearing in mind that the cross-section of a horn does not depend on time t, (7.390a) ≡ (7.400a), the dual horn wave equation (7.391b) can be written (7.401b):

$$\frac{\partial A}{\partial t}=0: \qquad \frac{\partial^2}{\partial t^2}(Av)-c_s^2\,A\frac{\partial}{\partial x}\left[\frac{1}{A}\frac{\partial}{\partial x}(Av)\right]=0, \qquad (7.401\text{a, b})$$

which coincides with the primal horn wave equation (7.391a) with the changes (7.402a–d):

$$A(x)v(x,t) \leftrightarrow p(x,t), \qquad A(x) \leftrightarrow \frac{1}{A(x)}. \qquad (7.402\text{a–d})$$

This proves (problem 383) **the duality principle for acoustic horns (Pyle, 1967):** *the bulk velocity, defined as the product of the acoustic velocity perturbation by the cross-sectional area (7.402a) satisfies the same horn wave equation (7.401b) ≡ (7.391a) as the pressure perturbation (7.402b) in* **the dual horn** *with inverse cross-sectional area (7.402c, d).*

Likewise multiplying (7.370b) by the cross-sectional area (7.403a) leads to (7.403b):

$$A(x)=b(x)\,h(x): \qquad \frac{\partial^2}{\partial t^2}(Av)-A\frac{\partial}{\partial x}\left[\frac{g}{b}\frac{\partial}{\partial x}(Av)\right]=0, \qquad (7.403\text{a, b})$$

which coincides with (7.370a) with the changes (7.404a–d):

$$A(x)v(x,t) \leftrightarrow \zeta(x,t), \qquad A(x) \leftrightarrow \frac{1}{A(x)}. \qquad (7.404\text{a–d})$$

This proves (problem 384) **the duality principle for water waves:** *the bulk velocity, that is, the longitudinal velocity multiplied by the cross-sectional area*

*(7.404a) satisfies the same wave equation (7.403b) ≡ (7.370a) that the surface eleva-tion (7.404b) in the **dual channel** with (7.404d) the inverse cross-sectional area (7.404c).*

By comparison of (7.382a, b), follows (problem 385) **the duality principle for electromagnetic waveguides:** *the electric (3.405a) and magnetic (3.405b) fields satisfy the same wave equation (7.382a) ≡ (7.382b) exchanging the dielectric permittivity (7.405c) by the magnetic permeability (7.405d):*

$$E(x,t) \quad \leftrightarrow \quad H(x,t), \quad \varepsilon(x) \quad \leftrightarrow \quad \mu(x). \qquad (7.405\text{a--d})$$

The duality principle also applies to elastic strings and rods (note 7.21).

NOTE 7.21: **Duality Principle for Elastic Strings and Rods**

Multiplying (7.344b) by the tangential tension that does not depend on time (7.406a) leads to (7.406b):

$$\frac{\partial T}{\partial t} = 0: \qquad \frac{\partial^2}{\partial t^2}(T\zeta') - T\frac{\partial}{\partial x}\left[\frac{1}{\sigma}\frac{\partial}{\partial x}(T\zeta')\right] = 0, \qquad (7.406\text{a, b})$$

which coincides with (7.343d) with the changes (7.407a–d):

$$T(x)\frac{\partial \zeta(x,t)}{\partial x} \quad \leftrightarrow \quad \zeta(x,t), \qquad T(x) \quad \leftrightarrow \quad \frac{1}{\sigma(x)}. \qquad (7.407\text{a--d})$$

This proves (problem 386) **the transversal duality principle for elastic string:** *the product of the tangential tension by the slope (7.407a) satisfies the same transverse wave equation (7.406b) ≡ (7.343d) as the transverse displacement (7.407b) for the dual string whose mass density (7.407d) is the inverse of the tension (7.407c).*

Multiplying (7.350b) by the torsional stiffness of the cross-section that does not depend on time t (7.408a) leads to (7.408b):

$$\frac{\partial C}{\partial t} = 0: \qquad \frac{\partial^2}{\partial t^2}(C\tau') - C\frac{\partial}{\partial x}\left[\frac{1}{I}\frac{\partial}{\partial x}(C\tau')\right] = 0, \qquad (7.408\text{a, b})$$

which coincides with (7.349e) with the changes (7.409a–d):

$$C(x)\frac{\partial \tau(x,t)}{\partial t} \quad \leftrightarrow \quad \tau(x,t), \qquad C(x) \quad \leftrightarrow \quad \frac{1}{I(x)}. \qquad (7.409\text{a--d})$$

This proves (problem 387) **the torsional duality principle for elastic rods:** *the product of the torsional stiffness of the cross-section by the rate-of-change of the torsion along the axis (7.409a) satisfies the same wave equation (7.408b) ≡ (7.349e)* *as the torsion (7.409b) in the dual rod whose moment of inertia of the cross-section, (7.409d), is the inverse of the torsional stiffness (7.409c).*

Multiplying (7.356b) by the Young modulus of the material, which may depend on position x but not on time t, (7.410a) leads to (7.410b):

$$\frac{\partial E}{\partial t} = 0: \qquad \frac{\partial^2}{\partial t^2}(ES) - E\frac{\partial}{\partial x}\left[\frac{1}{\sigma}\frac{\partial}{\partial x}(ES)\right] = 0, \qquad \text{(7.410a, b)}$$

which coincides with (7.355d) with the changes (7.411a–d):

$$E(x)S(x,t) \quad \leftrightarrow \quad u(x,t), \qquad E(x) \quad \leftrightarrow \quad \frac{1}{\sigma(x)}. \qquad \text{(7.411a–d)}$$

This proves (problem 388) **the longitudinal duality principle for an elastic rod**: *the product of the Young modulus of the material by the longitudinal strain, (7.411a), satisfies the same wave equation (7.410b) ≡ (7.355d) as the longitudinal displacement, (7.411b) in the dual rod whose mass density per unit length (7.411d) is the inverse of the Young modulus (7.411c).* The duality principle is useful (not needed) in inhomogeneous (homogeneous) media because distinct wave variables satisfy different (the same) wave equations [note 7.22 (7.25)].

NOTE 7.22: **Horn Wave Equation (Rayleigh, 1916; Webster, 1919)**

The horn wave equation for the acoustic pressure, (7.392b) [velocity (7.392c)] perturbations involves the following assumptions: (i) linear waves, that is, the perturbations of the mass density, (7.389a) [pressure (7.389b)], are small relative to the mean-state values and the velocity perturbation is small, (7.389c), compared with the sound speed (7.388b–d); (ii) the latter is constant, as well as other mean-state properties like mass density ρ_0 and pressure p_0; (iii) the wavelength is larger than the dimensions of the cross-section (7.365a, b), excluding the existence of transverse modes, so that only a fundamental longitudinal mode exists; (iv) the wave variables depend only on time t and axial position x, and are uniform over the cross-section for **quasi-one-dimensional waves**; (v) the cross-section depends on position x but not on time t (7.390a). Thus, the horn wave equations (7.392b, c) are linear second-order partial differential equations whose coefficients depend only on position x (note 7.1). This suggests (note 7.5) using *the spectra, (7.340a, b) for the acoustic pressure, (7.412a) [velocity (7.412b)], perturbation for sinusoidal sound waves with frequency ω:*

$$\{\tilde{p}(x;\omega), \tilde{v}(x;\omega)\} = \int\limits_{-\infty}^{+\infty} \{p(x;t), v(x;t)\}e^{-i\omega t}\, d\omega, \qquad \text{(7.412a, b)}$$

which satisfy, (problem 389), linear second-order ordinary differential equations whose coefficients are: (i) the constant sound speed, (7.388b–d); (ii) the lengthscale of variations in cross-section (7.392a) ≡ (7.413b), which may depend on position (7.413c) [(7.413d)]:

$$q' \equiv \frac{dq}{dx}; L = \frac{A}{A'}: \qquad \tilde{p}'' + \frac{1}{L}\tilde{p}' + \frac{\omega^2}{c_s^2}\tilde{p} = 0 = \tilde{v}'' + \left(\frac{\tilde{v}}{L}\right)' + \frac{\omega^2}{c_s^2}\tilde{v}, \qquad (7.413a–d)$$

where prime denotes derivative with regard to position (7.413a). The first-order derivatives in (7.413c, d) can be suppressed leading to the invariant form of the wave equation (note 7.23).

NOTE 7.23: **Invariant Form of the Horn Wave Equation**

The second-order linear ordinary differential equations (7.413c, d) can be put (note 5.8) in invariant form (5.242b) ≡ (7.414a, b):

$$\{\tilde{p}(x;\omega), \tilde{v}(x;\omega)\} = \{P(x;\omega), V(x;\omega)\}\exp\left\{-\frac{1}{2}\int^x L(\xi)d\xi\right\}, \qquad (7.414a, b)$$

introducing (5.242a) a factor (5.241c) ≡ (7.414c):

$$\frac{\tilde{p}(x;\omega)}{P(x;\omega)} = \frac{\tilde{v}(x;\omega)}{V(x;\omega)} = \exp\left\{-\frac{1}{2}\int^x \frac{A'(\xi)}{A(\xi)}d\xi\right\} = \exp\left\{-\frac{1}{2}\log[A(x)]\right\} = \frac{1}{\sqrt{A(x)}}, \qquad (7.414c)$$

which is the inverse square root of the cross-section. Thus, *the substitutions*:

$$\{p(x;t), v(x;t)\} = \int_{-\infty}^{+\infty} e^{-i\omega t}\{\tilde{p}(x;\omega), \tilde{v}(x;t)\}d\omega$$

$$= \frac{1}{\sqrt{A(x)}}\int_{-\infty}^{+\infty} e^{-i\omega t}\{P(x;\omega), V(x;\omega)\}d\omega, \qquad (7.415a, b)$$

*lead (problem 390) for the acoustic pressure (velocity) perturbations: (i) from the horn wave equation (7.392b) [(7.392c)], in space-time; (ii) to the spectra (7.413c) [(7.413d)] in space-frequency domain (7.412a, b) ≡ (7.415a); (iii) through the scaling (7.414a–c) on the inverse square root of the cross-section (7.415b) to the **invariant form** of the* *horn wave equation for (7.416a) [(7.416b)]* the **reduced pressure (velocity) perturbation spectrum:**

$$P'' + \left(\frac{\omega^2}{c_s^2} - \frac{1}{4L^2} + \frac{L'}{2L^2} \right) P = 0, \qquad V'' + \left(\frac{\omega^2}{c_c^2} - \frac{1}{4L^2} - \frac{L'}{2L^2} \right) V = 0. \qquad \text{(7.416a, b)}$$

The proof of (7.416a, b) follows (note 7.24).

NOTE 7.24: **Reduced Pressure and Velocity Perturbation Spectra**

The passage from (7.413c) [(7.413d)] to (7.416a) [(7.416b)] involves (7.415b) the substitutions (7.417a, b):

$$\left(A^{-1/2} \, \Phi \right)' = A^{-1/2} \left(\Phi' - \frac{A'}{2A} \Phi \right) = A^{-1/2} \left(\Phi' - \frac{\Phi}{2L} \right), \qquad \text{(7.417a)}$$

$$\left(A^{-1/2} \, \Phi \right)'' = A^{-1/2} \left(\Phi'' - \frac{\Phi'}{2L} + \frac{L'\Phi}{2L^2} - \frac{\Phi' A'}{2A} + \frac{\Phi A'}{4LA} \right)$$

$$= A^{-1/2} \left(\Phi'' - \frac{\Phi'}{L} + \frac{\Phi}{4L^2} + \frac{L'\Phi}{2L^2} \right), \qquad \text{(7.417b)}$$

which are used in (7.413c) [(7.413d)] with (7.418a) [(7.419a)] leading to (7.418b) [(7.419b)]:

$$\Phi \equiv P: \qquad 0 = A^{1/2} \left(\tilde{p}'' + \frac{1}{L} \tilde{p}' + \frac{\omega^2}{c_s^2} \tilde{p} \right)$$

$$= P'' - \frac{P'}{L} + \frac{L'P}{2L^2} + \frac{P}{4L^2} + \frac{1}{L}\left(P' - \frac{P}{2L} \right) + \frac{\omega^2}{c_s^2} P \qquad \text{(7.418a, b)}$$

$$= P'' + \left(\frac{\omega^2}{c_s^2} - \frac{1}{4L^2} + \frac{L'}{2L^2} \right) P,$$

$$\Phi \equiv V: \qquad 0 = A^{1/2} \left[\tilde{v}'' + \frac{\tilde{v}'}{L} + \left(\frac{\omega^2}{c_s^2} - \frac{L'}{L^2} \right) \tilde{v} \right]$$

$$= V'' + \left(\frac{L'}{2L^2} - \frac{1}{4L^2} \right) V + \left(\frac{\omega^2}{c_s^2} - \frac{L'}{L^2} \right) V \qquad \text{(7.419a, b)}$$

$$= V'' + \left(\frac{\omega^2}{c_s^2} - \frac{1}{4L^2} - \frac{L'}{2L^2} \right) V;$$

Note that (7.419b) uses the same transformations as (7.418b), proving the invariant form of the horn wave equation for the reduced acoustic pressure (7.418b) ≡ (7.416a) and velocity perturbation spectra (7.419b) ≡ (7.416b). Substituting (7.415a) in (7.389d) [(7.389f)] it follows that *in an acoustic horn with cross-section, which is a function of position but not of time (7.390a) ≡ (7.420a) hold (problem 391)* **the polarization relations** *for: (i) the sound pressure and velocity perturbation spectra (7.420b) [(7.421a) ≡ (7.421b)]:*

$$\frac{\partial A}{\partial t}=0: \qquad\qquad \tilde{v}(x;\omega)=-\frac{i}{\rho_0\omega}\frac{d\tilde{p}(x;\omega)}{dx}, \qquad\qquad (7.420a, b)$$

$$\tilde{p}(x;\omega)=-\frac{i\rho_0 c_s^2}{\omega A(x)}\frac{d}{dx}\left[A(x)\tilde{v}(x,t)\right]=-\frac{i\rho_0 c_s^2}{\omega}\left[\frac{d\tilde{v}(x;\omega)}{dx}+\frac{\tilde{v}(x;\omega)}{L(x)}\right];$$

$$(7.421a, b)$$

(ii) the reduced sound pressure and velocity perturbation spectra (7.415b) (7.422a, b) [(7.423a, b)]:

$$V(x;\omega)=-\frac{i}{\rho_0\omega}\sqrt{A(x)}\frac{d}{dx}\left[\frac{P(x;\omega)}{\sqrt{A(x)}}\right]=-\frac{i}{\rho_0\omega}\left[\frac{dP(x;\omega)}{dx}-\frac{P(x;\omega)}{2L(x)}\right],$$

$$(7.422a, b)$$

$$P(x;\omega)=-\frac{i\rho_0 c_s^2}{\omega\sqrt{A(x)}}\frac{d}{dx}\left[\sqrt{A(x)}\,v(x;\omega)\right]=\frac{i\rho_0 c_s^2}{\omega}\left[\frac{dV(x;\omega)}{dx}+\frac{V(x;\omega)}{2L(x)}\right].$$

$$(7.423a, b)$$

The simplest solution of (7.416a, b) is the ray approximation for high-frequency waves (note 7.26), which is an extension of waves in a uniform duct (note 7.25).

NOTE 7.25: **Classical Wave Equation in a Uniform Duct**

In the case of a homogeneous medium, the wave equation is the same for all variables; for example, for a uniform duct, that is, with constant cross-section (7.393a) both the acoustic pressure (velocity) perturbations satisfy the same classical wave equation (7.393b) [≡ (7.393c)]; the solution, for example, for the acoustic pressure perturbation is sinusoidal waves (7.424a) in time (position) with frequency ω (wavenumber k):

$$p_1^{\pm}(x,t)=B^{\pm}\exp\left[-i\left(\omega t\mp k x\right)\right]: \qquad \omega^2=c_s^2 k^2, \qquad k=\frac{\omega}{c_s}, \qquad (7.424a-c)$$

related (7.424c) by the dispersion relation (7.424b) of second-degree allowing for waves propagating in the positive p^+ (negative p^-) x-direction. Using (7.425a, b) in (7.420b) with constant cross-section in the linearized momentum equation (7.389d) specifies the acoustic velocity perturbation (7.425c) ≡ (7.425d):

$$\frac{\partial}{\partial t} \to -i\omega, \quad \frac{\partial}{\partial x} \to \frac{i\omega}{c_s} = ik: \quad v^{\pm}(x,t) = \frac{p^{\pm}(x,t)}{\rho_0 c_s} = \frac{B^{\pm}}{\rho_0 c_s} \exp\left[-i\left(\omega t \mp kx\right)\right].$$

$$(7.425a\text{--}d)$$

The duct of constant cross-section (7.426a) corresponds (7.392a) to an infinite lengthscale (7.426b), and thus, the pressure perturbation spectrum (7.413c), satisfies a linear harmonic oscillator equation (7.428c):

$$A_1 = const: \qquad L_1 = \infty; \qquad \tilde{p}_1'' + \frac{\omega^2}{c_s^2}\tilde{p}_1 = 0, \qquad (7.426a\text{--}c)$$

whose solution:

$$p_1^{\pm}(x,t) = B^{\pm}\exp\left(\pm i\frac{\omega}{c_s}x\right) = B^{\pm}\exp\left(\pm ikx\right), \qquad (7.427a, b)$$

agrees with the acoustic pressure perturbation (7.424a) ≡ (7.427a; 7.415a). From (7.420a; 7.427b) follows the acoustic velocity perturbation spectrum (7.428a):

$$\tilde{v}_1^{\pm}(x,t) = \pm\frac{k}{\rho_0\omega}B^{\pm}\exp\left(\pm ikx\right) = \pm\frac{B^{\pm}}{\rho_0 c_s}\exp\left(\pm i\frac{\omega x}{c_s}\right), \qquad (7.428a, b)$$

which also agrees with the acoustic velocity perturbation (7.425d) ≡ (7.428a; 7.415a). Thus, *in a duct of constant cross-section (7.426a) and hence (7.392a) infinite lengthscale (7.426b) holds (problem 392) the classical wave equation in space-time (6.819c, d) for the acoustic pressure (7.393b) [velocity (7.393c)] perturbations that have solutions (7.424a) [(7.425d)] compatible with the linearized equations of motion (7.389d, f) involving the frequency (7.415a) and the wavenumber (7.424c), which are related by the dispersion relation (7.424b). In the space-frequency domain (7.415a) the classical wave equation (7.393b) reduces to (2.54b) ≡ (7.426c), that of a harmonic oscillator, and the acoustic pressure (velocity) perturbation spectra, (7.427a, b) [(7.428a, b)] satisfy* **the polarization relations** *(7.429a) [(7.429b)]:*

$$\tilde{v}(x;\omega) = -\frac{i}{\rho_0\omega}\frac{d\tilde{p}(x;\omega)}{dx}, \qquad \tilde{p}(x;\omega) = -\frac{i\rho_0 c_s^2}{\omega}\frac{d\tilde{v}(x;\omega)}{dx}, \qquad (7.429a, b)$$

that also apply (7.420b) [need extension to (7.421b)] for a horn. The simplest case of acoustic propagation in a horn is the ray approximation for high-frequency waves (note 7.26) far above the cut-off frequency.

NOTE 7.26: Ray Approximation and Compactness Parameter

The invariant form of the horn wave equation for the reduced acoustic pressure perturbation spectrum (7.416a) reduces to the equation for the linear harmonic oscillator (2.54b) ≡ (7.430b) assuming (7.430a):

$$\frac{4\omega^2 L_2^2}{c_s^2} \gg 1: \qquad P_2'' + k^2 P_2'' = 0, \qquad P_2^{\pm}(x;\omega) = B^{\pm} e^{\pm ikx}, \qquad (7.430\text{a–c})$$

and leading to (7.430c). The condition (7.430a) is **the ray approximation**:

$$\omega_* = \frac{c_s}{2L}: \quad 1 \ll \varepsilon^2 \equiv \left(\frac{2\omega L_2}{c_s}\right)^2 = \left(2kL_2\right)^2 = \left(\frac{4\pi L_2}{\lambda}\right)^2 = \left(\frac{4\pi L_2}{c_s \tau}\right)^2 = \left(\frac{\omega}{\omega_*}\right)^2,$$

$$(7.431\text{a–g})$$

of large **compactness parameter** (7.431b) for high-frequency waves, (7.431c), stating alternatively that: (i) the product of the wavenumber (7.424c) by the lengthscale of variation of the cross-section (7.392a) is large (7.431d); (ii) the wavelength λ is small compared with the lengthscale (7.431e); (iii) the period τ is short compared with the time L/c_s taken to propagate one lengthscale at the sound speed (7.431f); (iv) the frequency is much higher (7.431g) than the **cut-off frequency** (7.431a) to be considered in the sequel (notes 7.27–7.30). Substituting (7.430c) in (7.415b) [and then in (7.420b)] it follows that *in the ray approximation (7.431a–g) the acoustic pressure (velocity) perturbation spectrum is given (problem 393) by (7.432a) [(7.432b)]:*

$$\tilde{p}_2^{\pm}(x;\omega) = \frac{B^{\pm}}{\sqrt{A(x)}} e^{\pm ikx}, \qquad \tilde{v}_2^{\pm}(x;\omega) = \frac{B^{\pm}}{\rho_0 c_s} \frac{e^{\pm ikx}}{\sqrt{A(x)}}\left(\pm 1 + \frac{i}{2kL}\right),$$

$$(7.432\text{a, b})$$

showing that: (i) the waves remain sinusoidal in time t (7.415a) [space (7.432a, b)] with frequency ω [wavenumber (7.424c)], propagating in opposite directions with amplitude modified by the inverse square root of the cross-sectional area; (ii) in an acoustic horn (Figure 7.11) the sound amplitude is smaller (larger) in the larger (smaller) cross-section; (iii) there is conservation of the product of the cross-sectional area by the square amplitude (7.433a) [(7.433b)]:

$$\left|\tilde{p}_2^{\pm}(x;\omega)\right|^2 = \frac{\left|B^{\pm}\right|^2}{A(x)} = \left(\rho_0 c_s\right)^2 \left|\tilde{v}_2(x;\omega)\right|^2; \qquad (7.433\text{a, b})$$

(iv) the reduced acoustic velocity perturbation spectrum (7.432b) has a small term $O(1/\varepsilon)$ in out-of-phase (7.431b–g) to the pressure, that does not affect the square of the amplitude (7.434b) in the ray approximation (7.434a):

$$4k^2 L_2^2 \gg 1: \quad \left(\rho_0 c_s\right)^2 A(x)\left|\tilde{v}_2^{\pm}(x;\omega)\right|^2 \left|B^{\pm}\right|^{-2} = \left|\pm 1 + \frac{i}{2kL}\right|^2 = 1 + \frac{1}{4k^2 L_2^2} \cong 1.$$

$$(7.434a, b)$$

This property of the ray approximation is considered together with the opposite compactness or scattering limit in the general theory of wave refraction in inhomogeneous media and diffraction by obstacles next (note 7.27).

NOTE 7.27: **Wave Refraction, Diffraction, and Scattering**

The conservation law (7.433a, b) valid in the ray approximation can be explained as follows: (i) the high-frequency waves are like sound rays with wavelength small compared with the lengthscale of variations of cross-section; (ii) thus, the wave reflection from the walls is negligible, and the acoustic horn acts as a **ray tube** along which the acoustic energy per unit length is conserved. The opposite limit to (note 7.25) the ray or high-frequency approximation (7.431d) = (7.435a) is the low-frequency or compactness limit of **scattering** (7.435c) when the wavelength is much larger than the lengthscale, for example, wave reflection and transmission (notes 7.44–7.52) at an abrupt change of cross-section:

$$\text{waves:} \quad \begin{cases} (2kL)^2 \gg 1: & \text{rays,} & (7.435a) \\ kL \sim 1 & \text{refraction/diffraction,} & (7.435b) \\ kL \ll 1 & \text{scattering} & (7.435c) \end{cases}$$

The intermediate and general case is compactness parameter of order unity applies to: (a) wave **refraction** in a steady inhomogeneous medium, when the wave period is comparable to the time taken to propagate one lengthscale of variation of properties of the medium; (b) wave **diffraction,** when the wavelength is comparable to the lengthscale of an obstacle (such as, the radius of a sphere) or obstacle has no lengthscale (for example, the edge of a semi-infinite plate or a wedge). The ray (or compactness) approximation can be taken to higher orders (notes 5.16–5.20). The ray (scattering) approximations are the opposite short (long) wavelength or high (low) frequency limits of the exact theory of wave refraction or diffraction, when: (ii) the wavelength can be comparable to the lengthscale; (ii) waves are no longer sinusoidal; (iii) an exact solution of the wave equation is needed. In the case of the horn wave equations, exact solutions: (i) exist in terms of elementary functions for only five shapes (notes 7.28–7.35); (ii) for all other shapes the exact solutions require non-elementary or special functions (notes 7.36–7.43).

NOTE 7.28: Self-Dual Duct: The Exponential Horn (Olson, 1930)

The invariant form of the horn wave equation for the acoustic pressure (velocity) perturbation spectrum (7.416a) ≡ (7.436a) [(7.416b) ≡ (7.437a)] shows that elementary exact solutions exist for the shapes with **constant invariant for the lengthscale (cross-section) (7.436b) [(7.437b)]**:

$$P'' + \left[\left(\frac{\omega}{c_s} \right)^2 - J^+ \right] P = 0 : \qquad J^+ = \frac{1 - 2L'}{4L^2} = \frac{2A''A - A'^2}{4A^2}, \qquad (7.436a, b)$$

$$v'' + \left[\left(\frac{\omega}{c_s} \right)^2 - J^- \right] v = 0 : \qquad J^- = \frac{1 + 2L'}{4L^2} = \frac{3A'^2 - 2A''A}{4A^2}; \qquad (7.437a, b)$$

In (7.436b) [(7.437b)], (7.392a) was used to obtain (7.438a) ≡ (7.436c) [(7.438b) ≡ (7.437c)]:

$$\frac{1 \mp 2L'}{4L^2} = \left(\frac{A'}{2A} \right)^2 \left[1 \mp 2 \left(\frac{A}{A'} \right)' \right] = \frac{A'^2}{4A^2} \mp \frac{A'^2}{4A^2} \left(2 - 2 \frac{A''A}{A'^2} \right). \qquad (7.438a, b)$$

The simplest case in both invariants (7.436b) ≡ (7.437b) coincide (7.439a), implying (7.438b) is a constant lengthscale (7.439c), that is, (7.439d) ≡ (7.392a) is an **exponential horn** (7.439e):

$$J_3^+ = J_3^- \rightarrow L_3' = 0 \rightarrow const = L_3 = \frac{A_3}{A_3'} \equiv \ell : \qquad A_3(x) = A(0) \exp \left(\frac{x}{\ell} \right). \qquad (7.439a-e)$$

*The exponential horn, (7.439e) is (problem 394) the only **self-dual duct** (7.402c, d) in the sense that the divergent (convergent) exponential horns [Figure 7.12a (b)] are inverses (7.440a), whose lengthscales have opposite signs (7.440b) leading to the same invariant (7.440c):*

$$A_3(x) = A(0)e^{x/\ell} \quad \leftrightarrow \quad \frac{1}{A_3(x)} = \frac{e^{-x/\ell}}{A(0)}, \qquad \ell \leftrightarrow -\ell, \qquad J_3^\pm = \frac{1}{4\ell^2}.$$

$$(7.440a-c)$$

Substitution of the invariants (7.440c) in the horn wave equations (7.436a; 7.437a) leads to a filtering function with cut-off-frequency (note 7.29).

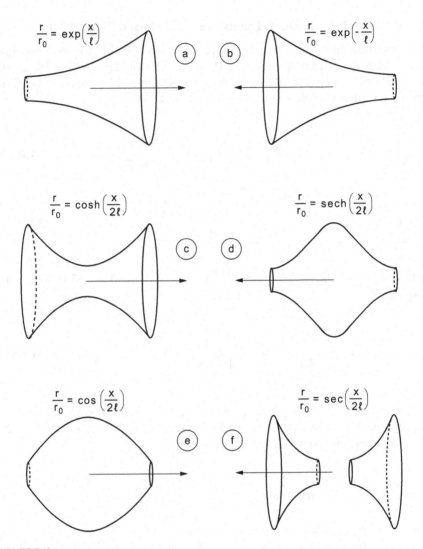

FIGURE 7.12
The horn wave equation has exact solutions in terms of elementary functions only for five shapes, of which: (I) three correspond to a filtering function, which excludes propagation below a cut-off frequency (Figure 7.13); (II) two correspond to a transparency function, which has no cut-off frequency and allows waves of all frequencies to propagate. The three cases (I) are: (I.1) the divergent (a) or convergent (b) exponential horn, which has a filtering function both for the acoustic velocity and pressure perturbations; (I.2/3) the catenoidal (c) [inverse catenoidal (d)] horn with a throat (bulge), which has a filtering function for the acoustic pressure (velocity) perturbation. The two cases (II) are the sinusoidal (e) [inverse sinusoidal (f)] horn, which is shaped like a single hump (a pair of baffles facing each other) and has a transparency function for the acoustic pressure (velocity) perturbation allowing propagation of all frequencies.

NOTE 7.29: Filtering Function and Cut-Off Frequency

In the case of the exponential horn (7.439e) the invariant forms (7.436b; 7.437b) of the horn wave equation (7.440c), both lead to a **filtering equation** (7.441b) = (7.441c) with cut-off frequency (7.431a) ≡ (7.441a):

$$\omega_* = \frac{c_s}{2\ell}: \qquad f''(x;\omega) = \left(\frac{1}{4\ell^2} - \frac{\omega^2}{c_s^2}\right) f(x;\omega) = \left(\frac{\omega_*^2 - \omega^2}{c_s^2}\right) f(x;\omega). \qquad (7.441\text{a–c})$$

*These designations arise because (problem 395) the solution of (7.441c) is a **filtering** **function** (Figure 7.13) that: (i) below the cut-off frequency (7.442a) has exponential growth or decay (7.442c) with scale (7.442b):*

$$\omega < \omega_*: \qquad K = \frac{\left|\omega^2 - \omega_*^2\right|^{1/2}}{c_s}: \qquad f^\pm(x;\omega) = \exp(\pm K x); \qquad (7.442\text{a–c})$$

(ii) at the cut-off frequency (7.443a) the filtering function is (7.443b) a linear function of the position (7.443c):

$$\omega = \omega_*: \qquad K = 0, \qquad f^\pm(x;\omega) = \{1, x\}; \qquad (7.443\text{a–c})$$

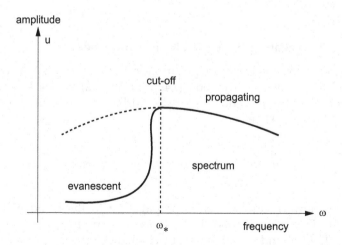

FIGURE 7.13
The acoustic pressure (velocity) perturbation in the exponential (Figure 7.12a, b) and also in the catenoidal (inverse catenoidal) horn [Figure 7.12c, d] has a filtering function (Figure 7.13) that: (i) allows propagating waves above the cut-off frequency; (ii) lead to decaying or divergent modes below the cut-off frequency; (iii) there is a smooth but rapid change between (i) and (ii) across the cut-off frequency.

(iii) above the cut-off frequency (7.444a) there are waves propagating in the positive and negative x-direction (7.444b):

$$\omega > \omega_*: \qquad\qquad f^\pm(x;\omega) = \exp(\pm i K x), \qquad\qquad (7.444\text{a, b})$$

*with **reduced wavenumber** (7.442b) ≡ (7.445b):*

$$K \equiv \frac{\sqrt{\omega^2 - \omega_*^2}}{c_s^2} \begin{cases} = \dfrac{\omega}{c_s} \equiv k & \text{if} & \omega^2 \gg \omega_*^2, & (7.445\text{a}) \\[2mm] < \dfrac{\omega}{c_s} \equiv k & \text{if} & \omega_* < \omega, & (7.445\text{b}) \\[2mm] 0 & \text{if} & \omega = \omega_*, & (7.445\text{c}) \\[2mm] = \pm i|K| & \text{if} & \omega = \omega_\alpha, & (7.445\text{d}) \end{cases}$$

that: (ii-1) coincides with the wavenumber (7.445a) ≡ (7.424c) in the ray limit of frequency much larger than the cut-off frequency; (iii-2) is smaller than the wavenumber at intermediate frequencies (7.445b); (iii-3) vanishes (7.445c) at the cut-off frequency (7.441a) when propagation becomes impossible; (iv) would be imaginary below the cut-off frequency (7.445d) when propagation is impossible, and the modes become (7.442a–c) unstable or evanescent (Figure 7.13). The filtering function appears both in the pressure and velocity perturbations in an exponential horn (note 7.30).

NOTE 7.30: **Propagating Waves and Monotonic Modes**

The reduced acoustic pressure perturbation spectrum (7.416a) coincides (7.439c) with the filtering function (7.436a) ≡ (7.437a) ≡ (7.441b) and using (7.415b) specifies the acoustic pressure perturbation spectrum (7.446) in an exponential horn (7.444a):

$$\tilde{p}_1^\pm(x;\omega) = B^\pm(\omega) \exp\left(-\frac{x}{2\ell}\right) f^\pm(x;\omega), \qquad (7.446)$$

with upper (lower) sign for waves propagating in the positive (negative) x-direction. The acoustic velocity and pressure perturbation spectra are related by (7.429a) and substitution of (7.446) specifies the acoustic velocity perturbation spectrum in an exponential horn (7.447):

$$\tilde{v}_3^\pm(x;\omega) = -\frac{i}{\rho_0\omega} B^\pm(\omega) \exp\left(-\frac{x}{2\ell}\right)\left[\frac{df^\pm(x;\omega)}{dx} - \frac{f^\pm(x;\omega)}{2\ell}\right], \qquad (7.447)$$

involving the spatial derivative (7.448a/b/c) of the filtering function, respectively, below (7.442a–c), at (7.443a–c) and above (7.444a, b) the cut-off frequency:

$$\frac{df^{\pm}(x;\omega)}{dx} = \begin{cases} \pm K \exp\left(\pm K x\right) & \text{if} & \omega < \omega_*, & (7.448a) \\ \{0,1\} & \text{if} & \omega = \omega_*, & (7.448b) \\ \pm i K \exp\left(\pm i K x\right) & \text{if} & \omega > \omega_\alpha. & (7.448c) \end{cases}$$

It has been shown that *the acoustic pressure (velocity) perturbation spectrum in an exponential horn (7.439e) with lengthscale (7.439d) is given (problem 396) by (7.446) [(7.447)] involving: (i) the mass density per unit volume (7.366a) of the mean state* ρ_0, *the sound speed (7.388b–d), and the cut-off frequency (7.441a) that appears in the reduced wavenumber (7.445a–d); (ii) the filtering function (7.442a–c; 7.443a–c; 7.444a, b) [and also its derivative (7.448a–c)]; (iii) the amplitudes* $B^{\pm}$ *apply respectively to waves propagating in the positive and negative x-directions.* The filtering function applies: (i) both to the acoustic pressure and the velocity perturbations in an exponential horn (notes 7.29–7.30); (ii)(iii) only to the acoustic pressure (velocity) perturbation in a catenoidal (inverse catenoidal) horn [note 7.31 (7.32)].

NOTE 7.31: Effective Filtering Wavenumber in a Catenoidal Horn (Salmon, 1946)

The invariant form of the horn wave equation for the acoustic pressure perturbation spectrum (7.416a) ≡ (7.436a) reduces to the filtering wave equation (7.441b) if the corresponding invariant (7.436b) is a constant (7.449a), leading to a first-order differential equation for the lengthscale (7.449b):

$$\frac{1}{4\ell^2} = J_4^+ = \frac{1-2L_4'}{4L_4^2}: \qquad 1 - \frac{L_4^2}{\ell^2} = 2L_4' = 2\frac{dL_4}{dx}. \qquad (7.449a, b)$$

The integration (7.450a) of (7.449b) shows that the lengthscale is (II.7.118b), a hyperbolic tangent (7.450b):

$$\frac{x}{2\ell} = \int\left(1-\frac{L_4^2}{\ell^2}\right)^{-1}\frac{dL_4}{\ell} = arc\tanh\left(\frac{L_4}{\ell}\right): \qquad L_4(x) = \ell\tanh\left(\frac{x}{2\ell}\right); \qquad (7.450a, b)$$

the constant of integration has been omitted in (7.418b) by placing the origin $x = 0$ at $L_4 = 0$. From (7.392a; 7.450b) follows (7.451):

$$2\frac{d}{dx}\left\{\log\left[\cosh\left(\frac{x}{2\ell}\right)\right]\right\} = \frac{1}{\ell}\tanh\left(\frac{x}{2\ell}\right) = \frac{1}{L_4(x)} = \frac{A_4'(x)}{A_4(x)} = \frac{d}{dx}\left\{\log\left[\frac{A_4(x)}{A_4(0)}\right]\right\},$$

$$(7.451)$$

implying the cross-section (7.452a):

$$A_4(x) = A_4(0)\cosh^2\left(\frac{x}{2\ell}\right) = \pi\left[r_4(x)\right]^2: \quad r_4(x) = r_4(0)\cosh\left(\frac{x}{2\ell}\right), \qquad (7.452a\text{--}c)$$

for an axisymmetric duct (7.452b) the radius is (Figure 7.12c) a catenoidal function of the length (7.452c).

Substituting (7.452a) in (7.414c) and noting that the reduced acoustic pressure perturbation spectrum is specified by the filtering function (7.416a) ≡ (7.441b) leads to (7.453) [(7.454)] for the acoustic pressure (velocity) perturbation spectrum:

$$\tilde{p}_4^\pm(x;\omega) = B^\pm(\omega)\,\text{sech}\left(\frac{x}{2\ell}\right)f^\pm(x;\omega), \qquad (7.453)$$

$$\tilde{v}_4^\pm(x;\omega) = -\frac{i}{\rho_0\omega}B^\pm(\omega)\,\text{sech}\left(\frac{x}{2\ell}\right)\left[\frac{df^\pm(x;\omega)}{dx} - \tanh\left(\frac{x}{2\ell}\right)\frac{f^\pm(x;\omega)}{2\ell}\right]; \qquad (7.454)$$

the passage from (7.453) to (7.454) uses (7.420a) and (II.7.103b). It has been shown that *in a catenoidal horn (Figure 7.12c), which is shaped like a "throat" with cross-sectional area (7.452a–c), and has lengthscale of variation of cross-section area (7.450b), the (problem 397) acoustic pressure (velocity) perturbation spectrum is given by (7.453) [(7.454)], involving the filtering function (7.442a–c; 7.443a–c; 7.444a, b) [and also its derivative (7.448a–c)].* From the acoustic reciprocity principle for horns (7.404a–d) follows that the filtering function specifies the reduced acoustic pressure (velocity) perturbation spectrum in [note 7.31 (7.32)] a catenoidal (inverse catenoidal) horn [Figure 7.12 c(d)].

NOTE 7.32: Acoustic Velocity in an Inverse Catenoidal Horn (Campos, 1984)

The filtering function (7.441b) ≡ (7.437a) also applies to the reduced acoustic velocity perturbation spectrum if the corresponding invariant (7.437b) is constant (7.455a) leading to the differential equation (7.455b) for the lengthscale:

$$\frac{1}{4\ell^2} = J_5 = \frac{1+2L_5'}{4L_5^2}: \qquad \frac{L_5^2}{\ell^2} - 1 = 2L_5' = 2\frac{dL_5}{dx}; \qquad (7.455a, b)$$

The integration (7.456a) of (7.455b) shows that the lengthscale is (II.7.124b) minus a hyperbolic tangent (7.456b):

$$\frac{x}{2\ell} = -\int\left(1-\frac{L_5^2}{\ell^2}\right)^{-1}\frac{dL}{\ell} = -arc\tanh\left(\frac{L_5}{\ell}\right): \quad L_5(x) = -\ell\tanh\left(\frac{x}{2\ell}\right). \qquad (7.456a, b)$$

The corresponding (7.392a) cross-sectional area (7.457):

$$-2\frac{d}{dx}\left\{\log\left[\cosh\left(\frac{x}{2\ell}\right)\right]\right\}=-\frac{1}{\ell}\tanh\left(\frac{x}{2\ell}\right)=\frac{1}{L_5(x)}=\frac{A_5'(x)}{A_5(x)}=\frac{d}{dx}\left\{\log\left[\frac{A_5(x)}{A_5(0)}\right]\right\},$$

(7.457)

is (7.458a) corresponding in the axisymmetric case (7.458b) to (7.458c):

$$A_5(x)=A_5(0)\,sech^2\left(\frac{x}{2\ell}\right)=\pi\left[r_5(x)\right]^2:\qquad r_5(x)=r_5(0)\,sech\left(\frac{x}{2\ell}\right),\qquad(7.458a\text{--}c)$$

which is an inverse catenoidal duct (Figure 7.12d) with the shape of a bulge.
Substituting (7.458a) in (7.414c) and using (7.437a) $\equiv$ (7.441b) leads to the acoustic velocity perturbation spectrum for the inverse catenoidal horn (7.459):

$$\tilde{v}_5^{\pm}(x;\omega)=D^{\pm}(\omega)\cosh\left(\frac{x}{2\ell}\right)f^{\pm}(x;\omega),$$

(7.459)

using (7.458b). The acoustic velocity and perturbation spectra in a horn are connected by the inverse relations (7.414b) and (7.428a, b).
Substituting (7.459; 7.458a) in (7.421a) specifies the acoustic pressure perturbation spectrum in an inverse catenoidal horn:

$$\tilde{p}_5^{\pm}(x;\omega)=-\frac{i\rho_0 c_s^2}{\omega}\cosh^2\left(\frac{x}{2\ell}\right)\frac{d}{dx}\left[sech^2\left(\frac{x}{2\ell}\right)\tilde{v}_5^{\pm}(x;\omega)\right]$$

$$=-\frac{i\rho_0 c_s^2}{\omega}\cosh^2\left(\frac{x}{2\ell}\right)\frac{d}{dx}\left[D^{\pm}(\omega)\,sech\left(\frac{x}{2\ell}\right)f^{\pm}(x;\omega)\right],$$

(7.460a, b)

which simplifies (II.7.103b) to:

$$\tilde{p}_5^{\pm}(x;\omega)=-\frac{i\rho_0 c_s^2}{\omega}D^{\pm}(\omega)\cosh\left(\frac{x}{2\ell}\right)\left[\frac{df^{\pm}(x;\omega)}{dx}-\tanh\left(\frac{x}{2\ell}\right)\frac{f^{\pm}(x;\omega)}{2\ell}\right].$$

(7.461)

Comparing (7.453; 7.459) [(7.454; 7.461)] leads to (7.462a) [(7.463a)]:

$$D^{\pm}(\omega)\tilde{p}_4^{\pm}(x;\omega)=sech^2\left(\frac{x}{2\ell}\right)B^{\pm}(\omega)\tilde{v}_5^{\pm}(x;\omega)=B^{\pm}(\omega)\frac{A_5(x)}{A_5(0)}\tilde{v}_5^{\pm}(x;\omega),$$

(7.462a, b)

$$B^{\pm}(\omega)\tilde{p}_5^{\pm}(x;\omega)=\left(\rho_0 c_s\right)^2 D^{\pm}(\omega)\cosh^2\left(\frac{x}{2\ell}\right)\tilde{v}_4^{\pm}(x;\omega)=\left(\rho_0 c_s\right)^2 D^{\pm}(\omega)\frac{A_5(x)}{A_5(0)}\tilde{v}_4^{\pm}(x;\omega),$$

(7.463a, b)

which are consistent with the acoustic duality principle (7.402a–d), stating that the acoustic pressure in a duct scales like the bulk velocity in the dual duct (7.462b) [(7.463b)]. It has been shown (problem 398) that *in an inverse catenoidal horn (Figure 7.12d), which is shaped like a "hump" with cross-sectional area (7.458a–c) and has the corresponding lengthscale (7.456b), the acoustic velocity (pressure) perturbation spectrum is given by (7.459) [(7.461)], involving the filtering function (7.442a–c; 7.443a–c; 7.444a, b) [and also its derivative (7.448a–c)] and the reduced wavenumber (7.445a–d).* Replacing real ℓ by an imaginary i ℓ parameter changes: (i) the filtering function to a transparency function as shown next (note 7.33); (ii) the catenoidal (inverse catenoidal) horn [note 7.30 (7.31)] to a sinusoidal (inverse sinusoidal horn) [note 7.33 (7.34)]. Taking into account the acoustic reciprocity principle (7.404a–d) it may be expected that the transparency function applies to the acoustic pressure (velocity) perturbation spectrum in a sinusoidal (inverse sinusoidal) horn [note 7.33 (7.34)].

NOTE 7.33: Transparency Function and Sinusoidal Horn (Nagarkar & Finch, 1971)

The change from real to imaginary parameter (7.464a) transforms the filtering wave equation (7.441b) to a **transparency equation** (7.464b):

$$\ell \to i\ell: \qquad g''(x;\omega) = -\left(\frac{\omega^2}{c_s^2} + \frac{1}{4\ell^2}\right)g(x;\omega), \qquad (7.464a, b)$$

*whose solution is (problem 399), a **transparency function** (7.465b) ensuring propagation of all frequencies as a linear harmonic oscillator (2.54c) with an **enhanced wavenumber** (7.465a):*

$$\bar{K} = \left|\frac{1}{4\ell^2} + \frac{\omega^2}{c_s^2}\right|^{1/2} = \frac{\sqrt{\omega^2 + \omega_*^2}}{c_s}: \qquad g^\pm(x;\omega) = B_\pm \exp(\pm i\bar{K}x). \qquad (7.465a, b)$$

The enhanced wavenumber: (i) coincides with the wavenumber (7.466b) at high-frequency (7.466a):

$$\omega^2 \gg \omega_*^2: \qquad \bar{K} = \frac{\omega}{c_s}; \qquad k < \bar{K}(\omega) \ge K_{min} = K(0) = \frac{1}{2\ell}. \qquad (7.466a–d)$$

(ii) is larger at intermediate frequencies (7.466c) and takes the minimum value at zero frequency (7.466d). The imaginary change of parameter (7.464a) applied to a catenoidal horn (7.452a) leads to a sinusoidal horn (7.467):

$$\frac{A_6(x)}{A_6(0)} = \cosh^2\left(\frac{x}{2i\ell}\right) = \left(\frac{e^{-ix/2\ell} + e^{ix/2\ell}}{2}\right)^2 = \cos^2\left(\frac{x}{2\ell}\right). \qquad (7.467)$$

From the acoustic reciprocity principle (7.402a–d) it should be expected that the transparency function (7.465a, b) applies to the acoustic pressure (velocity) perturbation spectrum in a sinusoidal (inverse sinusoidal) duct as shown next [note 7.32 (7.33)].

The invariant form of the horn wave equation for the reduced acoustic pressure perturbation spectrum (7.436a) ≡ (7.464b) coincides with the transparency equation, as for a harmonic oscillator if the corresponding invariant (7.436b) satisfies (7.468a) that is a differential equation for the lengthscale (7.468b):

$$-\frac{1}{4\ell^2} = J_6^+ = \frac{1-2L_6'}{4L_6^2}: \qquad\qquad 1+\frac{L^2}{\ell^2} = 2L_6' = \frac{dL_6}{dx}; \qquad (7.468a, b)$$

the integration (7.469a) of (7.468b) shows (II.7.113b), which is a lengthscale that is a circular cotangent (7.469b):

$$\frac{x}{2\ell} = \int\left(1+\frac{L_6^2}{\ell^2}\right)^{-1}\frac{dL_6}{\ell} = -arc\cot\left(\frac{L_6}{\ell}\right): \qquad L_6(x) = -\ell\cot\left(\frac{x}{2\ell}\right). \qquad (7.469a, b)$$

The corresponding (7.392a) cross-sectional area (7.470):

$$2\frac{d}{dx}\left[arc\cos\left(\frac{x}{2\ell}\right)\right] = -\frac{1}{\ell}\tan\left(\frac{x}{2\ell}\right) = \frac{1}{L_6(x)} = \frac{A_6'(x)}{A_6(x)} = \frac{d}{dx}\left\{\log\left[\frac{A_6(x)}{A_6(0)}\right]\right\},$$

$$\qquad (7.470)$$

is (7.471a) leading in the axisymmetric case (7.471b) to (7.471c) a sinusoidal horn [Figure 7.12e):

$$A_6(x) = A_6(0)\cos^2\left(\frac{x}{2\ell}\right) = \pi\left[r_6(x)\right]^2: \qquad r_6(x) = r_6(0)\cos\left(\frac{x}{2\ell}\right). \qquad (7.471a-c)$$

Substitution of (7.471a) and (7.465b) in (7.414c) specifies the acoustic pressure (velocity) perturbation spectra (7.472) [(7.473)]:

$$\tilde{p}_6^\pm(x;\omega) = B_\pm(\omega)\sec\left(\frac{x}{2\ell}\right)\exp\left(\pm i\bar{K}x\right), \qquad (7.472)$$

$$\tilde{v}_6^\pm(x;\omega) = -\frac{i}{\rho_0\omega}B_\pm(\omega)\sec\left(\frac{x}{2\ell}\right)\exp\left(\pm i\bar{K}x\right)\left[\pm i\bar{K}+\frac{1}{2\ell}\tan\left(\frac{x}{2\ell}\right)\right], \qquad (7.473)$$

where the passage from (7.472) to (7.473) uses (7.420a) and (II.7.103a). It has been shown that *a sinusoidal horn (Figure 7.12e), with cross-sectional area (7.471a–c)*

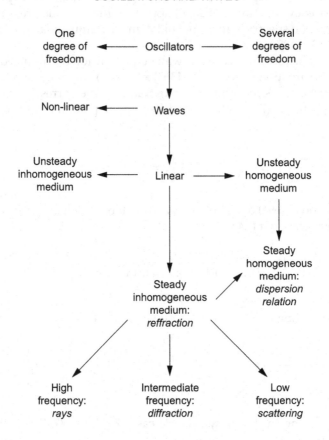

OSCILLATORS AND WAVES

DIAGRAM 7.3

The oscillators (waves) are specified by ordinary (partial) wave equations (Diagram 7.3) depending only on time (t) (also on position (x)). In the case of waves in a steady inhomogeneous medium, whose properties do not depend on time, the spectrum of a wave of fixed frequency depends only on position, like a spatial oscillator. The oscillators with several degrees-of-freedom (waves with several wave variables) lead to simultaneous systems of ordinary (partial) differential equations.

and lengthscale (7.469b) allows (problem 400) the propagation of all frequencies with enhanced wavenumber (7.465a; 7.466a–d) that appears in the acoustic pressure (7.472) [velocity (7.473)] perturbation spectra. It has been found (Nagarkar & Finch, 1971) that the mouth of the English horn, invented two centuries before, has a sinusoidal shape, which allows propagation of all frequencies.

NOTE 7.34: **Acoustics of the Inverse Sinusoidal Horn (Campos, 1985)**

The invariant form of the horn wave equation for the reduced acoustic velocity perturbation spectrum (7.437a) ≡ (7.464b) coincides with the transparency

TABLE 7.4

Comparison of Six Types of Waves

Cases	I	II	III	IV	V	VI
type	transversal	torsional	longitudinal	longitudinal	transversal	longitudinal
medium	elastic string	elastic rod	elastic rod	water channel	dielectric	acoustic horn
wave	transverse vibration	torsional oscillation	longitudinal vibration	longitudinal wave	electromagnetic wave	sound wave
note(s)	7.8–7.9	7.10	7.11	7.12–7.13	7.14–7.15	7.16–7.17
figure(s)	7.8a	7.8b	7.8c	7.8d, 7.9a–c	7.8e, 7.10	7.8f, 7.11a–c
main wave variable	(7.395a)	(7.395b)	(7.395c)	(7.395d)	(7.395f, g)	(7.395e)
dual wave variable	(7.396a)	(7.396b)	(7.396c)	(7.396d)	—	(7.396e)
inertia property	(7.397a)	(7.397b)	(7.397c)	(7.397d)	(7.397f)	(7.397e)
restoring property	(7.398a)	(7.398b)	(7.398c)	(7.398d)	(7.398f)	(7.398e)
phase speed	(7.399a)	(7.399b)	(7.399c)	(7.399d)	(7.399f)	(7.399e)
lengthscale of inhomogeneity	(7.400a)	(7.400b)	(7.400c)	(7.400d)	(7.400f, g)	(7.400e)
wave equation in space-time	(7.343a–d; 7.344a, b)	(7.349a–e; 7.350a, b)	(7.355a–d; 7.356a, b)	(7.370a, b)	(7.381a, b)	(7.391a, b)
in-phase speed and lengthscale	(7.348c, e)	(7.354a, b)	(7.360a, b)	(7.371b, e)	(7.384a, b)	(7.392b, c)
duality principle	(7.407a–d)	(7.409a–d)	(7.411a–d)	(7.404a–d)	(7.405a–d)	(7.402a–d)

Note: Comparison of the properties of six types of waves including; (i) type of medium; (ii) inertia and restoring effects; (iii) phase speed and length scale of inhomogeneity: (iv)–(v) dual wave variables and wave equations in space plus time or frequency domains; (vi) duality principle.

equation if the corresponding invariant (7.437b) satisfies (7.474a) leading to the differential equation (7.474b) for the lengthscale:

$$-\frac{1}{4\ell^2} = J_7 = \frac{1+2L_7'}{4L_7^2}: \qquad 1+\frac{L_7^2}{\ell^2} = -2L_7' = -2\frac{dL_7}{dx}; \qquad (7.474a, b)$$

the integration (7.475a) of (7.474b) shows that the lengthscale is (II.7.113b) minus a circular cotangent (7.475b):

$$\frac{x}{2\ell} = -\int\left(1+\frac{L_7^2}{\ell^2}\right)^{-1}\frac{dL_7}{\ell} = arc\cot\left(\frac{L_7}{\ell}\right): \qquad L_7(x) = \ell\cot\left(\frac{x}{2\ell}\right). \qquad (7.475a, b)$$

The corresponding cross-sectional area (7.476):

$$-2\frac{d}{dx}\left\{\log\left[\cos\left(\frac{x}{2\ell}\right)\right]\right\} = \ell\tan\left(\frac{x}{2\ell}\right) = \frac{1}{L_7(x)} = \frac{A_7'(x)}{A_7(x)} = \frac{d}{dx}\left\{\log\left[\frac{A_7(x)}{A_7(0)}\right]\right\},$$

$$(7.476)$$

is (7.477a) leading in the axisymmetric case (7.477b) to an inverse sinusoidal duct (7.477c):

$$A_7(x) = A_7(0)\sec^2\left(\frac{x}{2\ell}\right) = \pi[r_7(x)]^2: \qquad r_7(x) = r_7(0)\sec\left(\frac{x}{2\ell}\right), \qquad (7.477a\text{–}c)$$

which has the shape (Figure 7.12f) of a **pair of baffles**.

Substituting (7.477a) and (7.465b) in (7.414c) specifies the acoustic velocity perturbation spectrum (7.478).

$$v_7^{\pm}(x,t) = D_{\pm}(\omega)\cos\left(\frac{x}{2\ell}\right)\exp\left(\pm i\bar{K}x\right). \qquad (7.478)$$

The acoustic pressure perturbation spectrum follows substituting (7.477a) and (7.478) in (7.421a):

$$\tilde{p}_7^{\pm}(x;\omega) = -\frac{i\rho_0 c_s^2}{\omega}\cos^2\left(\frac{x}{2\ell}\right)\frac{d}{dx}\left[\sec^2\left(\frac{x}{2\ell}\right)\tilde{v}_7^{\pm}(x;\omega)\right]$$

$$(7.479a, b)$$

$$= -\frac{i\rho_0 c_s^2}{\omega}\cos^2\left(\frac{x}{2\ell}\right)\frac{d}{dx}\left[D_{\pm}(\omega)\sec\left(\frac{x}{2\ell}\right)\exp\left(\pm i\bar{K}x\right)\right],$$

which simplifies (II.7.103a) to:

$$\tilde{p}_7^{\pm}(x;\omega) = -\frac{i\rho_0 c_s^2}{\omega} D_{\pm}(\omega)\cos\left(\frac{x}{2\ell}\right)\exp\left(\pm i\bar{K}x\right)\left[\pm i\bar{K} + \frac{1}{2\ell}\tan\left(\frac{x}{2\ell}\right)\right].$$

(7.480)

Comparing (7.472; 7.478) [(7.473; 7.480)] leads to (7.481a) [(7.481b)]:

$$D_{\pm}(\omega)\tilde{p}_6^{\pm}(x;\omega) = \sec^2\left(\frac{x}{2\ell}\right)B_{\pm}(\omega)\tilde{v}_7^{\pm}(x;\omega) = B_{\pm}(\omega)\frac{A_7(x)}{A_7(0)}\tilde{v}_7^{\pm}(x;\omega),$$

(7.481a, b)

$$B_{\pm}(\omega)\tilde{p}_7^{\pm}(x;\omega) = \left(\rho_0 c_s\right)^2 D_{\pm}(\omega)\cos^2\left(\frac{x}{2\ell}\right)\tilde{v}_4^{\pm}(x;\omega) = \left(\rho_0 c_s\right)^2 D_{\pm}(\omega)\frac{A_6(x)}{A_6(0)}\tilde{v}_6^{\pm}(x;\omega),$$

(7.482a, b)

which is consistent (7.481b) [(7.482b)] with the acoustic duality principle (7.402a–d). It has been shown that (problem 401) *the acoustic velocity (pressure) perturbation spectrum is given by (7.478) [(7.480)] in terms of the enhanced wavenumber (7.465a; 7.466a–d), in an inverse sinusoidal horn (Figure 7.12f), which is shaped like a pair of "baffles" facing each other, with cross-sectional area (7.477a–c) and lengthscale (7.475b).* This completes the set of five duct shapes (Figures 7.12a–f) for which the horn wave equation has exact solution in terms of elementary functions (note 7.35).

NOTE 7.35: Elementary Solutions of the Horn Wave Equation (Campos, 1986)

There are only (Diagram 7.4) five cases (problem 402) of constant wave invariants (7.436b) [(7.437b)] leading to exact solutions of the horn wave equations in invariant form (7.436a) [(7.437a)] that are expressible in terms of elementary functions (Table 7.5), namely: (i) the exponential horn (7.483a) that has (notes 7.27–7.29) a filtering function (7.441a), both for the acoustic pressure and velocity perturbation spectra and is the only self-dual duct (Figure 7.12a, b); (ii)(iii) catenoidal (inverse catenoidal) duct (7.483b) [(7.483c)], which has [notes 7.30 (7.31)] filtering functions for the acoustic pressure (7.453)[(7.461)] and velocity (7.454)[(7.459)] perturbation spectra, and is shaped [Figure 7.12c, d)] like a smooth throat (bulge); (iv)–(v) the sinusoidal (inverse sinusoidal) duct (7.483d) [(7.483e)] that has [notes 7.30 (7.31)] a transparency function (7.464b) for the acoustic pressure (7.472) [(7.480)] and velocity

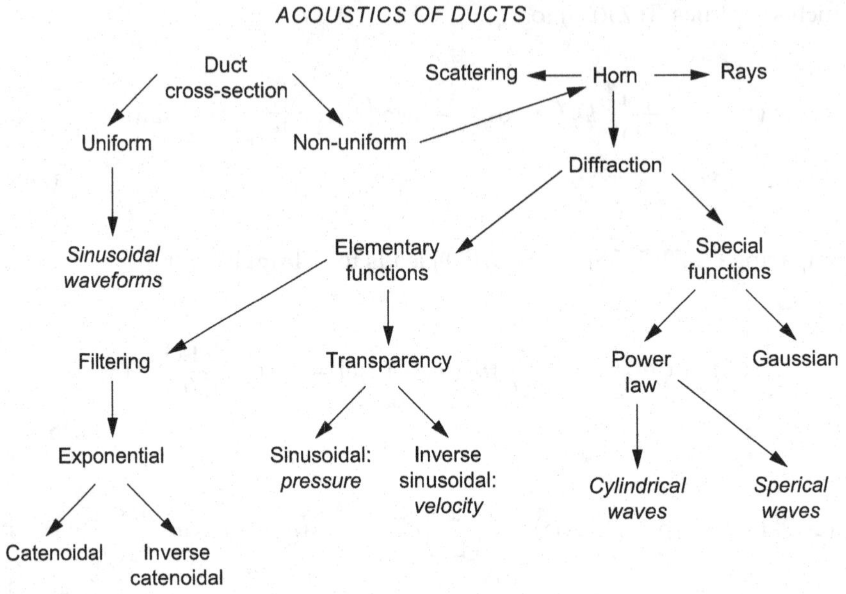

ACOUSTICS OF DUCTS

DIAGRAM 7.4
The acoustics of ducts includes the cases of uniform and non-uniform cross-sections. The acoustics of non-uniform ducts or horns may be considered: (i)/(ii) in the high (low) frequency approximations of sound rays (scattering); (iii) the intermediate case of diffraction requires exact solutions of the wave equations, including the nine duct shapes in the Table 7.5.

(7.473) [(7.478)] perturbation spectrum, and is shaped [Figure 7.12 e, f] like a hump (a pair of baffles):

$$\frac{A_{3-7}(x)}{A_{3-7}(0)} = \begin{cases} \exp\left(\dfrac{x}{2\ell}\right) & \text{if } J^+ = J^- = \dfrac{1}{4\ell^2}, & (7.483\text{a}) \\[2mm] \cosh\left(\dfrac{x}{2\ell}\right) & \text{if } J^+ = \dfrac{1}{4\ell^2} > 0, & (7.483\text{b}) \\[2mm] \operatorname{sech}\left(\dfrac{x}{2\ell}\right) & \text{if } J^- = \dfrac{1}{4\ell^2} > 0, & (7.483\text{c}) \\[2mm] \cos\left(\dfrac{x}{2\ell}\right) & \text{if } J^+ = -\dfrac{1}{4\ell^2} < 0, & (7.483\text{d}) \\[2mm] \sec\left(\dfrac{x}{2\ell}\right) & \text{if } J^- = -\dfrac{1}{4\ell^2} < 0. & (7.483\text{e}) \end{cases}$$

The filtering (7.442a–c; 7.443a–c; 7.444a, b) [transparency (7.465b)] function involves the reduced (7.445a–d) [enhanced (7.465a; 7.466a–d)] wavenumber. For all other duct shapes the exact solutions of the horn wave equations (7.436a; 7.437a) are not elementary and involve special functions, for example,

TABLE 7.5

Acoustics of Horns

Shape	Reference	Figure	Note	Cross-Sectional Area	Lengthscale	Acoustic Perturbation	
						Pressure	Velocity
*exponential**	Olson, 1930	7.12a, b	7.28–7.30	(7.440a)	(7.439c, d)	(7.446)	(7.447)
*catenoidal**	Salmon, 1946	7.12c	7.31	(7.452a–c)	(7.450b)	(7.453)	(7.454)
*inverse catenoidal**	Campos, 1984	7.12d	7.32	(7.458a–c)	(7.456b)	(7.459)	(7.461)
*sinusoidal***	Nagarkar & Finch, 1971	7.12e	7.33	(7.471a–c)	(7.469b)	(7.472)	(7.473)
*inverse sinusoidal***	Campos, 1986	7.12f	7.34	(7.477a–c)	(7.475b)	(7.478)	(7.480)
Gaussian	Bies, 1962	7.14	7.36–7.38	(7.484a)	(7.484b)	(7.487a, b)	(7.489)
power law	Ballantine, 1927	7.15a	7.39–7.41	(7.497a–c)	(7.497d)	(7.504)	(7.507)
wedge	cylindrical wave	7.15b	7.42–7.43	(7.508b)	(7.508c)	(7.508d)	(7.509b)
conical	spherical wave	7.15c	7.44–7.46	(7.513b)	(7.513c)	(7.515b)	(7.516)

* filtering function: (7.441a–c) (7.442a–c) (7.443a–c; 7.444a, b), (7.445a–d), (7.446a–d).

** transparency function: (7.464a, b), (7.465a, b), (7.466a–d).

Note: Acoustics of horns with nine different cross-sections and length scales, indicating the acoustic pressure and velocity perturbations in cases including: (i)(ii) elementary exact solutions involving filtering or transparency functions; (iii) solutions in terms of Hermite polynomials (Bessel functions) for Gaussian (power law) horns; (iv) the power law horns include, as particular cases, cylindrical and spherical waves.

Hermite polynomials (Bessel functions) for the Gaussian (power-law) horn [notes 7.36–7.38 (7.39–7.41)]. It may (may not) happen that the special functions take elementary forms, for example, this is not (is) the case [notes 7.42–7.43 (7.44–7.45)] for cylindrical (spherical) waves, which are the particular wedge-(cone-) shaped cases of power-law ducts.

NOTE 7.36: Gaussian Horn and Hermite Polynomials

A Gaussian horn (Figure 7.14a) has cross-section (7.484a), which leads to a lengthscale (7.484b) that varies inversely with distance:

$$A_8(x) = A_8(0)\exp\left(-\frac{x^2}{\ell^2}\right): \qquad L_8(x) = \frac{A_8(x)}{A_8'(x)} = -\frac{\ell^2}{2x}; \qquad (7.484a, b)$$

substitution in the horn wave equation (7.413c) for the acoustic pressure perturbation spectrum leads to a differential equation (7.485a):

$$\frac{d^2\tilde{p}}{dx^2} - \frac{2x}{\ell^2}\frac{d\tilde{p}}{dx} + \frac{\omega^2}{c_s^2}\tilde{p} = 0 \quad \leftrightarrow \quad \left\{\frac{d^2}{dy^2} - 2y\frac{d}{dy} + 2n\right\}H_n(y) = 0, \qquad (7.485a, b)$$

which is similar to the Hermite differential equation (III.1.206) ≡ (7.485b) of degree n. The change to a dimensionless independent variable (7.486a, b) leads to (7.486c):

$$y \equiv \frac{x}{\ell}; \quad \tilde{p}_8(x;\omega) = H_n(y): \qquad \left\{\frac{d^2}{dy^2} - 2y\frac{d}{dy} + \left(\frac{\omega\ell}{c_s}\right)^2\right\}H_n(x) = 0, \qquad (7.486a\text{–}c)$$

which is *(problem 403) a* **Hermite differential equation** *(7.486c)* ≡ *(7.485b) of order (7.487a) specified by one-half of the square of the* **Helmholtz number** *(7.487b), which is the frequency made dimensionless using the sound speed and length parameter:*

$$2n = \left(\frac{\omega_n\ell}{c_s}\right)^2 \equiv \Omega_n^2: \qquad \tilde{p}_8(x;\omega) = B(\omega)H_n\left(\frac{x}{\ell}\right), \qquad (7.487a, b)$$

leading to the acoustic pressure perturbation spectrum (7.487c). Using the differentiation formula for Hermite polynomials (III.1.204) ≡ *(7.488):*

$$H_n'(y) = 2nH_n(y) - H_{n+1}(y), \qquad (7.488)$$

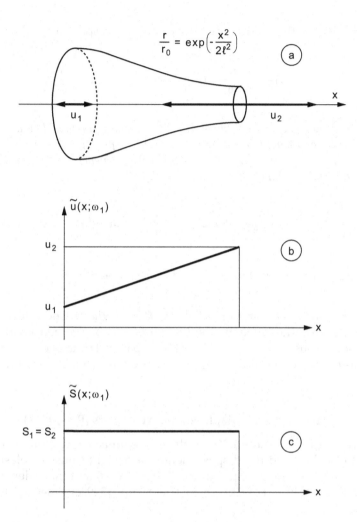

FIGURE 7.14

A horn whose cross-sectional area is a Gaussian function of the axial coordinate (*a*) has as an analogue a Gaussian elastic rod that acts as a displacement amplifier increasing the amplitude of small vibrations (Figure 7.11) at the wide base to larger vibrations at the narrow tip. The longitudinal displacement *u* as a function of the axial coordinate *x* is specified by Hermite polynomials of degree *n* for a set of discrete frequencies ω_n. The fundamental frequency ω_1 corresponds to a Hermite polynomial of first degree, implying that the corresponding (*b*) longitudinal displacement spectrum is a linear function of the axial coordinate; (*c*) the strain and stress spectra are constant along the length of the rod. This helps to prevent fracture or breaking of the tapered elastic rods used as displacement amplifiers in power tools, which operate close to resonance.

in (7.420b) leads to the acoustic velocity perturbation spectrum:

$$\tilde{v}_8(x;\omega) = -\frac{i}{\rho_0 \omega \ell} B(\omega)\left[2nH_n\left(\frac{x}{\ell}\right) - H_{n+1}\left(\frac{x}{\ell}\right)\right]. \qquad (7.489)$$

It has been shown that *in (problem 404) a Gaussian horn (Figure 7.14a) with cross-section (7.484a) and lengthscale (7.484b), the acoustic pressure (velocity) perturbation spectrum is specified by (7.487c) (7.489)] at the frequencies (7.487a) ≡ (7.490a) in terms of Hermite polynomials (III.1.18) ≡ (7.490b):*

$$\omega_n = \frac{c_s}{\ell}\sqrt{2n}: \qquad H_n(y) = (-)^n \exp(y^2)\frac{d^n}{dy^n}\left[\exp(-y^2)\right], \qquad (7.490a, b)$$

$$H_{0-4}(y) = \left\{ 1,\, 2y,\, 4y^2 - 2,\, 8y^3 - 12y,\, 16y^4 - 48y^2 + 12 \right\}, \qquad (7.491a-e)$$

with the first four degrees given by (III.1.19a–f) ≡ (7.491a–e). These results can be applied to the other analogue problems of quasi-one-dimensional waves in inhomogeneous media (notes 7.8–7.14), in particular, to the longitudinal vibrations of elastic rods (note 7.11) that are used as displacement amplifiers (note 7.37).

NOTE 7.37: **Elastic Rods as Displacement Amplifiers (Bies, 1962)**

The preceding results (note 7.36) for the Gaussian acoustic horn also apply (7.360a) to the longitudinal displacement of a straight Gaussian elastic rod with constant mass density per unit volume (7.345a) and mass density per unit length (7.345b) ≡ (7.492b) given (7.484a) by (7.492c) where (7.492a) is constant:

$$\sigma_0 = \rho A_7(0): \qquad \sigma(x) = \rho A_7(x) = \sigma_0 \exp\left(-\frac{x^2}{\ell^2}\right); \qquad E = const, \qquad (7.492a-d)$$

assuming also a homogeneous material with constant Young modulus (7.492d) leads to the frequencies (7.493a) similar to (7.490a), replacing: (i) the sound speed by the longitudinal wave speed (7.358b) leading to (7.493b):

$$\omega_n \ell = c_\ell \sqrt{2n} = \sqrt{\frac{2nE}{\sigma}}; \qquad \tilde{u}_n(x;\omega) = B(\omega) H_n\left(\frac{x}{\ell}\right), \qquad (7.493a-c)$$

(ii) the acoustic pressure perturbation spectrum (7.487b) ≡ (7.493c) by the spectrum of the longitudinal displacement of the elastic rod. The lowest

(7.494a) of the discrete set of frequencies (7.493b) is (7.494b), corresponding to the Hermite polynomial of degree 1 in (7.491b) ≡ (7.494c):

$$n=1: \qquad \omega_1 = \sqrt{\frac{2E}{\sigma}}, \qquad H_1(y)=2y, \qquad \left\{\frac{d^2}{dy^2} - 2y\frac{d}{dz} + 2\right\}H_1(y)=0,$$

$$(7.494a\text{–}d)$$

which is a solution (7.494d) of the Hermite differential equation (7.485b) of order one (7.494a); thus, to the **fundamental frequency** (7.494b) corresponds: (i) a longitudinal displacement spectrum (7.493c; 7.494c) that (Figure 7.14b) is a linear function of position (7.495a):

$$\tilde{u}_1(x;\omega_1)=2B(\omega_1)\frac{x}{L}; \qquad \tilde{S}_1(x;\omega_1) \equiv \frac{d}{dx}\left[\tilde{u}_1(x;\omega_1)\right] = \frac{2B(\omega_1)}{L} = const,$$

$$(7.495a, b)$$

(ii) the corresponding strain (7.495b) is uniform, which is independent of position. Thus, a Gaussian elastic rod oscillates at the fundamental frequency (7.494b) with uniform stress; this is desirable to avoid the risk of breakage of displacement amplifiers used in power tools (note 7.38).

NOTE 7.38: **Power Tools with Uniform Stress**

It has been shown that (problem 405) *an elastic rod with constant Young modulus (7.492d) and mass density per unit volume (7.492a, b), with (Figure 7.14a) a Gaussian cross-sectional area as a function of length (7.484a) with length-scale (7.484b) has a longitudinal displacement specified at the frequencies (7.490a) ≡ (7.493b) by (7.493c) the Hermite polynomials (7.490b) ≡ (7.491a–e). In particular, (problem 406) the Hermite polynomial (7.491b) ≡ (7.494c) of lowest non-zero degree (7.494a) corresponds to the frequency (7.494b) that leads to: (i) a longitudinal displacement spectrum (7.495a), which is a linear function of position (Figure 7.14b); (ii) the strain spectrum (7.495b) has constant amplitude (Figure 7.14c), and hence, also the stress spectrum.* The elastic rods with non-uniform cross-section are used as **displacement amplifiers** in power tools; a vibration (Figure 7.11) with small amplitude at the thick end of the tapering rod leads to a large amplitude at the thin end. Since the displacement amplifiers in power tools operate close to resonance there is the risk of breakage; this risk is minimized by operating at the frequency (7.494b), which leads to constant amplitude for the strain and stress spectra. The exact solution of the horn wave equation for Gaussian (power law) ducts falls outside the elementary exact solutions (note 7.35) and leads to special functions, namely, [notes 7.36–7.38 (7.39–7.46)] Hermite polynomials (Bessel functions). The power law horns (notes 7.39–7.41) include (Figure 7.15a) the wedge (cone) containing [Figure 7.15b, c] cylindrical (spherical) waves

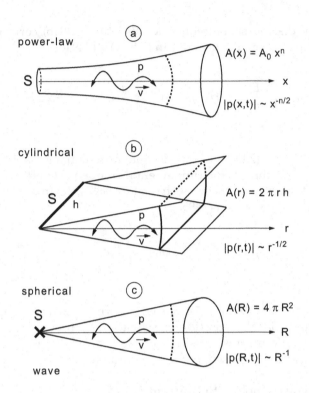

FIGURE 7.15
The sound waves in a horn with cross-sectional area (*a*) proportional to a power of the longi-tudinal coordinate $A \sim x^n$, include as particular cases $n = 1$ $(n = 2)$ a two-dimensional wedge (*b*) [cone (*c*)] containing a cylindrical (spherical) wave. In the far field, the ray approximation holds and the amplitude scales as $x^{-n/2}$, which is as $r^{-1/2}\left(R^{-1}\right)$ for a cylindrical (spherical) wave, so that the total energy flux across a cylinder (sphere) of radius $r(R)$ is constant. The scaling of the amplitude as $r^{-1/2}\left(R^{-1}\right)$ for a cylindrical (spherical) wave is valid only asymptotically at large radial distance compared with the wavelength (is valid exactly at all radial distances) because the cylindrical (spherical) wave is due to a line source along the axis (*b*) [a point source at the center (*c*)].

[notes 7.42–7.43 (7.44–7.46)]. In the latter case, the horn wave equation may be replaced by the classical wave equation extended from one (7.393c) to three-dimensions (7.496a):

$$\frac{1}{c_s^2}\frac{\partial^2 p}{\partial t^2} = \nabla^2 p \equiv \frac{\partial^2 p}{\partial x^2} + \frac{\partial^2 p}{\partial y^2} + \frac{\partial^2 p}{\partial z^2}; \qquad \text{(7.496a, b)}$$

replacing cartesian (7.496b) by cylindrical (spherical) coordinates (notes 7.45–7.46) with dependence only on the radial distance leads to cylindrical (spherical) waves.

NOTE 7.39: Power-Law Duct and Acoustic Rays in the Far Field

The duct with (Figure 7.15a) the power law cross-section (7.497a) corresponding in the axisymmetric case (7.497b) to the radius (7.497c) has lengthscale (7.497d) proportional to the distance:

$$A_9(x) = A_9(0)x^n = \pi\left[r_9(x)\right]^2: \qquad r_9(x) = r_9(0)x^{n/2}, \qquad L_9(x) = \frac{A_9(x)}{A_9'(x)} = \frac{x}{n}.$$

$$(7.497\text{a--d})$$

Substituting in the horn wave equation for the acoustic pressure perturbation spectrum (7.413c) leads to (7.498a):

$$\frac{d^2\tilde{p}}{dx^2} + \frac{n}{x}\frac{d\tilde{p}}{dx} + \left(\frac{\omega^2}{c_s}\right)^2 \tilde{p} = 0 \;\leftrightarrow\; \left\{z^2\frac{d^2}{dz^2} + z\frac{d}{dz} + z^2 - m^2\right\}H_m^{(1,2)}(z) = 0,$$

$$(7.498\text{a, b})$$

which is similar to a **Bessel differential equation** (7.498b), whose solutions are (9.573a) Hankel functions of the first $H^{(1)}$ and (second $H^{(2)}$) kind(s), corresponding, respectively, to waves propagating in positive (negative) z-direction. The last statement corresponds mathematically to the asymptotic scaling of Hankel functions for large variables, which is next shown to be equivalent physically to the ray approximation. The lengthscale (7.497d) of the power law horn (7.497a–c) increases with distance, and thus, the ray approximation (7.431d) ≡ (7.499a) holds in the far field (7.499b), which is beyond a distance that increases with the wavelength:

$$1 \ll (2kL_9)^2 = \left(\frac{4\pi x}{\lambda n}\right)^2: \qquad x^2 \gg \frac{16\pi^2\lambda^2}{n^2}; \qquad \tilde{p}_9^{\pm}(x;\omega) \sim x^{-n/2}\exp\left(\pm iKx\right);$$

$$(7.499\text{a--c})$$

the ray approximation (7.432a) applied to (7.497a) then specifies the asymptotic scaling of the acoustic pressure spectrum in the far field (7.499c). It has been shown that *the acoustic pressure spectrum (7.498a) in a power law duct (Figure 7.15a) with cross-sectional area (7.497a–c) and lengthscale (7.497d) scales (problem 407) like (7.499c) in the far field (7.499b), where the ray approximation holds (7.499a) for waves propagating in the positive and negative x-directions.* In order to obtain the acoustic pressure spectrum at all distances the horn wave equation (7.498a) is transformed into a Bessel differential equation (7.498b), leading to the solution in terms of Hankel functions (note 7.40) of which (7.499c) is the asymptotic limit.

NOTE 7.40: Sound in Power Law Ducts (Ballantine, 1927)

The transformation from the horn wave equation for the acoustic pressure spectrum (7.498a) to the Bessel differential equation (7.498b) requires three steps (i–iii) involving a change of (i) independent variable and (ii) dependent variable, and (iii) a choice of parameter. The new dimensionless independent variable (7.500a) is the axial distance multiplied (7.500b) by the wavenumber (7.424c) and leads (7.500c) the linear second-order differential equation (7.498a) with variable coefficients (7.500d):

$$z \equiv kx = \frac{\omega x}{c_s}, \qquad p_9(x;\omega) = G_n(z): \qquad \left\{ z^2 \frac{d^2}{dz^2} + nz\frac{d}{dz} + z^2 \right\} G_n(z) = 0,$$

$$(7.500a\text{–}d)$$

which differs from the Bessel differential equation (7.498b) mainly in involving the exponent n of the cross-sectional area (7.497a) in the coefficient of the first derivative in (7.500d). In order to eliminate this, a change (ii) of dependent variable is made (7.501a), implying (7.501b, c):

$$G_n(z) = z^a J_n(z): \quad G_n' = z^a\left(J_n' + \frac{a}{z} J_n \right), \quad G_n'' = z^a\left[J_n'' + \frac{2a}{z} J_n' + \frac{a(a-1)}{z^2} J_n \right],$$

$$(7.501a\text{–}c)$$

and leading from (7.500d) to (7.501d):

$$\left\{ z^2 \frac{d^2}{dz^2} + (n+2a)z\frac{d}{dz} + z^2 + a(a+n-1) \right\} J_n(z) = 0, \qquad (7.501d)$$

where the constant a may be chosen at will. The (iii) choice (7.502a) leads from (7.501d) to (7.502b):

$$a = \frac{1-n}{2}: \qquad \left\{ z^2 \frac{d^2}{dz^2} + z\frac{d}{dz} + z^2 - \left(\frac{n-1}{2} \right)^2 \right\} J_n(z) = 0, \qquad (7.502a, b)$$

which is (7.502b) $\equiv$ (7.498b), a Bessel equation of order (7.503a) with solutions (7.503b):

$$m = \frac{n-1}{2}: \qquad \tilde{p}_9(x;\omega) = G_n(z) = z^{(1-n)/2} H_m^{(1,2)}(z). \qquad (7.503a, b)$$

Substitution of (7.500a, b) in (7.503b) leads to the acoustic pressure perturbation spectrum (7.504):

$$\tilde{p}_9^{\pm}(x,\omega) = B^{\pm}(\omega)(kx)^{(1-n)/2} H_{(n-1)/2}^{(1,2)}(kx), \qquad (7.504)$$

where the Hankel functions of the first $H^{(1)}$ and (second $H^{(2)}$) kind(s), correspond to waves propagating in the positive (negative) x-direction. The asymptotic scaling of the Hankel functions for large radius is considered next (note 7.41).

NOTE 7.41: **Asymptotic Scaling of Hankel Functions**

Comparison of the exact acoustic pressure perturbation spectrum (7.503b) with its ray approximation (7.499c) in the far field (7.499a, b) of the power law horn (7.497a) leads to the asymptotic scaling of the Hankel functions of first (second) kinds as outward (inward) propagating waves (7.505b):

$$C_n^{\pm} = \sqrt{\frac{2}{\pi}} \exp\left(\pm i \frac{n\pi}{2} \pm \frac{i\pi}{4}\right): \qquad H_n^{(1,2)} \sim C_n^{\pm} z^{-1/2} e^{\pm iz}, \qquad (7.505a, b)$$

with a constant coefficient (7.505a) that depends (9.573d) on the order but not on the variable. Using the differentiation formula for cylinder functions, $(9.838c) \equiv (7.506)$, which include Hankel functions:

$$G_m'(z) = -G_{m+1}(z) + \frac{m}{z} G_m(z), \qquad (7.506)$$

in (7.503b) leads (7.420b) to the acoustic velocity perturbation spectrum (7.507):

$$\tilde{v}_9(x;\omega) = -\frac{ik}{\rho_0 \omega} \frac{d}{dz}[z^{(1-n)/2} H_{(n-1)/2}^{(1,2)}(z)] = \frac{i}{\rho_0 c_s} B^{\pm}(\omega) (k\,x)^{(1-n)/2} H_{(n+1)/2}^{(1,2)}(k\,x).$$

$$(7.507)$$

It has been shown that (problem 408) *in a horn with power law cross-section (7.497a–c) and lengthscale (7.497d) the acoustic pressure (velocity) perturbation spectrum is given by (7.504) [(7.507)] in terms of Hankel functions of the first $H^{(1)}$ and (second $H^{(2)}$) kind(s), which represent waves propagating in the positive (negative) x-direction.* The last statement will be confirmed next [notes 7.42–7.44 (7.45–7.46)] considering cylindrical (spherical) waves that correspond [Figure 7.15b (c)] to a wedge (cone) hence exponent $n = 1$ ($n = 2$).

NOTE 7.42: **Cylindrical Waves in a Two-Dimensional Wedge**

The case of *the power law duct (7.497a) with exponent (7.508a) corresponds (problem 409) to the cross-sectional area (7.508b) and lengthscale (7.508c) of a wedge (Figure 7.15b) with a **line source** at the edge generating **cylindrical waves**:*

$$n = 1: \qquad A_{10}(r) \sim r, \qquad L_{10}(r) = \frac{1}{r}, \qquad \tilde{p}_{10}^{\pm}(r;\omega) = B_{\pm}(\omega) H_0^{(1,2)}(k\,r), \qquad (7.508a–d)$$

corresponding (7.504) to an acoustic pressure perturbation spectrum (7.504) speci-
fied by Hankel functions of order zero. Using the differentiation formula (7.506) for
order zero (7.509a) shows that the acoustic velocity perturbation (7.420b) is specified
by Hankel functions of order one:

$$J_0' (z) = -J_1(z): \qquad \tilde{v}_{10}^{\pm}(r;\omega) = -\frac{ik}{\rho_0 \omega} \frac{d}{d(kr)}\left[B^{\pm}(\omega)H_0^{(1,2)}(kr)\right]$$

$$= \frac{i}{\rho_0 c_s} B^{\pm}(\omega) H_1^{(1,2)}(kr),$$

(7.509a, b)

corresponding to (7.507) with (7.508a). In (7.499a) the (problem 410) far field (7.510a)
the acoustic pressure (velocity) perturbations scale as (7.510b) [(7.510c)]:

$$r^2 \gg \frac{1}{4k^2} = \frac{\lambda^2}{16\pi^2}: \qquad \tilde{P}_{10}^{\pm}(r;\omega) \sim B^{\pm}(\omega)r^{-1/2}e^{\pm ikr},$$

(7.510a, b)

$$\tilde{v}_{10}^{\pm}(r;\omega) \sim \mp \frac{i}{\rho_0 c_s} B^{\pm}(\omega)r^{-1/2} e^{\pm ikr}.$$

(7.510c)

The asymptotic approximations (7.510b, c) to the Hankel functions (7.508d; 7.509b) correspond to the ray approximation (note 7.26) as confirmed (note 7.43) next.

NOTE 7.43: **Audible Range and Geometric Acoustics**

The **geometric acoustics** or ray approximation (note 7.26) is considered for cylindrical waves with audible frequencies. The audible range of frequencies is 20 Hz–20 kHz, with greater sensitivity of the human ear at middle frequencies. For a frequency (7.511a) the period is (7.511b) and the radian frequency (7.511c). Choosing (5.133c) ≡ (7.511d) for the sound speed at sea level leads to the wavelength (7.511e) and wavenumber (7.511f):

$$f = 1\ kHz, \qquad \tau = \frac{1}{f} = 10^{-3}s^{-1}, \qquad \omega = \frac{2\pi}{f} = 6.28 x 10^{-3} s^{-1}, \qquad (7.511a\text{–}c)$$

$$c_s = 341 ms^{-1}, \qquad \lambda = c_s \tau = 0.341\ m, \qquad k = \frac{2\pi}{\lambda} = 18.4\ m^{-1}; \qquad (7.511d\text{–}f)$$

$$4k^2r^2 \geq 10: \qquad r \geq \frac{\sqrt{10}}{2k} = \frac{\lambda\sqrt{10}}{4\pi} = 0.083\ m, \qquad (7.511g, h)$$

the ray approximation (7.510a) with a margin of about one order of magnitude (7.511g) then leads to the distance (7.511h) beyond which the ray approximation applies to cylindrical waves (7.510b, c).

The approximation (7.505a, b) to Hankel functions of order zero is (7.512a) applies to the acoustic pressure perturbation spectrum (7.508d):

$$H_0^{(1,2)}(z) \sim \sqrt{\frac{2}{\pi z}}\, e^{\pm i(z+\pi/4)}\; ; \qquad H_1^{(1,2)}(z) \sim \pm i \sqrt{\frac{2}{\pi z}}\, e^{\pm i(z+\pi/4)}, \qquad (7.512\text{a, b})$$

substituting (7.510b) in (7.420b) leads to the acoustic velocity perturbation (7.510c), which proves by comparison with (7.509b) that the asymptotic approximation to the Hankel functions of order one is, to within a multiplying constant, given by (7.512b) bearing in mind (7.509a). The coincidence of (7.512b) ≡ (7.512c):

$$H_1^{(1,2)}(z) \sim \pm i z^{-1/2} \exp\left[\pm i \left(z + \frac{\pi}{4} \right) \right] = z^{-1/2} \exp\left[\pm i \left(z + \frac{3\pi}{4} \right) \right], \qquad (7.512\text{c, d})$$

confirms (7.512d) ≡ (7.505a, b). The constant factor $\sqrt{2/\pi}\, e^{\pm i\pi/4}$ was introduced in (7.505a) and (7.512a, b) in agreement with the usual definition of Hankel functions; the term $O\left(r^{-3/2} \right)$ was omitted because it is of higher order, and similar terms are missing from (7.510b), so both (7.510b, c) are valid only to $O\left(r^{-3/2} \right)$. A similar method applies to spherical waves (note 7.44) with the important difference that the asymptotic approximation turns out to be exact and valid at all radial distances (note 7.45).

NOTE 7.44: Spherical Waves in a Conical Duct

The case of a power law duct (7.497a) with exponent (7.513a) corresponds (problem 411) to the cross-sectional area (7.513b) and lengthscale (7.513c) of a cone (Figure 7.15c) containing **spherical waves** *due to a* **point source** *at the vertex:*

$$n = 2: \quad A_{11}(R) \sim R^2, \quad L_{11}(R) = \frac{2}{R}, \quad \tilde{p}_{11}^{\pm}(R;\omega) = B^{\pm}(\omega)\,(kR)^{-1/2}\, H_{1/2}^{(1,2)}(kR),$$

$$(7.513\text{a--d})$$

leading to the acoustic pressure (7.504) ≡ (7.513d) [velocity (7.507) ≡ (7.514)] perturbation spectrum:

$$\tilde{v}_{11}^{\pm}(R;\omega) = -\frac{ik}{\rho_0 \omega} \frac{d}{d(kR)}\left[B^{\pm}(\omega)(kR)^{-1/2}\, H_{1/2}^{(1,2)}(kR) \right]$$

$$(7.514)$$

$$= \frac{i}{\rho_0 c_s}\, B^{\pm}(\omega)\,(kR)^{-1/2}\, H_{3/2}^{(1,2)}(kR).$$

The ray approximation (7.499a, b) applies in the far field (7.510a) ≡ (7.515a) and leads to the acoustic pressure perturbation (7.432a) ≡ (7.475b):

$$R^2 \gg \frac{\lambda^2}{16\pi^2}: \qquad\qquad \tilde{p}_{11}^\pm(R;\omega) = B^\pm(\omega)\,\frac{1}{R}\,e^{\pm ikR}; \qquad\qquad (7.515a, b)$$

substitution of (7.515b) in (7.420b) leads:

$$\tilde{v}_{11}^\pm(R;\omega) = -\frac{i}{\rho_0\omega}\frac{d}{dR}\left[\frac{B^\pm(\omega)}{R}e^{\pm ikR}\right] = \pm\frac{B^\pm(\omega)}{\rho_0 c_s}\frac{1}{R}\left(1\pm\frac{i}{kR}\right)e^{\pm ikR}, \qquad (7.516)$$

to the acoustic velocity perturbation (7.516). Although (7.515b) was obtained as an asymptotic approximation valid in the far field, it is in fact an exact result valid for all distances, as will be shown in the sequel (note 7.45); for this reason, the differentiation (7.420b) with regard to R in the passage from (7.515b) to (7.516) is exact, including in terms of higher order $O\left(R^{-2}\right)$. It has been shown that *in (problem 412) a conical horn (Figure 7.15c) corresponding (7.513a) to the cross-sectional area (7.513b) and length scale (7.513c) propagate spherical waves generated by a point source at the vertex, with acoustic pressure (velocity) perturbation (7.515b) [(7.516)] that: (i) both involve a monopole term decaying like* $O\left(R^{-1}\right)$; *(ii) a dipole term* $O\left(R^{-2}\right)$ *appears only in (7.516).* It remains to prove that (7.515b) is an exact solution of the horn wave equation for the pressure with cross-section (7.513b), and hence the Hankel functions of half-integer order (7.513d) reduce to elementary functions (note 7.46).

NOTE 7.45: **Wave Equation in Cylindrical/Spherical Coordinates**

The horn wave equation for the acoustic pressure (7.392b) with constant sound speed (7.388b–d) in the case of cylindrical (7.508c) [spherical (7.513c)] waves becomes (7.517a) ≡ (7.517b) [(7.518a) ≡ (7.518b)]:

$$c_s^2 \frac{\partial^2 p}{\partial t^2} = \frac{\partial^2 p}{\partial r^2} + \frac{1}{r}\frac{\partial p}{\partial r} = \frac{1}{r}\frac{\partial}{\partial r}\left(r\frac{\partial p}{\partial r}\right), \qquad (7.517a, b)$$

$$c_s^2 \frac{\partial^2 p}{\partial t^2} = \frac{\partial^2 p}{\partial R^2} + \frac{2}{R}\frac{\partial p}{\partial R} = \frac{1}{R^2}\frac{\partial}{\partial R}\left(R^2\frac{\partial p}{\partial R}\right). \qquad (7.518a, b)$$

These coincide with the classical wave equation (7.519a) ≡ (7.496a) ≡ (7.496b), where the Laplace operator in cylindrical (III.6.45b) ≡ (7.519b) [spherical (III.6.46b) ≡ (7.519c)] coordinates:

$$c_s^2 \frac{\partial^2 p}{\partial t^2} = \nabla^2 p: \qquad\qquad \nabla^2 \equiv \frac{1}{r}\frac{\partial}{\partial r}\left(r\frac{\partial}{\partial r}\right) + \frac{1}{r^2}\frac{\partial^2}{\partial\phi^2} + \frac{\partial^2}{\partial z^2}, \qquad (7.519a, b)$$

$$\nabla \equiv \frac{1}{R^2}\frac{\partial}{\partial R}\left(R^2\frac{\partial}{\partial R}\right) + \frac{\csc\theta}{R^2}\frac{\partial}{\partial \theta}\left(\sin\theta\frac{\partial}{\partial \theta}\right) + \frac{\csc^2\theta}{R^2}\frac{\partial^2}{\partial\phi^2}, \qquad (7.519c)$$

depends only on the distance $r(R)$ from the axis (origin). From (7.517a) [(7.518a)] follows that the acoustic pressure perturbation spectrum (7.412a) of a wave of frequency ω satisfies (7.480a) [(7.480b)]:

$$-\frac{\omega^2}{c_s^2}\tilde{p} = \frac{d^2\tilde{p}}{dr^2} + \frac{1}{r}\frac{d\tilde{p}}{dr}, \quad \frac{d^2\tilde{p}}{dR^2} + \frac{2}{R}\frac{d\tilde{p}}{dR}, \qquad (7.520a, b)$$

in agreement with (7.392a) for the lengthscale (7.508c) [(7.513c)] for cylindrical (spherical) waves. The radial dependence of cylindrical waves (7.520a) corresponds to a Bessel differential equation (7.498b) of order zero $m = 0$ leading to (7.508d). In the case of spherical waves (7.520b) instead of transforming to a Bessel differential equation, the elementary solution (7.515b) is obtained next (note 7.46).

NOTE 7.46: Ray Approximation and Asymptomatic Exact Waves

The acoustic pressure perturbation for spherical waves satisfies (7.518b) = (7.521b):

$$c_s^2\frac{\partial^2}{\partial t^2}\big[Rp(R,t)\big] = \left(R\frac{\partial^2}{\partial R^2} + 2\frac{\partial}{\partial R}\right)p(R,t) = \frac{\partial^2}{\partial R^2}\big[Rp(R,t)\big]. \qquad (7.521a, b)$$

Since (7.521b) ≡ (7.398b) is a plane wave equation for $Rp(R,t)$, it has solutions (7.424a) ≡ (7.522):

$$Rp(R,t) = B^{\pm}\exp(-i\omega t \pm ikR), \qquad (7.522)$$

whose spatial part coincides with (7.522) ≡ (7.515b), from which follows (7.516). Thus, (7.515b; 7.516), which were obtained in the ray approximation in the far field (7.515a), are actually exactly valid at all distances unlike in the cylindrical case (7.510a–c). The reason is that a spherical wave is due to a point source (Figure 7.15c), whereas a cylindrical wave is due to a uniform distribution of sources along a straight line (Figure 7.15b). The comparison of (7.513d) = (7.515b) shows that the Hankel function of order one-half scale is like an imaginary exponential divided by the variable:

$$H^{(1,2)}_{1/2}(z) = z^{-1}\exp(\pm iz). \qquad (7.523)$$

The properties of Hankel functions, which have been mentioned (7.505a, b; 7.506; 7.523), are usually established mathematically (section 9.7), and their relation with waves in inhomogeneous media has been highlighted here. The horn wave equation is of the second-order allowing waves propagating in opposite directions, for example, due to reflection at an impedance wall (note 7.47), which may also involve surface adsorption (note 7.48).

NOTE 7.47: Rigid and Impedance and Impedance Boundary Conditions

Consider (Figure 7.16) a wave of unit amplitude propagating in the positive x-direction (7.524a) that hits a wall at $x = 0$, and is reflected as a wave propagating in the negative x-direction (7.524b) whose amplitude is the **reflection coefficient** R:

$$\tilde{p}_I(x;\omega) = e^{ikx}, \tilde{p}_R(x;\omega) = Re^{-ikx}: \quad \tilde{p}(x;\omega) = \tilde{p}_I(x;\omega) + \tilde{p}_R(x;\omega) = e^{ikx} + Re^{-ikx},$$
(7.524a–c)

leading to the total pressure field (7.524c); in (7.524a–c) the factor $e^{-i\omega t}$ that is common to all terms has been omitted, because the frequency ω is conserved, and only the spatial dependence is of interest. In order to determine the reflection coefficient, it is necessary to have a **wall boundary condition** applied at $x = 0$. A **locally reacting or impedance wall** corresponds, as in chapter I.4, to proportional acoustic pressure and velocity perturbation spectra (7.525a), where the **impedance** may depend on frequency:

$$\tilde{p}(0;\omega) = Z(\omega)\tilde{v}(0;\omega); \quad \tilde{v}(0;\omega) = 0 \neq \tilde{p}(0;\omega): \quad Z = \infty;$$
$$\tilde{v}(0;\omega) \neq 0 = \tilde{p}(0;\omega): \quad Z = 0,$$
(7.525a–d)

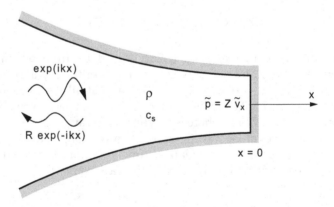

FIGURE 7.16
A sound wave in a horn incident on an impedance wall is partly reflected and partly adsorbed at the surface. Only in the extreme case of infinite impedance, corresponding to a rigid wall, is there total reflection and no surface adsorption.

a **rigid wall**, where the velocity is zero (7.525b), and the pressure is not (7.525c), corresponds to infinite impedance (7.525d); conversely, at a **pressure release interface** the impedance is zero (7.325f), allowing a non-zero velocity with zero pressure (7.325e).

Using the relation (7.420b) ≡ (7.526a) between acoustic velocity and pressure perturbation spectra leads to the **impedance boundary condition** (7.525a) ≡ (7.526b) = (7.526c):

$$\tilde{v}(x;\omega) = -\frac{i}{\rho_0\,\omega}\frac{d\tilde{p}(x;\omega)}{dx}: \quad 0 = \tilde{p}(0;\omega) - Z(\omega)\tilde{v}(0;\omega) = \tilde{p}(0;\omega) + \frac{iZ(\omega)}{\rho_0\,\omega}\tilde{p}'(0;\omega).$$

$$(7.526a\text{--}c)$$

Comparing (7.525a) with the relation (7.526b) between the pressure and the velocity perturbation spectra (7.527b) of a plane wave (7.527a):

$$\tilde{p}(0;\omega) = Be^{ikx}: \quad \tilde{v}(x;\omega) = -\frac{i}{\rho_0\,\omega}(ik)\tilde{p}(x;\omega) = \frac{k}{\rho_0\,\omega}\tilde{p}(x;\omega)$$

$$= \frac{\tilde{p}(x;\omega)}{\rho_0\,c_s}, \quad Z_0 = \rho_0\,c_s,$$

$$(7.527a\text{--}c)$$

shows *that (problem 413) the impedance (7.527c) of a plane wave (7.527a) is the product of the mass density by the sound speed. The specific impedance, defined (7.528a) as the ratio of the impedance to that (7.527c) of a plane wave:*

$$z(\omega) \equiv \frac{Z(\omega)}{\rho_0 c_s}: \quad 0 = \tilde{p}(0;\omega) + \frac{ic_s}{\omega}z(\omega)\tilde{p}'(0;\omega), \qquad (7.528a, b)$$

appears in (problem 414) the impedance boundary condition (7.485a) ≡ (7.528b).

NOTE 7.48: **Wave Reflection and Surface Adsorption at an Impedance Wall**

The spatial derivative of the total (7.524c), which is incident (7.524a) plus reflected (7.524b), pressure perturbation spectrum is (7.529):

$$\tilde{p}'(x;\omega) = ik\left(e^{ikx} - Re^{-ikx}\right). \tag{7.529}$$

Substituting (7.524c; 7.529) in the impedance boundary condition (7.528b) leads to (7.530a), specifying: (i) the reflection coefficient (7.530b):

$$1 + R = -\frac{ic_s z}{\omega}ik(1-R) = z(1-R); \quad R = \frac{z-1}{z+1}, \quad S \equiv 1 - R = \frac{2}{z+1},$$

$$(7.530a\text{--}d)$$

(ii) also to the **surface adsorption coefficient** (7.530d), which is defined as the difference (7.530c) between the unit amplitude of the incident wave (7.524a) and the amplitude R of the reflected wave (7.524b). The simplest case is a rigid wall (7.525d) ≡ (7.531a) for which there is **total reflection** (7.531b) and no adsorption (7.531c):

$$z = \infty: \qquad R = 1, \quad S = 0, \quad e^{-ikx}\,\tilde{p}_I(x;\omega) = 1 = e^{ikx}\,\tilde{p}_R(x;\omega), \qquad (7.531\text{a–d})$$

because the incident and reflected waves (7.524a, b) have the same amplitude and opposite phases (7.531d).

In general, the impedance Z is complex (7.532a) with the **reactance (inductance)** as the real X (imaginary Y) part, leading to reflection (7.532b) [absorption (7.532c)] coefficients:

$$z = X + iY: \qquad R = \frac{X - 1 + iY}{X + 1 + iY}, \qquad S = \frac{2}{X + 1 + iY}, \qquad (7.532\text{a–c})$$

which are also complex (7.533a, c) [(7.534a, b)]:

$$R = \frac{(X - 1 + iY)(X + 1 - iY)}{(X + 1 + iY)(X + 1 - iY)} = \frac{X^2 + Y^2 - 1 + 2iY}{(X + 1)^2 + Y^2} = |R|\,e^{i\phi}, \qquad (7.533\text{a–c})$$

$$S = \frac{2X + 2 - 2iY}{(X + 1)^2 + Y^2} = |S|\,e^{i\phi}, \qquad (7.534\text{a, b})$$

implying changes of amplitude (7.535a) [(7.535b)] and phase (7.535c) [7.535d)]:

$$\{|R|, |S|\} = \frac{\left\{(X - 1)^2 + Y^2, 4\right\}}{(X + 1)^2 + Y^2}, \qquad \tan\{\phi, \psi\} = \left\{\frac{2Y}{X^2 + Y^2 - 1}, -\frac{Y}{X + 1}\right\}. \qquad (7.535\text{a–d})$$

It has been shown that (problem 415) *the reflection of a plane wave (7.524a–c) at wall (7.528b) with specific impedance (7.528a) leads to complex reflection (7.532b) [surface adsorption (7.532c)] coefficients, whose amplitude (7.535a) [(7.535b)] and phase (7.535c) [(7.535d)] depend on the reactance X and inductance Y. In the case (7.531d) of a rigid wall (7.531a), there is total reflection (7.531b) and no surface adsorption (7.531c).* If two impedance walls are present, standing modes form between them (note 7.49) that may have volume absorption (note 7.50) in addition to surface adsorption.

NOTE 7.49: Standing Modes between Impedance Walls

Suppose that in addition (7.528b) ≡ (7.536a), the wall (Figure 7.16) at $x = 0$ with specific impedance z_1, there is also (7.536b) another wall (Figure 7.17) at $x = a$ with specific impedance z_2:

$$\tilde{p}(0;\omega) + \frac{ic_s}{\omega} z_1 \tilde{p}'(0;\omega) = 0 = \tilde{p}(a;\omega) + i\frac{c_s}{\omega} z_2 \tilde{p}'(a;\omega). \qquad (7.536a, b)$$

The reflection coefficient in the total acoustic pressure perturbation (7.524a–c) satisfies two relations, namely, (7.537a) ≡ (7.530b) [(7.537b)] arising from the first (7.536a) [second (7.536b)] impedance wall boundary condition:

$$1 + R = z_1(1 - R), \qquad e^{ika} + Re^{-ika} = z_2\left(e^{ika} - Re^{-ika}\right). \qquad (7.537a, b)$$

The reflection coefficient, (7.538a) ≡ (7.530c) [(7.538b)], specified by (7.537a) [(7.537b)]:

$$\frac{z_1 - 1}{z_1 + 1} = R = \frac{z_2 - 1}{z_2 + 1}e^{2ika}: \qquad (z_1 - 1)(z_2 + 1) = e^{2ika}(z_2 - 1)(z_1 + 1), \qquad (7.538a–c)$$

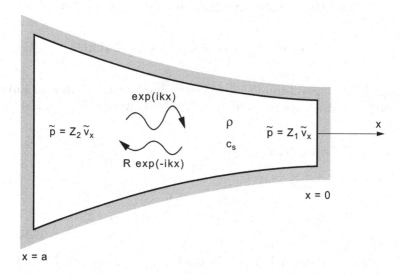

FIGURE 7.17
An acoustic horn blocked by two walls with possibly different impedances leads by double reflection (Figure 7.16) to standing modes trapped between the two walls. If the walls are rigid, the natural modes are the same as for an elastic string (Figure 7.8a) fixed at two ends (Figure 7.17). In the case of one or two impedance walls as reflectors: (i) there is no total reflection, so the reflection coefficient need not be unity and may include a phase change; (ii) the natural wavenumbers are complex with the real (imaginary) part specifying the wavelength (amplification or attenuation in the axial direction) of the normal modes.

must be the same, leading to (7.538c), whose roots specify the wavenumbers of the standing modes. In the case of two rigid walls (7.539a, b), the wavenumbers of standing modes satisfy (7.538c), which reduces to (7.539c):

$$z_1 = \infty = z_2: \quad \exp(2ika) = 1 = \exp(2i\pi n); \quad k_n = \frac{\pi n}{a}, \quad \lambda_n = \frac{2\pi}{k_n} = \frac{2a}{n}. \quad (7.539\text{a–e})$$

the wavenumbers (7.539d) correspond to wavelengths, (7.539e) $\equiv$ (6.818a), of standing modes between rigid walls at a distance a. In the general case of one or two impedance walls, the wavenumbers of normal modes are complex (note 7.50) leading to wave amplification or attenuation in addition to surface adsorption as for the reflection, transmission, and absorption/adsorption of light in a lens (chapter I.22).

NOTE 7.50: **Amplification or Attenuation of Normal Modes**

In the general case of one or two impedance walls, the wavenumber is complex (7.540a):

$$k = \alpha + i\beta: \qquad \exp(i2ka) = \exp(i2a\alpha)\exp(-2\beta a), \qquad (7.540\text{a, b})$$

so (7.540b) that: (i) the real part specifies the wavelength (7.539d) $\equiv$ (7.540a):

$$\lambda = \frac{2\pi}{\alpha} = \frac{2\pi}{\mathrm{Re}(k)}: \quad \left|\exp(i2ka)\right| = \exp(-2\beta a) = \exp\left[-2a\,\mathrm{Im}(k)\right]; \quad (7.541\text{a, b})$$

(ii) the imaginary part leads (7.541b) to **wave amplification (attenuation)** if it is negative (positive). The amplification (7.540b) is given (7.538c) by (7.542a–d):

$$\exp(-2\beta a) = \left|\exp(i2ka)\right| = \frac{|z_1 - 1||z_2 + 1|}{|z_1 + 1||z_2 - 1|} = \frac{|X_1 - 1 + iY_1||X_2 + 1 + iY_2|}{|X_1 + 1 + iY_1||X_2 - 1 + iY_2|}$$

$$= \left|\frac{(X_1 - 1)^2 + Y_1^2}{(X_1 + 1)^2 + Y_1^2} \frac{(X_2 + 1)^2 + Y_2^2}{(X_2 - 1)^2 + Y_2^2}\right|^{1/2}.$$

$$(7.542\text{a–d})$$

The wavelength of normal modes (7.541a) is given (7.538c) by (7.543a–c):

$$2a\alpha = \frac{4\pi a}{\lambda} = \arg(z_1 - 1) + \arg(z_2 + 1) - \arg(z_1 + 1) - \arg(z_2 - 1)$$

$$= arc\tan\left(\frac{Y_1}{X_1 - 1}\right) + \arg\tan\left(\frac{Y_2}{X_2 + 1}\right) - arc\tan\left(\frac{Y_1}{X_1 + 1}\right) - arc\tan\left(\frac{Y_2}{X_2 - 1}\right),$$

$$(7.543\text{a–c})$$

completing the specification of the complex wavenumber (7.540a). It has been shown that *plane waves (7.524a–c) reflected between walls at $x = 0 (x = a)$ with (7.536a) [(7.536b)] impedances $z_1 (z_2)$ lead to (problem 416) standing modes with complex wavenumbers (7.538c) whose (7.540a, b): (i) real part (7.543a–c) specifies the wavelength (7.541a); (ii) the imaginary part (7.542a–d) determines (7.541b) the amplification (attenuation) if it is negative (positive). The reflection (surface adsorption) coeffcient (7.538a) [(7.530d)] can be calculated in terms of the first impedance z_1, as in (7.533a–c; 7.535a, c) [(7.534a, b; 7.535b, d)].* The opposite case to the ray approximation (notes 7.25–7.27) is the scattering limit (note 7.51), when the wavelength is much larger than the lengthscale of variation of the cross-section, so that area changes are abrupt, as the matching of ducts with different cross-sections.

NOTE 7.51: Incident, Reflected, and Transmitted Waves

Consider two ducts (Figure 7.18) with different cross-sectional areas $A_1 (A_2)$ containing fluids with different mass densities $\rho_1 (\rho_2)$ and sound speeds $c_1 (c_2)$. An incident wave (7.544b) with unit amplitude and wavenumber

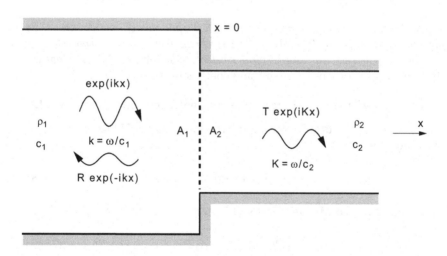

FIGURE 7.18
The opposite limits of sound wave diffraction in a horn (Figures 7.11–7.15) are the ray (scattering) approximation for high (low) frequency or short (long) wavelength [Figures 5.24–5.25 (7.16–7.19)]. An example of scattering is sound reflection and transmission at (Figure 7.18), which is the junction of two tubes such that: (i) the change of cross-sectional area is abrupt on a wavelength scale, and appears as a discontinuity between the area A_1 before the junction and A_2 after the junction; (ii) the fluid may have before (after) the junction different mass densities $\rho_1 (\rho_2)$ and sound speeds $c_1 (c_2)$. The reflection (transmission) coefficient is larger (smaller) if the change is: (i) from a larger A_1 to a smaller $A_2 < A_1$ area; (ii) from a medium with small $\rho_1 c_1$ to a larger $\rho_2 c_2 > \rho_1 c_1$ plane wave impedance.

(7.544a) gives rise to: (i) a reflected wave (7.544c) with the same wavenumber (7.544a) whose amplitude is the reflection coefficient R:

$$k = \frac{\omega}{c_1}: \qquad \tilde{p}_I(x;\omega) = e^{ikx}, \qquad \tilde{p}_R(x;\omega) = R e^{-ikx}, \qquad \text{(7.544a, b)}$$

$$K = \frac{\omega}{c_2}: \qquad\qquad \tilde{p}_T(x;\omega) = T e^{iKx}, \qquad\qquad \text{(7.545a–c)}$$

(ii) a transmitted wave (7.545b) with wavenumber (7.545a), whose amplitude is the transmission coefficient T. At the junction (7.546a) the: (i) pressures must balance (7.546b); (ii) the flow rate, which equals the area multiplied by the velocity, must also balance (7.546c):

$$x = 0: \quad p_I(0;\omega) + \tilde{p}_R(0;\omega) = \tilde{p}_T(0;\omega), \quad A_1\left[\tilde{v}_I(0;\omega) - \tilde{v}_R(0;\omega)\right] = A_2\, \tilde{v}_T(0;\omega).$$
$$\text{(7.546a–c)}$$

The relation between the acoustic pressure and the velocity perturbation spectra (7.527b) substituted in (7.546c) leads to (7.547):

$$\rho_2\, c_2\, A_1\left[\tilde{p}_I(0;\omega) - \tilde{p}_R(0;\omega)\right] = \rho_1\, c_1\, A_2\, \tilde{p}_T(0;\omega). \qquad \text{(7.547)}$$

Thus, *the two acoustic matching conditions at the junction of the two tubes (7.546a) may be expressed (problem 417) alternatively in terms of the acoustic pressure (7.546b) and the velocity (7.546c) [or derivative of the pressure (7.547)], leading to the same reflection and transmission coefficients (note 7.52).*

NOTE 7.52: **Reflection and Transmission Coefficients at a Junction of Ducts**

At a junction of ducts substituting the three elements (7.544b, c; 7.545b) of the total pressure:

$$\tilde{p}(x;\omega) = p_I(x;\omega) + p_R(x;\omega) + p_T(x;\omega) = e^{ikx} + R e^{-ikx} + T e^{iKx}, \qquad \text{(7.548a, b)}$$

in the **matching conditions** (7.546b) [(7.547)] leads to (7.549a) [(7.549b)]:

$$1 + R = T, \qquad \rho_2\, c_2\, A_1(1-R) = \rho_1\, c_1\, A_2\, T = \rho_1\, c_1\, A_2(1+R), \qquad \text{(7.549a–c)}$$

which implies (7.549c). From (7.549c) [(7.549a)] follow the reflection (7.550b) [transmission (7.550c)] coefficients:

$$\tilde{Z} = \frac{\rho_2 c_2 A_1}{\rho_1 c_1 A_2}: \qquad R = \frac{\tilde{Z}-1}{\tilde{Z}+1}, \qquad T = \frac{2\tilde{Z}}{\tilde{Z}+1}, \qquad \text{(7.550a–c)}$$

in terms of the **overall impedance** (7.550a). It has been shown that *a plane wave with unit amplitude incident (7.544a, b) at the junction of two ducts (Figure 7.18)* *gives rise (problem 418) to reflected (7.544a, c) [transmitted (7.545a, b)] waves whose amplitudes are the reflection (7.550b) [transmission (7.550c)] coefficients. Both are determined by the overall impedance (7.550a) ≡ (7.551c):*

$$\bar{Z}_{01} = \rho_1 c_1, \qquad \bar{Z}_{02} = \rho_2 c_2: \qquad \qquad \tilde{Z} = \frac{A_1}{A_2} \frac{\bar{Z}_{02}}{\bar{Z}_{01}}, \qquad (7.551\text{a–c})$$

which is given by: (i) the ratio of the cross-sectional areas of the ducts of incidence A_1 (transmission A_2); (ii) multiplied by the ratio of plane wave impedances (7.527c) of media of transmission (7.551b) to that of incidence (7.551a). The reflection and transmission coefficients (note 7.52) can be used to determine the scattering matrix (note 7.53), which specifies the linear relation between the pairs of acoustic waves propagating towards and away from the abrupt change of cross-section on the two sides.

NOTE 7.53: Scattering Matrix for an Abrupt Change of Cross-Section

Consider an abrupt change of cross-section in a duct (Figure 7.19); the acoustic pressure perturbation spectra of waves propagating in the positive (negative) x-direction in the first $p_1^+ \left(p_1^- \right)$ and second $p_2^+ \left(p_2^- \right)$ ducts, are related linearly through the **scattering matrix** (7.552a):

$$\begin{bmatrix} p_1^- \\ p_2^+ \end{bmatrix} = \begin{bmatrix} R^+ & T^- \\ T^+ & R^- \end{bmatrix} \begin{bmatrix} p_1^+ \\ p_2^- \end{bmatrix} = \begin{bmatrix} S_{11} & S_{12} \\ S_{21} & S_{22} \end{bmatrix} \begin{bmatrix} p_1^+ \\ p_2^- \end{bmatrix}, \qquad (7.552\text{a, b})$$

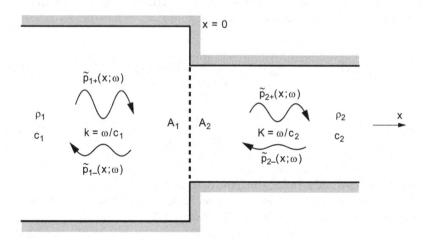

FIGURE 7.19
Considering pairs of sound waves propagating in the positive (negative) x-direction in the first $p_1^+ \left(p_1^- \right)$ and second $p_2^+ \left(p_2^- \right)$ ducts, the corresponding acoustic pressure perturbation spectra are related by a scattering matrix, consisting of a pair of reflection and transmission coefficients with inverse impedances.

whose components (7.552b) may be interpreted as follows: (i) a wave propagating in the first duct in the positive direction towards the junction p_1^+ gives rise by reflection R^+ (transmission T^+) to two waves propagating in the first (second) duct away from the junction in the negative (positive) x-direction p_2^- (p_2^+); (ii) a wave propagating in the second duct in the negative x-direction towards the junction p_2^- gives rise by transmission T^- (reflection R^-) to two waves propagating in the first (second) duct away from the junction in the negative (positive) x-direction p_1^- (p_2^+).

From (i) and (ii) it follows that all four components of the scattering matrix (7.552b) can be determined by considering separately a wave incident on the junction from each side. In the case (i) of a wave incident on the junction from the first duct (7.544b) the reflected (7.544c) [transmitted (7.545b)] waves specify two components (7.553a) [(7.553b)] of the scattering matrix:

$$S_{11} = R^+ = \frac{\tilde{p}_R(x;\omega)}{\tilde{P}_I(x;\omega)} = R e^{-i2Kx} = \frac{\rho_2 c_2 A_1 - \rho_1 c_1 A_2}{\rho_2 c_2 A_1 + \rho_1 c_1 A_2} e^{-i2kx}, \qquad (7.553a)$$

$$S_{21} = T^+ = \frac{\tilde{p}_T(x;\omega)}{\tilde{P}_I(x;\omega)} = T e^{i(K-k)x} = \frac{2\,\rho_2\,c_2 A_1}{\rho_2 c_2 A_1 + \rho_1 c_1 A_2} e^{i(K-k)x}, \qquad (7.553b)$$

where (7.550a–c) were used. The first column of the scattering matrix (7.551b) is given by (7.553a, b) and the second column is similar (7.554b, d) with: (i) interchange of the indices (7.554a) for the ducts; (ii) reversal of the wavenumbers and directions of propagation (7.513c):

$$(1,2) \quad \leftrightarrow \quad (2,1): \qquad S_{12} = T^- = \frac{2\,\rho_1 c_1 A_2}{\rho_1 c_1 A_2 + \rho_2 c_2 A_1} e^{i(K-k)x}, \qquad (7.554a, b)$$

$$(k,K) \quad \leftrightarrow \quad \{-K,-k\}: \qquad S_{22} = R^- = \frac{\rho_1 c_1 A_2 - \rho_2 c_2 A_1}{\rho_1 c_1 A_2 + \rho_2 c_2 A_1} e^{i2Kx}. \qquad (7.554c, d)$$

This completes (7.553a, b; 7.554b, d) the determination of the scattering matrix (7.552b), which consists of two reflection functions (7.553a; 7.554d) and two transmission functions (7.553b; 7.554b) (note 7.54).

NOTE 7.54: **Pairs of Reflection and Transmission Functions**

It has been shown that (problem 419) *the acoustic pressure perturbation of sound waves propagating in the positive (negative) direction before p_1^+ (p_1^-) and after p_1^+ (p_1^-)*

*an abrupt change of cross-section of a duct (Figure 7.19) are related linearly (7.552b)
by the scattering matrix (7.553a, b; 7.554b, d) ≡ (7.555):*

$$
S_{ij} = \begin{bmatrix} \dfrac{\rho_2 c_2 A_1 - \rho_1 c_1 A_2}{\rho_1 c_1 A_2 + \rho_2 c_2 A_2} e^{-i2kx} & \dfrac{2\rho_1 c_1 A_2}{\rho_1 c_1 A_2 + \rho_2 c_2 A_2} e^{i(K-k)x} \\ \dfrac{2\rho_2 c_2 A_1}{\rho_1 c_1 A_2 + \rho_2 c_2 A_2} e^{i(K-k)x} & \dfrac{\rho_1 c_1 A_1 - \rho_2 c_2 A_1}{\rho_1 c_1 A_2 + \rho_2 c_2 A_1} e^{i2Kx} \end{bmatrix},
\tag{7.555}
$$

*which consists of two pairs of **reflection and transmission functions** (7.552a) ≡
(7.556):*

$$
\begin{bmatrix} R^+ & T^- \\ T^+ & R^- \end{bmatrix} = \frac{1}{\tilde{Z}+1} \begin{bmatrix} (\tilde{Z}-1) e^{-2ikx} & 2 e^{i(K-k)x} \\ 2\tilde{Z} \, e^{i(K-k)x} & (1-\tilde{Z}) e^{i2Kx} \end{bmatrix},
\tag{7.556}
$$

*involving the (7.550a–c) and the wavenumbers in the first (7.544a) [second (7.545a)]
duct before (after) the junction. The constant coefficients in the second column of the
scattering matrix (7.556) are obtained from the first column (7.557b, c) by using the
inverse of the impedance (7.557a):*

$$
\tilde{Z} \to \frac{1}{\tilde{Z}}: \quad |S_{11}| = |R^+| = \frac{\tilde{Z}-1}{\tilde{Z}+1} \to |S_{22}| = |R^-| = \frac{\frac{1}{\tilde{Z}}-1}{\frac{1}{\tilde{Z}}+1} = \frac{1-\tilde{Z}}{1+\tilde{Z}},
\tag{7.557a, b}
$$

$$
|S_{21}| = |T^+| = \frac{2\tilde{Z}}{\tilde{Z}+1} \to |S_{12}| = |T^-| = \frac{\frac{2}{\tilde{Z}}}{\frac{1}{\tilde{Z}}+1} = \frac{2}{1+\tilde{Z}},
\tag{7.557c}
$$

because the ducts are interchanged relative to the direction of wave incidence.

NOTE 7.55: Wave Refraction: Ray, Scattering, and Diffraction

The simplest case I (Diagram 7.3, see page 128) of linear waves is for a steady
homogeneous medium for which: (I-i) all wave variables satisfy the same
wave equation that is a linear partial differential equation in space-time with
constant coefficients; (a-2) sinusoidal waves exist in space (time) with wavenumber (frequency) related by an algebraic dispersion relation. In the case
II (III) of linear waves in a steady inhomogeneous (unsteady homogeneous)
medium: (II, III-i) different wave variables satisfy different wave equations
that are linear partial differential equations whose coefficients depend on

position (time) but not on time (position); (II, III-ii) sinusoidal waves exist in time (space) with constant frequency (wavenumber), but there is no wavenumber (frequency) because the waves are not sinusoidal in space (time). In the case IV of linear waves in unsteady inhomogeneous media: (IV-i) the wave equation is a linear partial differential equation with coefficients depending on position and time; (IV-ii) there is neither frequency (nor wavenumber) because sinusoidal waves do not exist either in time (or in space).

Focusing on the case II of linear waves in steady inhomogeneous medium there is **refraction**, that is, the waves change in amplitude as they propagate (II-a, b). The two opposite limits of refraction are high (low) frequency waves, when the wavelength is small (large) compared with the lengths-cale of variation of properties of the medium leading to **geometrical rays (scattering)** with wavelength varying slowly (abruptly) along a ray path (when crossing the scatterer); (II-c) for intermediate frequencies, such that the wavelength is comparable to the lengthscales of variation of properties of the medium, the waves are not sinusoidal, no wavelength exists, and the **diffraction** is specified by exact solutions of the wave equation. *The classification of refraction* (problem 420) *into rays/diffraction/scattering at respectively high/intermediate/low frequencies applies to short/comparable/long wavelengths relative to: (i) the lengthscale of variation of proportion of properties of an inhomogeneous medium; (ii) the size of a rigid or impedance obstacle present in the otherwise free-wave field.* The oscillators (waves) differ in depending only on time (also in position) leading to ordinary (partial) differential equations, that is, with one (more than one) independent variable. Concerning the dependent variables, waves can have several, for example, the acoustic pressure and velocity perturbations for sound. Likewise, the oscillators with one (several) **degrees-of-freedom** [chapters 2 and 4 (8)] have one (more) dependent variables, leading to single (simultaneous systems) of ordinary differential equations [chapters 1, 3, and 5 (7)].

Conclusion 7

The family of curves (Figure 7.1) tangent to vector field $\vec{X}$, may be specified by the intersection of two families of surfaces (Figure 7.2); the two parameters C_1, C_2 specify one curve through each point in three-dimensional space. For example, the radial vector fields specify all straight lines through the origin (Figure 7.3), which can be obtained as the intersections of two families of planes passing through two distinct coordinate axis. Another example is a vector field tangent to a family of parabolas (Figure 7.4), which can be obtained by the intersection of a family of parabolic cylinders by a family of planes oblique relative to the generators. Unlike the problem of finding the curves tangent to a vector field, which always has a solution, the problem of finding a family of orthogonal surfaces (Figure 7.6) has a solution if the vector field has zero helicity. If the vector field has non-zero helicity, then (Figure 7.7) on each arbitrary family of surfaces lies a family of curves orthogonal to the vector field. The set of families of curves, for all possible surfaces (Figure 7.7), forms a normal surface (Figure 7.6), if vector field has zero helicity. The existence of a normal surface depends on: (i) either the conditions immediate integrability for the vector field; (ii) or on the existence of a parallel vector field obtained by multiplication by an integrating factor that satisfies the conditions of immediate integrability. The proof of the sufficiency of the condition of immediate integrability uses Stokes theorem (Figure 7.5) for a regular surface D with area element supported on a closed loop ∂D with tangential displacement dx_n; if the surface D is regular, that is, has continuous normal bivector, the boundary curve ∂D is regular and has continuous tangent vector (Figure 7.5).

The family of curves tangent to a vector field (Figures 7.1–7.4) is the solution of an autonomous system of ordinary differential equations. A single (simultaneous system of) ordinary differential equation(s) is reducible to an autonomous system. Analogies between the solution of a single (a simultaneous system of) ordinary differential equation(s) exist, for example, (Table 7.1) in the cases for which a characteristic polynomial (a matrix of polynomials), namely constant and homogeneous coefficients; a characteristic polynomial (matrix of polynomials) also exists for a single (simultaneous system of) finite difference equation(s). The ordinary (partial) differential equations (Table 7.2) have one (more than one) independent variable(s) (Diagram 7.2) and can (Diagram 7.3) represent oscillators (waves). An example of this relation is the case of one-dimensional linear waves in steady inhomogeneous media: (i) that are described by linear partial differential equations in space-time; (ii) since the medium is steady, the coefficients do not depend on time and a Fourier representation exists, corresponding to sinusoidal waves in time whose frequency is conserved; (iii) this leads to an ordinary differential equation in the remaining variable, namely, the position, as a spatial oscillator, whose coefficients are non-uniform if the medium is inhomogeneous. The differential equations can be combined (Diagram 7.2) with other types of equations (Diagram 7.1). The acoustics of horns (Diagram 7.4 and Table 7.5) is one example of quasi-one-dimensional propagation (Table 7.3) in inhomogeneous media (Table 7.4, see page 129).

Six analogous cases of quasi-one-dimensional waves in inhomogeneous media (Tables 7.2 and 7.3) are given: (i) transverse vibrations of an elastic string (Figure 7.8a); (ii)(iiii) longitudinal (torsional) vibrations of an elastic rod [Figure 7.8b(c)]; (iv)(v) hydraulic or water (electromagnetic) waves [Figures 7.8d and 7.9 (7.8e and 7.10)] along a channel (waveguide); (vi) sound waves in a horn, which is a duct of varying cross-section (Figure 7.8f). Considering in more detail (Table 7.4 and Diagram 7.2) the acoustics of horns, the refraction effects of the inhomogeneous medium on waves can be considered over the whole frequency range by means of three approaches: (I)(II) rays (scattering) at high (low) frequency; (III) diffraction at intermediate frequencies. High-frequency for (I) rays means that the wavelength is small compared with the lengthscale of variation of the cross-sectional section of the horn; the waves remain sinusoidal in space, and since reflection from the walls is negligible (Figure 7.11) the amplitude is smaller (larger) in wider (narrower) sections. The low frequencies correspond to the opposite limit of (II); scattering the wavelength is large compared with the lengthscale, and the changes in cross-section are abrupt, for example, in the reflection and transmission of sound at the junction of two ducts (Figures 7.18–7.19). Sound reflection and surface adsorption can occur at an impedance wall (Figure 7.16); between two impedance walls exist standing modes (Figure 7.17), which may be spatially amplified or attenuated. At intermediate frequencies, neither the ray (I) nor the scattering (II) approximations hold, because the lengthscale of variation of the properties of the medium comparable to the wavelength, and the waves are not sinusoidal in general; exact solutions of the appropriate wave equation are needed in diffraction theory. In the case of the horn wave equation, exact solution in terms of elementary functions exist in five cases: (III.i) three cases are the exponential convergent or divergent, the catenoidal and inverse catenoidal horns, (respectively in Figures 7.12a–d) for which there is (Figure 7.13) a filtering function, excluding propagation below a cut-off frequency; (III.ii) two cases are the sinusoidal (inverse sinusoidal) horns [Figure 7.12 e(f)], for which there is a transparency function allowing the propagation of all frequencies. For all other duct shapes, the exact solutions of the horn waves equations involve (III.iii) special functions, for example, Hermite polynomials (Bessel functions) for Gaussian (power law) horns [Figure 7.14 (7.15)]. The two most important particular cases of power law horns (Figure 7.15a) are cylindrical (spherical) waves [Figure 7.15b(c)] in a wedge (cone) due to a line (point) source at the edge (vertex).

8

Oscillations with Several Degrees-of-Freedom

The theory of oscillators, amplifiers, and deformations involves (chapter 2) a linear second-order system with or without damping and forcing with one degree-of-freedom. It can be generalized in four directions: (i) non-linear oscillations (chapter 4), associated with non-linear restoring or damping forces; (ii) higher-order systems, such as fourth-order, for example, (chapter 6) the transverse deflection of one (two) dimensional elastic bodies with bending stiffness, including bars (plates); (iii) systems with several degrees-of-freedom, such as multidimensional oscillators (chapter 8) with inertia, damping, resilience, and forcing; (iv) systems with several independent variables, leading to partial differential equations (notes 7.1 to 7.55 and 8.1 to 8.17), such as waves depending on position (x) and time (t), or deformations depending on several spatial coordinates. A case has already been presented involving all four (i) to (iv) features: the strong bending and stretching of a plate (section 6.9) involves two fourth-order partial differential equations depending on two spatial coordinates coupling non-linearly the transverse deflection and the stress function. The present section concerns second-order linear oscillators with or without damping and forcing (sections 8.1–8.2) in two dimensions first (sections 8.3–8.6), then N-dimensional chains (sections 8.7–8.8) and transmission lines (section 8.9) with infinite dimension.

The vibrations with small amplitude of a one-dimensional oscillator are (chapter 2) an example of the solution of a linear ordinary differential equation (chapter 1) in the cases of free or forced oscillations. Very often, vibrating systems have more than one degree-of-freedom, for example, rigid bodies supported on springs and dampers, or associations of quasi-stationary electrical circuits; in most cases, these degrees-of-freedom interact (chapter 8) and the multidimensional oscillator is described by a set of simultaneous ordinary differential equations (chapter 7). An oscillator with N degrees-of-freedom (chapter 8.1) has N modal frequencies, and each degree-of-freedom generally consists of a linear superposition of oscillations at all these frequencies (chapter 8.2). It is possible to find a linear combination of the original degrees-of-freedom, which eliminates all modal frequencies but one; thus, a set of modal coordinates exist, each oscillating at one modal frequency, and leading to one of a set of N decoupled ordinary differential equations (chapter 8.2). The modal coordinates are found *a posteriori* after solving the oscillator problem, and they occur *a priori* only for decoupled systems. If an N-dimensional oscillator is forced at an externally applied frequency, it will oscillate with constant amplitudes and phase in the presence of damping; in the absence of damping, the amplitude of oscillation is still constant except if the applied frequency is close (equal) to a natural frequency, and beats (resonance) occur. In the case of an N-dimensional oscillator, it is possible (section 8.3) to have: (i) internal beats (resonance) if two natural frequencies are close (equal); (ii) externally forced multiple beats (resonance) if the applied frequency is close (equal) to several coincident modal frequencies.

The methods of study of N-dimensional linear oscillators with damping and forcing are similar to the one-dimensional case (chapter 2), replacing one dependent variable by N variables, and single coefficients by matrices of coefficients. In order to illustrate the properties of N-dimensional oscillators with a minimum of algebra, it is sufficient to consider a coupled two-dimensional oscillator (sections 8.3–8.5) of which one example is the vibration absorber (section 8.6). A particular class of N-dimensional systems leading to a banded matrix, with all terms zero except for the diagonal and some parallel lines, are chains in which each element is connected only to the preceding and following, for example, a chain of radioactive disintegration (sequence of oscillators) consisting of first- (second-) order system [section 8.7 (8.8)]. An infinite chain becomes a transmission line (section 8.9), which may allow passage with constant amplitude within a frequency band and causes signal reflection outside the "band pass"; this problem leads to finite difference equations instead of ordinary differential equations.

8.1 Balance of Forces, Energy, and Dissipation

The multidimensional oscillator involves several degrees-of-freedom in the inertia force that is balanced by: (i) external applied forces depending on time (subsection 8.1.1); (ii)(iii) restoring (friction) forces depending on position (velocity) and leading [subsection 8.1.2 (8.1.3)] to the potential (dissipation) function. The restoring, friction, inertia, and applied forces (power of the forces, including the potential and dissipation functions) appear in the momentum (energy) equation [subsection 8.1.5 (8.1.6)] and apply both to decoupled and simultaneous oscillators (subsection 8.1.4). The energy equation specifies the total energy, that is, the sum of the kinetic and potential energies (subsection 8.1.6).

8.1.1 Restoring, Friction, Inertial and Applied Forces

For an N-dimensional (1a) oscillator with coordinates x_r, the **equations of motion** state that the inertial force, equal to the product of constant (8.1b) mass m_r and acceleration $\ddot{x}_r$, equals the sum (8.1c) of other forces:

$$r,s,\ell,n = 1,...,N; \quad m_r = \text{const}: \qquad m_r\,\ddot{x}_r = h_r\left(\dot{x}_s\right) + j_r\left(x_s\right) + F_r\left(t\right), \qquad \text{(8.1a–c)}$$

namely: (i) the friction force, which depends on the velocity $\dot{x}_r$: (ii) the restoring force, which depends on the position x_r; (iii) the external force, which depends on time t. The motion of the oscillator is specified by the coordinates as a solution of the system of M ordinary differential equations (8.1a, b), involving not only position, that is, a twice continuously differentiable function of time (8.2a), but also velocity (8.2b) and acceleration (8.2c):

$$x_r\left(t\right) \in D^2\left(|R\right): \qquad \dot{x}_r \equiv \frac{dx_r}{dr}, \qquad \ddot{x}_r \equiv \frac{d\dot{x}_r}{dt} = \frac{d^2 x_r}{dt^2}. \qquad \text{(8.2a–c)}$$

The condition (8.2a) implies that the acceleration (8.2c) is a continuous function of time and excludes collisions. A particular case is linear restoring (friction) forces [subsection 8.1.2 (8.1.3)].

8.1.2 Linear Restoring Force and Quadratic Potential

The **restoring force** depends on position, and if it has continuous second-order derivatives near the origin (8.3a), it can be expanded in a MacLaurin series to first-order (I.23.34b) ≡ (8.3b):

$$j_r\left(x_s\right) \in C^2\left(|R^N\right): \quad j_r\left(x_s\right) = j_r\left(0\right) + \sum_{s=1}^{N} x_s \frac{\partial j_r}{\partial x_s} + O\left(x_r x_s\right), \quad j_r\left(0\right) = 0, \qquad \text{(8.3a–c)}$$

where: (i) if the origin $x_i = 0$ is a position of equilibrium, the force there is zero (8.3c); (ii) for a linear oscillator, performing vibrations with small amplitude, the quadratic and high-order terms are negligible; (iii) thus, only the middle term is left, specifying a restoring force that is a linear function of position (8.4a):

$$j_r = -\sum_{s=1}^{N} k_{rs} x_s, \qquad\qquad k_{ij} \equiv -\left(\frac{\partial j_r}{\partial x_s}\right)_{\bar{x}=0}, \qquad \text{(8.4a, b)}$$

with the coefficients specifying a **resilience matrix** (8.4b), whose component k_{rs} is the force on the r-th particle due to a unit displacement of the s-th particle and is specified by minus the derivatives of the restoring force with regards to the coordinates evaluated at the position of equilibrium. A force is conservative if it is the gradient (8.5a) of a potential energy (8.5b):

$$j_r = -\frac{\partial \Phi_m}{\partial x_r}, \qquad d\Phi_m = \sum_{r=1}^{N} \frac{\partial \Phi_m}{\partial x_r} dx_r = -j_r \, dx_r; \qquad (8.5a, b)$$

in case of linear restoring force (8.4b), the force is always conservative (8.6b) because it derives from a quadratic potential (8.6a):

$$\Phi_m(x_\ell) = \frac{1}{2} \sum_{r,s=1}^{N} k_{rs} \, x_r \, x_s: \qquad -\frac{\partial \Phi_m}{\partial x_r} = -\sum_{s=1}^{N} k_{rs} \, x_s = j_r. \qquad (8.6a, b)$$

The coefficients of the quadratic potential (8.6a) ≡ (8.7c) form the resilience matrix (8.4b), which may be symmetrized (8.7a) ≡ (8.7b):

$$\bar{k}_{rs} \equiv \frac{k_{rs} + k_{sr}}{2} = \bar{k}_{sr}: \quad \Phi_m(x_\ell) = \frac{1}{4} \sum_{r,s=1}^{N} (k_{rs} + k_{sr}) \, x_r \, x_s = \frac{1}{2} \sum_{r,s=1}^{N} \bar{k}_{rs} \, x_r \, x_s, \qquad (8.7a\text{--}d)$$

without changing the potential (8.6a) ≡ (8.7c) ≡ (8.7d). The potential (8.7a) is defined to within an added constant, that is, taken to be zero (8.8b) at the equilibrium point at the origin:

stable equilibrium at $x_r = 0$: $\Phi(0) = 0,$ $\Phi(x_r \neq 0) > 0,$ (8.8a–c)

implying that the potential is positive (8.8c) in its neighborhood for stable equilibrium. Thus, *a linear restoring force (8.4a, b) is (problem 421) always conservative (8.5a, b), because it derives from a quadratic potential (8.6a) ≡ (8.7c, d), where the coefficients form a symmetric (8.7a, b) resilience matrix that must be positive-definite in order that the potential (8.8c) has a minimum of zero (8.8b) at the position of stable equilibrium (8.8a) at the origin.*

8.1.3 Friction Force and Dissipation Function

The **restoring (friction) force** is a function of position (8.3b) [velocity (8.9b)] and if it has a continuous second-order derivative (8.3a) [(8.9a)] near the origin, it can be expanded in a MacLaurin series (8.3b) [(8.9b)] to first-order:

$$h_r(\dot{x}_s) \in C^2(|R^N|): \quad h_r(\dot{x}_j) = h_r(0) - \sum_{s=1}^{N} \mu_{rs} \dot{x}_s + O(\dot{x}, \dot{x}_s), \quad h_r(0) = 0, \qquad (8.9a\text{--}c)$$

where: (i) the first term on the right-hand side (r.h.s.) is the **static friction** at zero velocity, and it is assumed to be zero (8.9c); (ii) for small velocities, the second and higher-order terms are negligible; (iii) the remaining term specifies a **kinematic friction force** that is a linear function (8.10a) of the velocity (8.2b):

$$h_r = -\sum_{s=1}^{N}\mu_{rs}\,\dot{x}_s, \qquad \mu_{rs} = -\left(\frac{\partial h_r}{\partial \dot{x}_s}\right)_{\dot{x}_\ell=0}, \qquad (8.10\text{a, b})$$

with the **friction matrix** (8.9b) as coefficients. Minus the work per unit time or **activity** or **power** of the friction force specifies a **dissipation function** (8.11a):

$$\Psi_m = -\sum_{s=1}^{N}h_r\frac{dx_r}{dt}; \qquad \Psi_m = \sum_{r,s=1}^{N}\mu_{rs}\,\dot{x}_r\,\dot{x}_s \geq 0, \qquad (8.11\text{a, b})$$

for a linear kinematic friction (8.10a), the dissipation function (8.11a) is quadratic (8.10b) and hence: (i) the friction matrix can be made symmetric (8.12a), as for the resilience matrix (8.7a, b); (ii) it must be positive definite (8.11b), so that the friction force does negative work, that is, dissipates energy (8.11a):

$$\mu_{rs} = \mu_{rs}; \qquad N = 1: \qquad h_1\left(\dot{x}_1\right) = -b_{11}\,\dot{x}_1, \qquad j_{11}\left(x_1\right) = -k_{11}\,x_1, \qquad (8.12\text{a–d})$$

for example, in a one-dimensional case (8.12b), the friction (restoring) force (8.12c) [(8.12d)] is opposite and proportional to the velocity (displacement) through the scalar kinematic friction (resilience). Thus, *minus the activity or power of the friction force specifies (problem 422) a dissipation function (8.11b) that cannot be negative; a kinematic friction force linear (8.10a) on the velocity (8.2b), corresponds to a quadratic dissipation function (8.11b), whose coefficients are a symmetric (8.12a, b) positive definite friction matrix (8.10b).* The same signs in the linear the restoring (8.4a) [friction (8.10a)] force opposite to the displacement (velocity), together with opposite signs for the corresponding potential (8.5a, b) [dissipation function (8.11a)] lead to quadratic forms (8.7d) [(8.11b)] with symmetric (8.7a, b) [(8.12a)] positive-definite coefficients, specifying the resilience (8.4b) [friction (8.10b)] matrix.

8.1.4 Coupled and Decoupled Equations of Motion

Substituting (8.4a) and (8.10a) into (8.1a, b), leads to *(problem 423) the equation of motion for an N-dimensional linear oscillator with damping and forcing, which is a simultaneous system of N differential equations (8.13a):*

$$m_r\,\ddot{x}_r + \sum_{s=1}^{N}\left(\mu_{rs}\,\dot{x}_s + k_{rs}\,x_s\right) = F_r\left(t\right); \qquad m_r\,\ddot{x}_r + \mu_r\,\dot{x}_r + k_r\,x_r = F_r\left(t\right), \qquad (8.13\text{a, b})$$

the system is decoupled (8.13b), if the resilience (8.14a) [and friction (8.14b)] matrix:

$$\left\{ k_{rs}, \mu_{rs} \right\} = \delta_{rs} \left\{ k_r, \mu_r \right\}, \qquad \delta_{rs} \equiv \begin{cases} 0 & \text{if} & r \neq s, \\ 1 & \text{if} & r \neq s, \end{cases} \qquad \text{(8.14a–c)}$$

*equals the product of a **resilience (friction) vector** by the **identity matrix** (8.14c). In the particular (general) case of decoupled (coupled) forced N-dimensional oscillator, the resilience vector k_r (matrix k_{rs}) and the friction vector μ_r (matrix μ_{rs}) matrices are both diagonal (non-diagonal) and lead to a restoring/friction force that depends only on the same coordinate (8.15a, b)/velocity (8.16a, b) [can depend on all coordinates (8.4a)/velocities (8.10a)]:*

$$k_{rs} = k_r \, \delta_{rs}: \qquad j_r = -k_r \, x_r, \qquad \Phi_m = \frac{1}{2} \sum_{r=1}^{N} k_r \left(x_r \right)^2, \qquad \text{(8.15a–c)}$$

$$\mu_{rs} = \mu_r \, \delta_{rs}; \qquad h_r = -\mu_r \, \dot{x}_s, \qquad \Psi_m = \sum_{r=1}^{N} \mu_r \left(\dot{x}_r \right)^2; \qquad \text{(8.16a–c)}$$

the corresponding potential/dissipation function is a sum of squares (8.15c)/(8.16c) [a positive definite quadratic form (8.7d; 8.8c)/(8.11b)]. The decoupled N-dimensional oscillator corresponds to N separate one-dimensional oscillators, which have already been considered (chapter 2); it will be shown in the sequel (section 8.2) that an N-dimensional coupled oscillator is always the superposition of N decoupled one-dimensional oscillators, like the natural integrals of a simultaneous system of differential equations (section 7.4). In order to help interpret these and other results, first is considered the energy balance (subsection 8.1.5) that follows from the equations of motion (subsection 8.1.3).

8.1.5 Activity/Power and Work of the Applied Forces

The **activity** or **power**, which is the work per unit time of the external applied forces, is specified by (8.17a):

$$\frac{dW}{dt} = \sum_{r=1}^{N} F_r(t) \, \frac{dx_r}{dt} = \sum_{r=1}^{N} \left(m_r \, \ddot{x}_r - h_r - j_r \right) \dot{x}_r, \qquad \text{(8.17a, b)}$$

where in (8.17b) was used, the equation of motion (8.1b) without restriction on any of the forces. In (8.17b), the dissipation function (8.11b) may be introduced leading to (8.18):

$$\frac{dW}{dt} - \Psi_m = \sum_{r=1}^{N} \left(m_r \, \ddot{x}_r \, \dot{x}_r - j_r \, \dot{x}_r \right), \qquad \text{(8.18)}$$

where on the r.h.s. appear: (i) the time derivative (8.19c) of the kinetic energy (8.19a), under the assumption that mass is independent of time (8.19b):

$$E_v = \frac{1}{2} \sum_{r=1}^{N} m_r (\dot{x}_r)^2, \qquad \dot{m}_r = 0: \qquad \frac{dE_v}{dt} \equiv \dot{E}_v = \sum_{r=1}^{N} m_r \ddot{x}_r \dot{x}_r; \qquad (8.19a\text{--}c)$$

$$j_r = -\frac{\partial \Phi_m}{\partial x_r}: \qquad \frac{d\Phi_m}{dt} = \sum_{r=1}^{N} \frac{\partial \Phi}{\partial x_r} \frac{dx_r}{dt} = -\sum_{r=1}^{N} j_r \dot{x}_r, \qquad (8.20a, b)$$

(ii) for a conservative restoring force (8.5a) ≡ (8.20a), the time derivative of the potential (8.20b). Substituting (8.19c, 8.20b) in (8.18) follows:

$$\frac{dW}{dt} - \Psi_m = \frac{dE}{dt}, \qquad E = E_v + \Phi_m = \sum_{r=1}^{N} \frac{1}{2} m_r (\dot{x}_r)^2 + \Phi_m, \qquad (8.21a, b)$$

the **energy balance** (8.21a) stating that (problem 424) the work unit time of the external applied forces (8.17a) minus the dissipation function (8.11a) due to the friction forces, equals the rate of change with time (8.21a) of the **total energy** (8.21b), specified by the sum of: (i) the kinetic energy (8.19a); (ii) the potential (8.20a) of the conservative restoring forces. If the work of the external applied forces is balanced by dissipation (8.22a) the total energy is conserved (8.22b):

$$\sum_{r=1}^{N} F_r \, dx_r = dW = \Psi_m \, dt = -\sum_{r=1}^{N} h_r \, dx_r \rightarrow \quad \text{const} = E = \sum_{r=1}^{N} \left[\frac{1}{2} m_r (\dot{x}_r)^2 + \Phi_m \right];$$

$$(8.22a, b)$$

in the particular case of linear restoring force (8.4a) ≡ (8.23a) the potential is a quadratic function of the coordinates (8.7d) as the kinetic energy (8.19a) is a quadratic function of the velocity (8.2b), and the total energy (8.21b) is specified by (8.23b):

$$j_r = -\sum_{s=1}^{N} k_{rs} x_s: \qquad 2 E = \sum_{r=1}^{N} m_r (\dot{x}_r)^2 + \sum_{r,s=1}^{N} k_{rs} x_r x_s. \qquad (8.23a, b)$$

In particular, an oscillator without damping or forcing has constant total energy, for linear or non-linear oscillations. All of these results assume that the mass is independent of time (8.1b) ≡ (8.19b).

8.1.6 Kinetic, Potential, and Total Energies

The preceding results from (8.17a, b) to (8.22a, b) apply to the general case of non-linear restoring and friction forces in (8.1a) and (8.23a, b) and assumes a linear restoring force (8.4a). If in addition the friction force is also linear (8.10a), the work per unit time of the applied external forces is given by:

$$
A \equiv \frac{dW}{dt} = \sum_{r=1}^{N} F_r\, \dot{x}_r = \sum_{r=1}^{N} m_r\, \ddot{x}_r\, \dot{x}_r - \sum_{r,s=1}^{N} \left(\mu_{rs}\, \dot{x}_s + k_{rs}\, x_s \right) \dot{x}_r
$$

$$
= \Psi_m + \frac{1}{2} \frac{d}{dt} \left[\sum_{r=1}^{N} m_r \left(\dot{x}_r \right)^2 + \sum_{r,s=1}^{N} k_{rs}\, x_r\, x_s \right] = \Psi_m + \frac{dE}{dt},
$$

(8.24a–e)

which agrees with (8.21a) ≡ (8.24e). In (8.24d) were used the differentiations (8.25) [(8.26a–c)] of the kinetic (8.18a) [potential (8.7d)] energy:

$$
\dot{E}_v = \frac{1}{2} \frac{d}{dt} \left[\sum_{r=1}^{N} m_r \left(\dot{x}_r \right)^2 \right] = \sum_{r=1}^{N} m_r\, \dot{x}_r\, \ddot{x}_r ,
$$

(8.25)

$$
\dot{\Phi} = \frac{1}{2} \frac{d}{dt} \left[\sum_{r,s=1}^{N} \left(k_{rs}\, x_r\, x_s \right) \right] = \frac{1}{2} \sum_{u,s=1}^{N} k_{rs} \left(\dot{x}_r x_s + x_r\, \dot{x}_s \right)
$$

$$
= \frac{1}{2} \sum_{r,s=1}^{N} \left(k_{rs} + k_{sr} \right) \dot{x}_r x_s = \sum_{r,s=1}^{N} \overline{k}_{rs} \dot{x}_r x_s ;
$$

(8.26a–d)

the latter (8.26d) uses the symmetry (8.7a, b) of the resilience matrix. *In the particular case of (problem 425) a decoupled linear oscillator (8.14a–c) ≡ (8.27a) the total energy (8.21b) ≡ (8.27b):*

$$
k_{rs} = k_r\, \delta_{rs}: \qquad 2E = \sum_{r=1}^{N} \left[m_r \left(\dot{x}_r \right)^2 + k_r \left(x_r \right)^2 \right],
$$

(8.27a, b)

is a sum of squares both for the kinetic (8.19a) [potential (8.15c)] energies, which equal one-half of the mass (resilience) multiplying the square of the velocity (displacement) summed for all N degrees-of-freedom leading to separate equations of motion (8.13b). In the case of simultaneous oscillators, the potential (8.6a) [dissipation (8.11b) functions corresponding to the restoring (8.4a) [friction (8.10a)] forces, which are linear functions of the position (8.2a) [velocity (8.2b)], involve cross-terms in the symmetric resilience (8.7a, b) [friction (8.12a)] matrices; the mass vector in the kinetic energy (8.19a) corresponds to a diagonal mass matrix, which may be generalized to a non-diagonal mass matrix (section 8.2).

8.2 Modal Frequencies, Damping, Coordinates, and Forces

The mass, friction, and resilience matrices (subsection 8.2.1) appear in the damping and oscillation matrices (subsection 8.2.2), and specify the equations of motion around a position of stable equilibrium (subsection 8.2.3) that are considered for free (forced) cases [subsections 8.2.3–8.2.8 (8.2.9–8.2.16)]. The free oscillations, that is, in the absence of external applied forces and without (with) friction [subsection 8.2.4 (8.2.5)] specify the modal frequencies (dampings) and hence, the corresponding modal coordinates (subsection 8.2.6). The physical coordinates are (subsection 8.2.8) linear combination of the modal coordinates with coefficients determined by initial and compatibility conditions (subsection 8.2.7). The physical (modal) coordinates in the case of forcing without (with) damping are associated with the applied (modal) external forces (subsection 8.2.9) and matrix (diagonal) dispersion operators (subsection 8.2.10) in the coupled (decoupled) equations of motion (subsection 8.2.11). The sinusoidal forcing (subsection 8.2.12) leads to a modal matrix (subsection 8.2.13), which applies without (with) damping [subsection 8.2.14 (8.2.16)] using physical or modal coordinates (subsection 8.2.15).

8.2.1 Mass, Damping, and Oscillation Matrices

The simultaneous equation of motion (8.13a) for the multidimensional linear oscillator with friction and forcing can be generalized to (8.28):

$$\sum_{s=1}^{N} \left(m_{rs}\,\ddot{x}_s + \mu_{rs}\,\dot{x}_s + k_{rs}\,x_s \right) = F_r(t), \tag{8.28}$$

where, in addition to the resilience (8.4a, b) and friction (8.10a, b) matrices, a **mass or inertia matrix** was introduced, which appears symmetrically (8.29a) in the kinetic energy (8.19a) generalized to (8.29b):

$$m_{rs} = m_{sr}: \qquad\qquad E_v = \frac{1}{2}\sum_{r,s=1}^{N} m_{rs}\,\dot{x}_r\dot{x}_s. \tag{8.29a, b}$$

The original kinetic energy (8.19a) and equation of motion (8.13a) correspond to a diagonal mass matrix (8.30a), with the masses along the diagonal:

$$m_{rs}\, m_{rs} = m_r\, \delta_{rs}; \quad Det(m_{r,s}) \neq 0; \quad \sum_{\ell=1}^{N} m_{r\ell}\, \tilde{m}_{\ell s} = \delta_{rs}, \quad (8.30a\text{–}c)$$

a non-diagonal mass matrix may arise when discretizing a continuous system, such as an elastic body or a fluid flow, and if it has a non-zero determinant (8.30b) there is an inverse mass matrix (8.30c). Multiplying the generalized equation of motion (8.28) by the inverse mass matrix (8.30c) leads to (8.31a) with explicit accelerations:

$$\ddot{x}_r + \sum_{s=1}^{N} \left(2\, \lambda_{rs}\, \dot{x}_s + \omega_{rs}^2\, x_s \right) = f_r: \quad \left\{2\, \lambda_{rs}\,,\, \omega_{rs}^2\,,\, f_r \right\} \sum_{\ell=1}^{n} \equiv \tilde{m}_{r\ell} \left\{\mu_{\ell s}\,,\, k_{\ell s}\,,\, F_\ell \right\}.$$

$$(8.31a\text{–}d)$$

Thus, *the equations of motion (problem 426) for a generalized linear multidimensional oscillator with friction and forcing (8.28) involve the three* **system matrices,** *namely mass (8.29a, b), friction (8.10a, b), and resilience (8.4a, b); these matrices can be rewritten with explicit accelerations (8.31a) by premultiplication by the inverse mass matrix (8.30b, c) that leads, respectively, to the* **damping (oscillation) matrices (8.31b) [(8.31c)]** *and to the* **reduced external force (8.31d).** *In the case of a diagonal mass matrix (8.30a)* ≡ *(8.32a) the damping (oscillation) matrices (8.32b) [(8.32c)] and the reduced external force (8.32d) follow from the friction (resilience) matrices and external force dividing by the masses:*

$$m_{rs} = m_r \delta_{rs}: \quad \left\{2\lambda_{rs}\,,\, \omega_{rs}^2\,,\, f_r \right\} = m_r^{-1} \left\{\mu_{r,s}\,,\, k_{rs}\,,\, F_r \right\}, \quad (8.32a\text{–}d)$$

$$\ddot{x}_r + 2\lambda_r\, x_r + \omega_r^2\, x_r = f_r\,, \quad (8.32e)$$

and the kinetic energy (8.29b) [equation of motion (8.31a)] simplify to (8.19b) [(8.32e)]. The generalized equation of motion (8.28) in the form (8.31a) with explicit accelerations is used in the following discussion of undamped (damped) free [subsections 8.2.2–8.2.4 (8.2.5–8.2.8)] and forced [subsections 8.2.14–8.2.15 (8.2.9–8.2.13, 8.2.16)] oscillations.

8.2.2 Friction, Oscillation, and Dispersion Matrices

The unforced (8.34a) simultaneous system of linear differential equations with constant coefficients (8.31a) implies that the displacements are exponential functions of time (8.33a) leading (8.2b) [(8.2c)] to the velocity (8.33b) [acceleration (8.33c)]:

$$q_r(t) = E_r\, e^{\xi t}: \qquad \dot{q}_r(t) = \xi E_r\, e^{\xi t} = \xi q_r(t), \qquad \ddot{q}_r(t) = \xi^2 q_r(t). \qquad (8.33a\text{–}c)$$

Substituting (8.33a–c) in the unforced (8.34a) equations of motion (8.31a) leads to (8.34b) ≡ (8.34c):

$$f_r = 0: \qquad 0 = \ddot{q}_r + \sum_{s=1}^{N}\left(2\lambda_{rs}\dot{q}_s + \omega_{rs}^2\, q_s\right) = \sum_{s=1}^{N}\left(\delta_{rs}\xi^2 + 2\lambda_{rs}\xi + \omega_{rs}^2\right)q_s, \qquad (8.34a\text{–}c)$$

where appears (8.34c) ≡ (8.35b), the **dispersion matrix** (8.35a):

$$P_{rs}(\xi) \equiv \delta_{rs}\,\xi^2 + 2\lambda_{rs}\,\xi + \omega_s^2: \qquad 0 = \sum_{s=1}^{N} P_{rs}(\xi)\, q_s(t). \qquad (8.35a, b)$$

A non-trivial solution requires that the displacements cannot be all zero (8.36a) and thus, the determinant of the displacement matrix be zero (8.36b):

$$\{q_1(t),\dots,q_N(t)\} \ne \{0,\dots,0\}: \qquad 0 = P_{2N}(\xi) \equiv Det\left[P_{rs}(\xi)\right] \equiv \prod_{n=1}^{2N}\{\xi - \xi_n\}.$$

$$(8.36a\text{–}c)$$

Thus, *the vanishing of the determinant of the dispersion matrix (8.36b) specifies (problem 427) the **dispersion polynomial** (8.36c) whose roots ξ_n determine the modes (8.33a).* The modal coordinates are considered next for unforced (8.34a) or **free motion** without damping, which leads to decoupled (simultaneous) oscillations [subsection (8.2.3) (8.2.4)].

8.2.3 Free Undamped Decoupled Oscillations

The multidimensional decoupled (8.32e) oscillator with neither forcing (8.37a) nor friction (8.37b) leads to the equation of motion (8.37c):

$$F_r = 0 = \lambda_r: \qquad \ddot{x}_r + \omega_r^2\, x_r = 0, \qquad \omega_r \equiv \sqrt{\frac{k_r}{m_r}}, \qquad (8.37a\text{–}d)$$

showing that each coordinate oscillates independently of the others at a natural frequency (8.37d); the displacement (2.56a) ≡ (8.38b):

$$q_r(t) = A_r \cos(\omega_r\, t) + B_r \sin(\omega_r\, t) = C_r \cos(\omega_r t - \alpha_r), \qquad (8.38a, b)$$

involves two arbitrary constants of integration A_r, B_r in (8.38a), which may be replaced (1.80; 1.79a–d) by amplitude C_r and phase α_r in (8.38b), both determined from initial conditions (2.56b, c; 2.57a, b). In the decoupled case, the system of differential equations (8.37c) has: (i) dispersion matrix (8.39a), which is diagonal; (ii) thus, its determinant (8.39b) is the product of diagonal elements; (iii) the roots of the dispersion relation (8.39b) are the roots of each factor (8.39c):

$$P_{rs}\left(\xi\right)=\left(\xi^2 + \omega_r^2\right)\delta_{rs}, \qquad P_{2N}\left(\xi\right)=\prod_{r=1}^{N}\left(\xi^2 + \omega_r^2\right), \qquad \xi = \pm i\omega_r; \qquad (8.39\text{a–c})$$

(iv) each pair of conjugate imaginary roots (8.39c) leads to a displacement (8.40):

$$x_r\left(t\right)= C_r^+\, e^{+i\omega_r t} + C_r^-\, e^{-i\omega_r t} = A_r \cos\left(\omega_r t\right) + B_r \sin\left(\omega_r t\right), \qquad (8.40)$$

which coincides with (8.38a) ≡ (8.38b) ≡ (8.40), using an alternate set $C_r^{\pm}$ of arbitrary constants that are related by (8.41a, c) [(8.41b, d)]:

$$A_r = C_r^+ + C_r^- = C_r \cos\alpha_r, \qquad\qquad B_r = i\left(C_r^+ + C_r^-\right) = C_r \sin\alpha_r, \qquad (8.41\text{a–d})$$

to the arbitrary constants $\left(A_r, B_r\right)\left[\left(C_r, \alpha_r\right)\right]$ in (8.38a) [(8.38b)]. In the decoupled case, each coordinate can be treated separately; that is not the case for simultaneous oscillations (subsection 8.2.4).

8.2.4 Modal Frequencies of Undamped Oscillations

In the case of simultaneous oscillations (8.31a) ≡ (8.42c) without forcing (8.42a) and damping (8.42b):

$$F_r = 0 = \lambda_{rs}: \qquad 0 = \ddot{x}_r + \sum_{s=1}^{N}\omega_{rs}^2\, x_s = \sum_{s=1}^{N}\left(\delta_{rs}\,\xi^2 + \omega_{rs}^2\right) x_s, \qquad (8.42\text{a–c})$$

the dispersion matrix (8.35a) is not diagonal (8.43a) and the dispersion relation (8.36b) shows (8.43a) that $-\xi^2$ are the eigenvalues of the oscillation matrix (8.43c):

$$P_{rs}\left(\xi\right)= \xi^2\,\delta_{rs} + \omega_{rs}^2, \qquad 0 = Det\left(\omega_{rs}^2 + \xi^2\,\delta_{rs}\right)=\prod_{\ell=1}^{N}\left(\xi^2 + \omega_\ell^2\right). \qquad (8.43\text{a–c})$$

Thus: (i) the origin has been taken as a position of equilibrium where the restoring force vanishes (8.3c); (ii) for a linear restoring force (8.4a) the quadratic potential (8.7d) is zero (8.8b) at the equilibrium position; (iii) the equilibrium position is **stable** if it is a minimum (8.8a) of the potential; (iv) the potential is positive (8.8c) in the neighborhood of the equilibrium position; (v) this requires that the resilience matrix (8.4b), which can be symmetrized (8.7a), be positive-definite; (vi) the mass matrix is also symmetric (8.29a) and positive-definite since the kinetic energy (8.29b) must be positive for non-zero velocity; (vii) the oscillation matrix (8.32c) is also positive-definite because it is the product of the inverse of (vi) by (v), which are both positive-definite matrices; (viii) therefore, the eigenvalues $-\omega_\ell^2$ must be positive (8.44a); (ix) the roots of the dispersion relation (8.43c) are conjugate imaginary (8.44b):

$$\omega_\ell^2 > 0; \qquad \xi = \sqrt{-\omega_\ell^2} = \pm i\omega_\ell: \qquad q_\ell(t) = C_\ell \cos(\omega_\ell t - \alpha_\ell), \qquad \text{(8.44a–c)}$$

(x) the corresponding **modal coordinates** (8.44c) are oscillations with constant amplitude and phase and natural frequency ω_ℓ. It has been proved that *the unforced (8.42a) undamped (8.42b) linear motion (8.42c) around a position of stable equilibrium consists (problem 428) of modal coordinates corresponding to oscillations (8.44c) with constant amplitude and phase and **natural frequencies** (8.43c), which are the square root of the modulus of the eigenvalues of the oscillation matrix (8.43a), which is the product (8.31c) of the inverse of the mass matrix (8.29a, b) by the resilience matrix (8.4a, b). The modal frequencies are specified equivalently as the modulus or imaginary part of the roots of the dispersion relation (8.43c), specified by the vanishing of the determinant (8.43b) of the dispersion matrix (8.43a), that is, the dispersion matrix (8.35a) without damping (8.42b).* In the presence of friction (subsection 8.2.5), there are both modal frequencies and dampings.

8.2.5 Modal Dampings of Decaying Oscillations

Returning to the equations of motion (8.31a) without forcing (8.45a), but retaining friction, leads to the free damped oscillations (8.45b):

$$f_r = 0: \qquad \ddot{x}_r + \sum_{s=1}^{N} \left(2\,\lambda_{rs}\,\dot{x}_s + \omega_{rs}^2\,x_s \right) = 0. \qquad \text{(8.45a, b)}$$

The full dispersion matrix (8.35a), including restoring and friction terms, has real coefficients, and so does the dispersion relation (8.36b) that is a polynomial (8.36c) of degree $2N$. The roots can be real or complex conjugate pairs (8.46a–d):

$$0 = \operatorname{Det}\left(\xi^2\,\delta_{rs} + 2\,\xi\,\lambda_{rs} + \omega_{rs}^2 \right) \equiv P_{2N}(\xi)$$

$$= \prod_{\ell=1}^{N} \left(\xi + \lambda_\ell + i\bar{\omega}_\ell \right)\left(\xi + \lambda_\ell - i\bar{\omega}_\ell \right) = \prod_{\ell=1}^{N} \left(\xi - \xi_\ell^+ \right)\left(\xi - \xi_\ell^- \right). \qquad \text{(8.46a–d)}$$

The complex conjugate roots (8.46d) $\equiv$ (8.47a) correspond to the natural integrals (8.47b) $\equiv$ (8.47c):

$$\xi_\ell^\pm = -\lambda_\ell \pm i\bar{\omega}_\ell: \qquad q_\ell^\pm(t) = \exp\left(\xi_\ell^\pm t\right) = \exp\left(-\lambda_\ell t\right)\exp\left(\pm i\bar{\omega}_\ell t\right), \qquad (8.47\text{a–c})$$

which are equivalent to the modal coordinates:

$$q_\ell^\pm(t) = C_\ell \exp\left(-\lambda_r t\right)\cos\left(\bar{\omega}_\ell t - \alpha_\ell\right), \qquad (8.48)$$

and add damping relative to (8.44c).

Thus, *the unforced (8.45a) linear simultaneous oscillator with damping (8.45b) has (problem 429) the modal coordinates (8.48) whose* **modal frequencies (dampings)** *are minus the real part (the positive imaginary part) of the roots (8.46a–d) $\equiv$ (8.49c) of the determinant (8.49b) of the* **modal-decay matrix** *(8.49a):*

$$P_{rs}(\xi) = \xi^2 \delta_{rs} + 2\xi\,\lambda_{rs} + \omega_{rs}^2: \qquad P_{rs}(\xi) = \text{Det}\left\{P_{rs}(\xi)\right\}, \qquad 0 = P_{2N}\left(-\lambda_\ell \pm i\bar{\omega}_\ell\right), \qquad (8.49\text{a–c})$$

which is the dispersion matrix (8.35a) involving the damping (8.31b) and oscillation (8.31c) matrices. Thus, the motion is: (i) damped (amplified) if the real part is negative (positive), and the amplitude is constant if the real part is zero. In the preceding analysis, the case of multiple roots of the dispersion relation (8.35b) that would lead to the appearance in the modal coordinates of factors involving powers of time (8.50b) has been excluded:

$$\gamma = 0, \ldots, \beta - 1: \qquad q_{\ell,\gamma}(t) = C_{\ell,\gamma}\, t^\gamma\, e^{-\lambda_\ell t}\cos\left(\bar{\omega}_\ell t - \alpha_\ell\right), \qquad (8.50\text{a, b})$$

for a root of multiplicity β in (8.50a). These factors cannot occur in the undamped case $\lambda_\ell = 0$, because they would lead to displacements increasing as powers of time, which is incompatible with the conservation of energy (subsection 8.1.6). Multiple roots and powers of time can occur for damped $\lambda_\ell > 0$ or amplified $\lambda_\ell < 0$ motion, since the exponentials always dominate the powers, that is, the limit (8.51a):

$$\lim_{t \to \infty} t^\gamma\, e^{-\lambda_\ell t} = \begin{cases} 0 & \text{if} \quad \lambda_\ell < 0, & (8.51\text{a}) \\ \infty & \text{if} \quad \lambda_\ell > 0, & (8.51\text{b}) \end{cases}$$

is zero (infinity) for any power γ in the case of damping (8.51a) [amplification (8.51b)]. The case of multiple roots of the characteristic polynomial has been considered for simultaneous systems of linear differential equations with constant coefficients (sections 7.4–7.5) and only distinct roots are considered next (subsection 8.2.6) for the modal coordinates associated with modal frequencies and dampings.

8.2.6 Modal Coordinates and Oscillation Frequencies

Each modal coordinate, corresponding to the pair (8.47c), is associated with a pair of complex conjugate roots (8.47a, b) of the dispersion relation (8.46a–d), and satisfies a separate linear second-order differential equation (8.52a–d):

$$
\begin{aligned}
0 &= \left\{ \left(d/dt - \xi_\ell^+ \right)\left(d/dt - \xi_\ell^- \right) \right\} q_\ell(t) \\
&= \left\{ \left(d/dt + \lambda_\ell - i\bar{\omega}_\ell \right)\left(d/dt + \lambda_\ell + i\bar{\omega}_\ell \right) \right\} q_\ell(t) \\
&= \left\{ \left(d/dt + \lambda_\ell \right)^2 + \bar{\omega}_\ell^2 \right\} q_\ell(t) \\
&= \left\{ d^2/dt^2 + 2\lambda_\ell \, d/dt + \lambda_\ell^2 + \bar{\omega}_\ell^2 \right\} q_\ell(t),
\end{aligned}
\tag{8.52a–d}
$$

which involves (8.52d) ≡ (8.53b), the damping λ_ℓ and **oscillation frequency** (8.53a):

$$
\omega_\ell \equiv \left| \left(\bar{\omega}_\ell \right)^2 + \left(\lambda_\ell \right)^2 \right|^{1/2} : \qquad \ddot{q}_\ell + 2\lambda_\ell \, \dot{q}_\ell + \omega_\ell^2 \, q_\ell = 0.
\tag{8.53a, b}
$$

Thus, *each modal coordinate has (problem 430) a decoupled motion (8.53b) consisting of an oscillation (8.54b):*

$$
\bar{\omega}_\ell = \left| \left(\omega_\ell \right)^2 - \left(\lambda_\ell \right)^2 \right|^{1/2} : \qquad q_\ell(t) = C_\ell \exp\left(-\lambda_\ell t \right) \cos\left(\bar{\omega}_\ell t - \alpha_\ell \right),
\tag{8.54a, b}
$$

with amplitude C_ℓ, phase α_ℓ, damping λ_ℓ, and oscillation frequency (8.54a) ≡ (2.105c). The oscillation frequency: (i) generally involves the damping (8.53a); (ii) for **weak damping** *(8.5a) much smaller than the modal frequency:*

$$
\left(\lambda_\ell \right)^2 \ll \left(\omega_\ell \right)^2 : \qquad \bar{\omega}_\ell = \omega_\ell, \qquad q_\ell(t) = C_\ell \, e^{-\lambda_\ell t} \cos\left(\omega_\ell t - \alpha_\ell \right),
\tag{8.55a–c}
$$

the oscillation frequency coincides with the natural frequency (8.55b) in the modal coordinate (8.55c). The modal coordinates q_ℓ are used next (subsection 8.2.7) to specify the physical coordinates x_r.

8.2.7 Relation between the Physical and Modal Coordinates

The modal coordinates (8.54b) form a set of decoupled (8.53b) linearly independent solutions of the unforced (8.45a) equations of motion (8.45b).

The general integral of (8.45b) of the equations of motion for the original **physical coordinates** is a linear combination of the modal coordinates (8.56a):

$$x_r(t) = \sum_{\ell=1}^{N} Q_{r\ell}\left(\xi_n^{\pm}\right) q_\ell(t) = \sum_{\ell=1}^{N} Q_{r\ell}\left(-\lambda_n \pm i\bar{\omega}_n\right) q_\ell(t), \qquad \text{(8.56a, b)}$$

where the **transformation matrix** $Q_{r\ell}$ does not depend on time and can depend only (8.56b) on the modal frequencies and dampings. The N^2 components of the transformation matrix are not all independent; because they must satisfy **compatibility relations** obtained substituting (8.56b) in the unforced equations of motion (8.45b) leading to (8.57a):

$$0 = \sum_{s,\ell=1}^{N} \left(\delta_{rs}\,\ddot{q}_\ell + 2\,\lambda_{rs}\,\dot{q}_\ell + \omega_{rs}^2\,q_\ell\right) Q_{r\ell}(\xi), \qquad \text{(8.57a)}$$

$$= \sum_{s,\ell=1}^{N} \left(\delta_{rs}\,\xi^2 + 2\lambda_{rs}\,\xi + \omega_{rs}^2\right) Q_{r\ell}(\xi)\,q_\ell(t), \qquad \text{(8.57b)}$$

$$= \sum_{s,\ell=1}^{N} P_{rs}(\xi)\,Q_{r\ell}(\xi)\,q_\ell(t), \qquad \text{(8.57c)}$$

where: (i) in (8.57b) was used (8.33b, c); (ii) in (8.57c) appears the dispersion matrix (8.35a). Since the modal coordinates (8.54) are linearly independent functions of time, it follows from (8.57c) that *(problem 431) the product of the dispersion (8.35a) and transformation (8.56a) matrices evaluated for the eigenvalues is zero (8.58a):*

$$0 = \sum_{s=1}^{N} P_{rs}\left(\xi_n\right) Q_{r\ell}\left(\xi_n\right); \qquad \sum_{s=1}^{N} P_{rs}\left(\xi_n\right)\bar{P}_{s\ell}\left(\xi_n\right) = \delta_{r\ell}\,P_{2N}\left(\xi_n\right) = 0, \qquad \text{(8.58a–c)}$$

the product of the dispersion matrix by its co-factors (8.58b) equals the identity matrix multiplied by the determinant, which is zero (8.58c) since the eigenvalues are its roots (8.36b, c). The comparison of (8.58a) ≡ (8.58b, c) shows that *(problem 432) the compatibility relations state that the transformation matrix coincides (8.59a) with matrix of co-factors (8.58b) of the dispersion matrix (8.35a) evaluated for the eigenvalues:*

$$Q_{r\ell}\left(\xi_n^{\pm}\right) = \bar{P}_{r\ell}\left(-\lambda_n \pm i\omega_n\right): \qquad x_r(t) = \sum_{\ell=1}^{N} \bar{P}_{r\ell}\left(-\lambda_n \pm i\omega_n\right) q_\ell(t), \qquad \text{(8.59a, b)}$$

to within a set of multiplying constants that can be incorporated in the amplitudes C_ℓ of the modal coordinates (8.55c); the matrix (8.59a) relates (8.56b) the physical to the modal coordinates (8.59b). From (8.59b; 8.55c) follows the general unforced motion (subsection 8.2.8), which is the general integral of the unforced equations of motion (8.45b), satisfying the compatibility conditions, to which can be applied the initial conditions.

8.2.8 Compatibility Relations and Initial Conditions

Substituting the modal coordinates (8.55c) in the relation (8.59b) with the physical coordinates specifies the latter (8.60):

$$x_r(t) = \sum_{\ell=1}^{N} \overline{P}_{r\ell}(-\lambda_n \pm i\omega_n) C_\ell\, e^{-\lambda_\ell t} \cos(\overline{\omega}_\ell t - \alpha_\ell), \qquad (8.60)$$

showing that *the general unforced multidimensional oscillation satisfying the linearized equations of motion (8.45b) is (problem 433) a superposition of N oscillations: (i) with natural frequency (damping), which is the modulus of the imaginary (minus the real) part (8.61a) [(8.61b)] of the eigenvalues (8.47a):*

$$\omega_\ell = \pm \mathrm{Im}\left(\xi_\ell^\pm\right) = \left| \mathrm{Im}\left(\xi_\ell^\pm\right) \right|, \qquad \lambda_\ell = -\mathrm{Re}\left(\xi_\ell^\pm\right), \qquad (8.61a, b)$$

which are the roots of the dispersion relation (8.46a–d); (ii) the dispersion relation is specified by the vanishing of the determinant of the dispersion matrix (8.35a); (iii) the dispersion matrix involves the damping (8.32b) and oscillation (8.32c) matrices, which are specified by the mass (8.29a, b), friction (8.10a, b) and resilience (8.4a, b) matrices; (iv) the oscillation frequency (8.54a) is generally affected by the damping, and coincides with the natural frequency (8.55b) only for weak damping (8.55a); (v) the co-factors (8.58b) of the dispersion matrix (8.35a) ensure that the compatibility relations among the physical coordinates are satisfied; (vi) the displacements (8.60) imply (8.2b) the velocities (8.62):

$$\dot{x}_r(t) = -\sum_{\ell=1}^{N} P_{r\ell}(-\lambda_n \pm i\omega_n) C_\ell\, e^{-\lambda_\ell t}\left[\lambda_\ell \cos(\omega_\ell t - \alpha_\ell) + \omega_\ell \sin(\omega_\ell t - \alpha_\ell) \right];$$

$$(8.62)$$

(vii) the 2N arbitrary constants are the amplitudes C_ℓ and phases α_ℓ which can be determined from 2N compatible and non-redundant **initial conditions**, *for example, specifying the initial displacements (8.63a, b) and velocities (8.64a, b):*

$$x_{r0} \equiv x_r(0) = \sum_{\ell=1}^{N} P_{r\ell}(-\lambda_n \pm i\omega_n) C_\ell \cos\alpha_\ell, \qquad (8.63a, b)$$

$$\dot{x}_{r0} \equiv \dot{x}_r(0) = -\sum_{\ell=1}^{N} P_{r\ell}\left(-\lambda_n \pm i\omega_n\right)C_\ell\left(\lambda_\ell\cos\alpha_\ell - \omega_\ell\sin\alpha_\ell\right). \qquad \text{(8.64a, b)}$$

The modal coordinates can be applied both to the free (forced) motion [subsections 8.2.2–8.2.8 (8.2.9–8.2.14)] leading in the latter case to the modal forces.

8.2.9 Physical/Modal Coordinates and Forces

The relation (8.59b) from the natural to the physical coordinates can be inverted by multiplication (8.65a) by the dispersion matrix (8.35a) and use (8.58b) of the determinant in (8.65b, c):

$$\sum_{r=1}^{N} P_{sr}(\xi)x_r(t) = \sum_{\ell,r=1}^{N} P_{sr}(\xi)\bar{P}_{r\ell}(\xi)q_\ell(t) = \sum_{\ell,r=1}^{N} \delta_{s\ell}\,P_{2N}(\xi)\,q_\ell(t) = P_{2N}(\xi)\sum_{r=1}^{N} q_s(t).$$

$$\text{(8.65a–c)}$$

Thus, *the transformation from (problem 434) the physical to the modal coordinates (8.65c) ≡ (8.66c) involves the dispersion matrix (8.35a) divided by its determinant (8.36b):*

$$P_{2N}(\xi) \neq 0 \quad \Leftrightarrow \quad \xi \neq \xi_n: \qquad q_\ell(t) = \frac{1}{P_{2N}(\xi)}\sum_{r=1}^{N} P_{\ell r}(\xi)x_r(t), \qquad \text{(8.66a–c)}$$

and is valid for non-zero determinant (8.66a), that is, (8.36c) excludes the eigenvalues (8.66b); the restriction (8.66a) ≡ (8.66b) on the "inverse relation" (8.66c, d) does not apply to the direct relation (8.59b) from the natural to the physical coordinates. The work of the external applied forces on the physical coordinates (8.67a) can be used to define the **modal forces** (8.67b) that perform the same work on the modal coordinates:

$$\sum_{r=1}^{N} F_r\,dx_r = dW = \sum_{\ell=1}^{N} G_\ell\,dq_\ell; \qquad \sum_{r=1}^{N} F_r\,dx_r = \sum_{r,\ell=1}^{N} F_r\,\bar{P}_{r\ell}\,dq_\ell, \qquad \text{(8.67a–c)}$$

substitution of (8.59b) in (8.67a) leads to (8.67c), which compared with (8.67b) shows that *the transformation from physical to modal forces (8.68a) is specified (problem 435) by the matrix of co-factors (8.58c) of the dispersion matrix (8.35a):*

$$G_\ell(t) = \sum_{r=1}^{N} \bar{P}_{\ell r}\left(-\lambda \pm i\omega_n\right)F_r(t); \qquad F_r(t) = \frac{1}{\bar{P}_{2N}(\xi)}\sum_{\ell=1}^{N} P_{\ell r}(\xi)\,G_\ell(\xi), \qquad \text{(8.68a, b)}$$

*which is the same as the transformation (8.59b) from modal to physical coordinates. Conversely, the inverse (8.68b) of (8.68a) shows that the transformation from modal to physical forces is the same as the transformation (8.66c) from physical to modal coordinates, involving the dispersion matrix divided by its determinant. The reason for this **duality** (8.59a) ≡ (8.68a) and (8.66c) ≡ (8.68b) is that the displacement (force) is a contravariant (covariant) vector (note III.9.7), so that the work of the forces is an **invariant,** that is the same (8.67a, b) in terms of physical and modal coordinates and forces.* The physical (modal) coordinates are associated with the non-diagonal (diagonal) dispersion operator (subsection 8.2.10) and together with the physical (modal) forces specify the coupled (decoupled) equations of forced, damped oscillations (subsection 8.2.10).

8.2.10 Matrix and Diagonal Dispersion Operators

The coupled (decoupled) multidimensional oscillator (8.45b) [(8.53b)] exchanges (problem 436) the physical (modal) coordinates (8.69a) for the free motion with (8.69b):

$$
x_r(t) \quad \leftrightarrow \quad q_\ell(t), \qquad P_{rs}\left(\frac{d}{dt}\right) \quad \leftrightarrow \quad \delta_{rs} Q_s\left(\frac{d}{dt}\right), \qquad \text{(8.69a, b)}
$$

matrix (diagonal) dispersion operator (8.70a) [(8.70b)]:

$$
P_{rs}\left(\frac{d}{dt}\right) \equiv \frac{d^z}{dt^2} + 2\lambda_{rs}\frac{d}{dt} + \omega_{rs}^2, \qquad Q_r\left(\frac{d}{dt}\right) = \delta_{rs}\left(\frac{d^2}{dt^2} + 2\lambda_s\frac{d}{dt} + \omega_s^2\right),
$$

$$
\text{(8.70a, b)}
$$

which coincides with the dispersion matrix (8.35a) [(8.71c)]:

$$
\frac{d}{dt}\left(e^{\xi t}\right) = \xi e^{\xi t}: \qquad \xi \quad \leftrightarrow \quad \frac{d}{dt}, \qquad Q_{r\ell}(\xi) = \delta_{r\ell}\left(\xi^2 + 2\lambda_\ell \xi + \omega_\ell^2\right), \qquad \text{(8.71a–c)}
$$

replacing the eigenvalue by a time derivative (8.71b) for an exponential solution (8.71a). The tensor invariant form (note III.9.7) of the coupled equations of motion with explicit acceleration is (8.31a) ≡ (8.72c):

$$
f_r \quad \leftrightarrow \quad g_\ell: \qquad g_\ell(t) = \sum_{r=1}^{N} \overline{P}_{\ell r} f_r(t): \qquad \sum_{s=1}^{N}\left\{P_{rs}\left(\frac{d}{dt}\right)\right\} x_s(t) = f_r(t), \qquad \text{(8.72a–c)}
$$

*where the transformation from physical to modal coordinates shows that: (i) the coordinates form a contravariant vector (III.9.314b) ≡ (8.66c); (ii) the external forces (8.68a) and **reduced modal forces** (8.72a) form (8.72b) ≡ (III.9.316b) a covariant* *vector; (iii) the non-diagonal dispersion operator (8.70a) in (8.72c) is a covariant tensor with transformation law (III.9.320) ≡ (8.73) similar to the forces (8.68a) ≡ (8.72b):*

$$\sum_{r,s=1}^{N} \overline{P}_{\ell r}\left(\xi\right) P_{rs}\left(\frac{d}{dt}\right) \overline{P}_{sn}\left(\xi\right) = \delta_{\ell n} Q_{\ell}\left(\frac{d}{dt}\right), \tag{8.73}$$

and diagonalizes to the decoupled dispersion operator. The diagonalization of the dispersion operator (subsection 8.2.10) together with the modal forces (subsection 8.2.9) leads to decoupled equations for damped and forced oscillations (subsection 8.2.11).

8.2.11 Decoupled Damped and Forced Oscillations

The passage from (problem 437) the physical to modal coordinates (8.69a; 8.59b; 8.66c) and reduced forces (8.72a, b; 8.74a) transforms the equations of forced damped oscillations from coupled (8.31a) to decoupled (8.74b):

$$f_r\left(t\right) = \frac{1}{P_{2N}\left(\xi\right)} \sum_{\ell=1}^{N} P_{\ell r}\left(\xi\right) x_r\left(t\right): \qquad \ddot{q}_\ell + 2\lambda_\ell \dot{q}_\ell + \omega_\ell^2 = g_\ell\left(t\right), \tag{8.74a, b}$$

implying that: (i) the dispersion matrix (8.35a) is diagonalized (8.75b) into N dispersion relations:

$$P_{rs} \leftrightarrow Q_{rs}: \quad Q_{rs}\left(\xi\right) = \left(\xi^2 + 2\lambda_s \xi + \omega_s^2\right)\delta_{rs}; \quad \lambda_{rs} \leftrightarrow \lambda_s \delta_{rs}, \quad \omega_{rs}^2 \leftrightarrow \omega_s^2 \delta_{rs},$$
$$\tag{8.75a–d}$$

(iii) hence the damping (8.31b) [oscillation (8.31c)] matrices are replaced by the modal dampings (8.75c) [frequencies (8.75d)], which appear in the oscillation frequencies (8.54a). The proof of the decoupled equations of damped forced oscillation (8.74b) generalizing the unforced case (8.53a, b) is made in three steps: (i) the coupled equations of motion in physical coordinates (8.31a) specify the reduced physical force that is substituted in the reduced modal force (8.72b) leading to (8.76a); (ii) the physical coordinates are expressed in terms of modal coordinates by (8.59b) leading to (8.76b):

$$g_\ell\left(t\right) = \left\{\sum_{r,s=1}^{N} \overline{P}_{\ell r}\left(\xi\right) P_{rs}\left(\frac{d}{dt}\right)\right\} x_s\left(t\right) = \left\{\sum_{r,s,m=1}^{N} \overline{P}_{\ell r}\left(\xi\right) P_{rs}\left(\frac{d}{dt}\right) \overline{P}_{sn}\left(\xi\right)\right\} q_n\left(t\right)$$
$$\tag{8.76a–e}$$

$$= \left\{\delta_{\ell n} Q_\ell\left(\frac{d}{dt}\right)\right\} q_n\left(t\right) = \left\{Q_\ell\left(\frac{d}{dt}\right)\right\} q_\ell\left(t\right) = \ddot{q}_\ell + 2\lambda_\ell \dot{q}_\ell + \omega_\ell^2 q_\ell,$$

(iii) the operator in curly brackets in (8.76b) is (8.73) the diagonal dispersion operator (8.70b) leading to (8.76c), which simplifies (8.76d) to (8.76e) ≡ (8.74b). QED. The preceding results lead to the following *(problem 438) method for forced linear damped simultaneous oscillations (8.31a): (i) obtain the dispersion matrix (8.35a), its determinant (8.36b) and co-factors (8.58b); (ii) transform the physical to the reduced modal forces (8.72b); (iii) solve the decoupled forced modal reduced equations (8.74b); (iv) transform back to the physical coordinates (8.59b).* An alternative for forced oscillations is to solve directly (subsections 8.2.12–8.2.16) the coupled equations of motion (8.28).

8.2.12 Forcing with Bounded Fluctuation in a Finite Time Interval

A forcing function of time with bounded fluctuation (subsection I.27.9.5) in a finite interval (8.77a) can be represented (subsection II.5.7.6) by a Fourier series (II.5.168b) ≡ (8.77b) with period τ in (8.77c) and coefficients (I.5.169c) ≡ (8.77d):

$$0 \le t \le \tau: \qquad F_r(t) = \sum_{k=-\infty}^{+\infty} C_{rk}\, e^{i2\pi kt/\tau}, \qquad (8.77\text{a, b})$$

$$F_r(t+\tau) = F_r(t): \qquad C_{rk} = \frac{1}{\tau}\int_0^\tau F_r(t)\, e^{-i2\pi kt/\tau}\, dt. \qquad (8.77\text{c, d})$$

The forcing of a linear damped multidimensional oscillator (8.28) satisfies the principle of superposition (subsection III.7.6.2), which states that the displacement due to a superposition of forcings equals the sum of the displacements for each forcing. Thus, it is sufficient to consider one term of (8.77b), which is the forcing (8.78b) at an applied frequency (8.78a):

$$\omega_a = \frac{2\pi k}{\tau}: \qquad F_r(t) = G_r \cos(\omega_a t) = \mathrm{Re}\!\left(G_r\, e^{i\omega_a t}\right), \qquad (8.78\text{a–c})$$

and the complex representation of real quantities (section I.3.6) is used (8.78c), leading to a modal matrix (subsection 8.2.13).

8.2.13 Modal Matrix for Sinusoidal Forcing

Substituting the **sinusoidal forcing** (8.78c) in the equations of motion (8.28) for the linear damped oscillator:

$$x_s(t) = H_s\, e^{i\omega_a t}: \qquad \sum_{S=1}^{N}\left(m_{rs}\,\ddot{x}_s + \mu_{rs}\,\dot{x}_s + \omega_{rs}^2\, x_s\right) = G_r\, e^{i\omega_a t}, \qquad (8.79\text{a, b})$$

the displacement sought as (8.79a) an oscillation the same applied frequency and amplitudes to be determined. Substitution of (8.79a) in (8.79b) leads to (8.80):

$$G_r e^{i\omega_a t} = e^{i\omega_a t} \sum_{s=1}^{\infty} H_s \left(k_{rs} + 2 i \mu_{rs} \omega_a - m_{rs} \omega_a^2\right). \qquad (8.80)$$

Bearing in mind (8.81a) from (8.80) follows the relation (8.81b) between the amplitudes of forcing and displacement:

$$e^{i\omega_a t} \neq 0: \quad G_r = \sum_{s=1}^{N} H_s M_{sr}(\omega_a), \quad M_{rs}(\omega) \equiv k_{rs} + 2 i \mu_{rs} \omega - m_{rs} \omega^2, \qquad (8.81\text{a--c})$$

where (8.81c) is the **modal matrix** involving the resilience, damping, and mass matrices. Comparing (8.81c) with (8.35a; 8.31b, c) it follows that *(problem 439) the modal matrix (8.81c) equals (8.82a) the product of the mass matrix by the dispersion matrix (8.35a) and thus, has (8.36a–c) the same eigenvalues (8.82b, c):*

$$M_{rs}(\omega) = \sum_{\ell=1}^{N} m_{r\ell} P_{\ell s}(\omega): \qquad M_{2N}(\xi_n) = Det\left[M_{rs}(\xi_n)\right] = 0. \qquad (8.82\text{a--c})$$

Using (8.83a) the inverse modal matrix (8.83b), the amplitudes of the displacements are expressed in terms of the amplitudes of the forcing by (8.83c):

$$\sum_{\ell=1}^{N} M_{r\ell} \tilde{M}_{r\ell} = \delta_{rs}, \qquad \tilde{M}_{r\ell} = \frac{\bar{M}_{rs}}{M_{2N}}: \qquad H_r = \sum_{s=1}^{N} G_s \frac{\bar{M}_{rs}(\omega_a)}{M_{2N}(\omega_a)}. \qquad (8.83\text{a--c})$$

The relation (8.75c) is substituted in (8.79a) to specify the displacements of a sinusoidally forced linear multidimensional oscillator:

$$x_r(t) = \text{Re}\left\{\frac{e^{i\omega_a t}}{M_{2N}(\omega_a)} \sum_{s=1}^{N} \bar{M}_{rs}(\omega_a) G_s\right\}, \qquad (8.84)$$

which is considered next [subsections 8.2.14 (8.2.15)] in the undamped case using physical (modal) coordinates and forces.

8.2.14 Undamped Multidimensional Sinusoidal Forcing

The sinusoidal forcing (8.85b) of a linear multidimensional oscillator (8.79b) in the undamped case (8.85a):

$$\mu_{rs} = 0: \qquad \sum_{s=1}^{N}\left(m_{rs}\,\ddot{x}_s + \omega_{rs}\,x_s\right) = G_s\, e^{i\omega_a t}, \qquad (8.85a, b)$$

leads (problem 440) to the displacements (8.86c), similar to (8.84) for the undamped (8.86a) modal matrix (8.81c):

$$N_{rs}(\omega) = k_{rs} + m_{rs}\,\omega^2;\ \omega_a \neq \omega_n: \qquad x_r(t) = \mathrm{Re}\left\{\frac{e^{i\omega_a t}}{N_{2N}(\omega_a)}\sum_{s=1}^{N}G_s\,\bar{N}_{rs}(\omega_a)\right\},$$

$$(8.86a\text{–}c)$$

in the non-resonant case, when (8.86b) the applied frequency does not coincide with any of the modal frequencies. In the resonant case (8.87a), when the applied frequency equals one of the modal frequencies the displacements are given by (8.87b):

$$\omega_a = \omega_n: \qquad x_r(t) = \lim_{\omega \to \omega_a}\mathrm{Re}\left\{\frac{e^{i\omega t}}{\partial N_{2N}(\omega)/\partial\omega}\sum_{s=1}^{N}G_s\,\bar{N}_{rs}(\omega)\right\}$$

$$(8.87a\text{–}c)$$

$$= \mathrm{Re}\left\{\frac{e^{i\omega_a t}}{N'_{2N}(\omega_a)}\sum_{s=1}^{N}G_s\left[\bar{N}'_{2N}(\omega_a) + i\,t\,\bar{N}_{rs}(\omega_a)\right]\right\},$$

consisting (8.87c) of two terms: (i) one with constant amplitude involving the derivative with regards to the frequency of the matrix of co-factors of the undamped modal matrix (8.86a); (ii) the latter undamped modal matrix appears in the second term with an amplitude increasing linearly with time. The passage from non-resonant (8.86a, b) to the resonant (8.87a, b) forcing uses (section I.19.8) the L'Hôspital rule (I.19.35) as an alternative to the method in subsection 2.7.3. This alternative can be justified more simply using modal coordinates (subsection 8.2.15).

8.2.15 Beats and Resonant and Non-Resonant Forcing

The sinusoidal forcing (problem 441) of a linear multidimensional undamped (8.88a) oscillator can be decoupled (8.88b) using modal coordinates and forces (8.72b):

$$\lambda_\ell = 0: \qquad \ddot{q}_\ell + \omega_\ell^2\, q_\ell = \mathrm{Re}\left(g_\ell\, e^{i\omega_a t}\right), \qquad (8.88a, b)$$

leading to three cases for the displacement:

$$q_\ell(t) = \begin{cases} \mathrm{Re}\left\{\dfrac{g_\ell}{\omega_\ell^2 - \omega_a^2}e^{i\omega_a t}\right\} & \text{if} \quad \omega_a \neq \omega_\ell, & (8.89a) \\[4mm] \dfrac{g_\ell}{2\omega_\ell\,\varepsilon}\sin(\varepsilon t)\sin(\omega_\ell t) & \text{if} \quad \omega_a = \omega_\ell + \varepsilon, & (8.89b) \\[4mm] \dfrac{g_\ell}{2\omega_\ell}t\sin(\omega_\ell t) & \text{if} \quad \omega_a = \omega_\ell, & (8.89c) \end{cases}$$

*namely: (i) an oscillation with constant amplitude (8.89a) in the non-resonant case of applied frequency not close to the modal frequency; (ii) if the applied and modal frequencies are close $\varepsilon \ll \omega_a - \omega_\ell$ there are **beats** (8.89b), that is, oscillations at the modal frequency ω_ℓ with **sinusoidal amplitude modulation** at the small difference frequency $\varepsilon = \omega_a - \omega_\ell$; (iii) in the **resonant limit** $\varepsilon \to 0$ when the applied and modal frequencies coincide (8.89c) the amplitude increases linearly with time. The three cases of modal sinusoidal forcing (i)(ii)(iii) are the same as for a one-dimensional oscillator (subsections 2.7.1–2.7.2; 2.7.5–2.7.6; 2.7.3–2.7.4).*

The undamped resonant displacement (8.89c) due to sinusoidal forcing can be obtained by three methods: (i) the method used in subsection 2.7.3; (ii) the limit of beats (8.89b) for coincident frequencies leads to (8.90b) $\equiv$ (8.89c):

$$\lim_{\zeta \to 0}\frac{\sin\zeta}{\zeta} = 1: \qquad \frac{g_\ell}{2\,\omega_\ell}\sin(\omega_\ell t)\lim_{\varepsilon \to 0}\frac{\sin(\varepsilon t)}{\varepsilon} = \frac{g_\ell t}{2\omega_\ell}\sin(\omega_\ell t), \qquad (8.90a, b)$$

using (8.90a); (iii) the use of the L'Hôspital rule, as in the passage from (8.86a, b) to (8.87a–c), which is justified next. From a forced oscillation (8.89a) may be subtracted a free oscillation with the same amplitude leading to (8.91):

$$q_\ell(t) = \frac{g_\ell}{\omega_\ell^2 - \omega_a^2}\left[\cos(\omega_a t) - \cos(\omega_\ell t)\right]. \qquad (8.91)$$

In the resonant limit (8.92a) $\equiv$ (8.92b), both the numerator and denominator of (8.91) have simple zeros, and the indetermination of type 0:0 is lifted (subsection I.19.8) using the L'Hôspital rule (I.19.38), which leads to (8.92c) $\equiv$ (8.92d):

$$\varepsilon = \omega_a - \omega_\ell \to 0 \Leftrightarrow \quad \omega_a \to \omega_\ell: \quad q_\ell(t) = \lim_{\omega_a \to \omega_\ell}\frac{g_\ell}{-2\,\omega_a}\frac{\partial}{\partial\omega_a}\left[\cos(\omega_a t) - \cos(\omega_\ell t)\right]$$

$$= \frac{g_\ell}{2\,\omega_\ell}\lim_{\omega_a \to \omega_\ell}t\sin(\omega_a t) = \frac{g_\ell t}{2\omega_\ell}\sin(\omega_\ell t),$$

$$(8.92a–e)$$

which proves (8.92e) ≡ (8.89c). The physical (modal) coordinates [subsection 8.9.14 (8.9.15)] may be used not only for undamped but also for damped forcing (subsection 8.2.16).

8.2.16 Forcing of a Damped Multidimensional Oscillator

The sinusoidal forcing of a damped linear multidimensional oscillator (8.79b) leads (problem 442) to oscillations with constant amplitude (8.84) in all cases, with the resonant case distinguished from the non-resonant case only by replacing the applied with the modal frequency (8.92b). In terms of modal coordinates (8.74b) the sinusoidal forcing (8.93a):

$$\ddot{q}_\ell + 2\,\lambda_\ell \dot{q}_\ell + \bar{\omega}_\ell^2\, q_\ell = \mathrm{Re}\!\left(g_\ell\, e^{i\omega_a t}\right)\!: \qquad q_\ell(t) = \mathrm{Re}\left\{\frac{g_\ell\, e^{i\omega_a t}}{\bar{\omega}_\ell^2 - \omega_a^2 + 2\,i\lambda_\ell \omega_a}\right\}, \qquad \text{(8.93a, b)}$$

leads to the modal displacements (8.93b), which simplify to (8.94b) in the resonant case (8.94a):

$$\omega_a = \bar{\omega}_\ell\!: \qquad\qquad q_\ell(t) = \mathrm{Re}\left\{-i\,\frac{g}{2\lambda_\ell \omega_\ell}\, e^{i\omega_\ell t}\right\}. \qquad\qquad \text{(8.94a, b)}$$

In all cases of damped forcing, resonant (8.94a, b) [non-resonant (8.93a, b)] the amplitude is constant, and the phase ϕ is $0 < \phi < \pi/2\,(\phi = \pi/2)$.
 The use of modal coordinates (problem 443) diagonalizes (8.95a, b, c) the potential (8.7a–d)/kinetic (8.29a, b) energies and dissipation function (8.11a, b) per unit mass:

$$\{\Phi, E_v, \Psi\} = \sum_{\ell=1}^{N}\left\{\frac{1}{2}\dot{q}_\ell^2, \frac{1}{2}\big(\bar{\omega}_\ell\, q_\ell\big)^2, -2\lambda_\ell\, \dot{q}_\ell^2\right\}\!: \qquad \frac{dW}{dt} \equiv \sum_{\ell=1}^{N} g_\ell\, \dot{q}_\ell = \dot{\Phi} + \dot{E}_v - \Psi,$$

$$\text{(8.95a–d)}$$

and leads to a diagonalized (8.95d) energy balance (8.21a, b) using modal forces; the latter (8.95d) follows (8.96a) from (8.74b):

$$\frac{dW}{dt} = \sum_{\ell=1}^{N}\dot{q}_\ell\big(\ddot{q}_\ell + 2\lambda_\ell\, \dot{q}_\ell + \bar{\omega}_\ell^2\, q_\ell\big) = \frac{d}{dt}\left\{\sum_{\ell=1}^{N}\frac{1}{2}\Big[\dot{q}_\ell^2 + \big(\omega_\ell\, q_\ell\big)^2\Big]\right\} - \sum_{\ell=1}^{N} 2\lambda_\ell\, \dot{q}_\ell^2,$$

$$\text{(8.96a, b)}$$

as shown by the coincidence of (8.96d) ≡ (8.95a–d). *Diagram 8.1 summarizes (problem 444), the three cases of coupled (decoupled) free multidimensional oscillations: (case I) free undamped oscillations (8.59b) [(8.44c)] with modal frequencies*

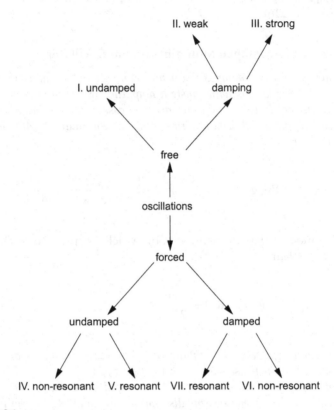

CLASSIFICATION OF OSCILLATIONS

DIAGRAM 8.1
The classification of oscillations applies both in one (several) dimensions [chapter 2(8)] and uses the same criteria: (i) free (forced) in the absence (presence) of external forces; (ii) undamped (damped) in the absence (presence) of dissipation. The damping is weak (strong) if much smaller (comparable) to the modal frequency. Amplification can be seen as negative damping. The sinusoidal forcing is non-resonant (resonant) if the applied frequency does not (does) coincide with a modal frequency. Beats occur at the undamped transition from non-resonant to resonant response.

(8.43b, c); (cases II/III) free damped oscillations (8.59b) [(8.54b)] with modal damp-ings (8.49c) and oscillation frequency for strong (8.54a) [weak (8.55a, b)] damp-ing. In addition there are four cases of forced oscillations without (with) resonance: (cases IV/V) undamped forced oscillations without (8.86c) [with (8.87c)] resonance if the applied frequency does not (8.86b) [does (8.87a)] equal an oscillation frequency using physical coordinates; (cases VI/VII) damped forced oscillations without (8.93b) [with (8.94a, b)] resonance using modal coordinates. The simplest illus-tration of a multidimensional simultaneous oscillator (section 8.1) is the two-dimensional coupled oscillator (section 8.3), which can be considered (section 8.2) in unforced (forced) cases [section 8.4 (8.5)].

8.3 Coupled Circuits and Electromechanical Simulations

The simplest case of the general theory (sections 8.1–8.2) of the damped
N-dimensional free (forced) oscillator [section 8.4 (8.5)] is two-dimensional
(section 8.3). Three examples are given of equivalent coupled circuits, such
that each allows an electromechanical simulation (subsections 8.3.4–8.3.5) of
the other two. The three analogous two-dimensional oscillators are: (i) two
masses with two applied forces connected to each other and to two fixed
walls by three pairs of springs and dampers (subsection 8.3.1); (ii) two electrical circuits consisting of distinct selfs, resistors, capacitors, and batteries
with a common branch with a resistor and a capacitor (subsection 8.3.2);
(iii) the suspension of a two-wheeled vehicle. The particular cases of the latter include: (iii-a) a diatomic molecule represented by two masses at a fixed
distance; (iii-b) a homogeneous rod acted by forces and moments that can
perform heave (and pitch) oscillations, that is, vertical (rotatory) displacements (subsection 8.3.3). The analogy among the three circuits applies to
different physical coordinates (subsection 8.3.4) and the associated mass,
friction, and resilience (damping and oscillation) matrices, which specify the
modal (dispersion) matrix (subsection 8.3.5).

8.3.1 Two Masses Linked by Three Spring-Damper Units

The first example (Figure 8.1a) concerns two masses m_1, m_2 connected to rigid
walls by two spring-damper sets connected to each other through a third
spring-damped set. The equations of motion (8.97a, b):

$$m_1\ddot{x}_1 + \mu_1\dot{x}_1 - \mu_3(\dot{x}_2 - \dot{x}_1) + k_1 x_1 - k_3(x_2 - x_1) = F_1(t), \qquad (8.97a)$$

$$m_2\ddot{x}_2 + \mu_2\dot{x}_2 - \mu_3(\dot{x}_1 - \dot{x}_2) + k_2 x_2 - k_3(x_1 - x_2) = F_2(t), \qquad (8.97b)$$

take into account that the middle damper (spring) connects the two damped
oscillators near the walls through the difference of velocities (displacements).
The equations of motion (8.97a, b) ≡ (8.98a, b) can be rewritten with the separate oscillators on the left-hand side (l.h.s.) and coupling and forcing terms
on the right-hand side (r.h.s.):

$$m_1\ddot{x}_1 + (\mu_1 + \mu_3)\dot{x}_1 + (k_1 + k_3)x_1 = F_1(t) + \mu_3\dot{x}_2 + k_3 x_2, \qquad (8.98a)$$

$$m_2\ddot{x}_2 + (\mu_1 + \mu_3)\dot{x}_2 + (k_2 + k_3)x_2 = F_2(t) + \mu_3\dot{x}_1 + k_3 x_1, \qquad (8.98b)$$

and the middle spring-damper set acting on both oscillators. The equations
of motion (8.97a, b) ≡ (8.98a, b) include external forces $F_{1,2}(t)$ applied to the

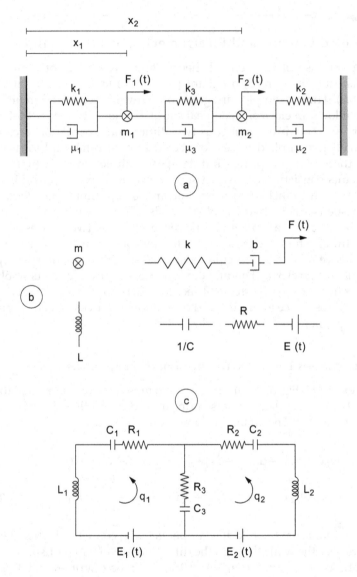

FIGURE 8.1
The analogy (b) between mass (self), spring (condenser), damper (resistor), and mechanical (electromotive) force allows the simulation of (a) a mechanical circuit consisting of masses, springs, dampers forced by external forces by (c) an electrical circuit consisting of selfs, capacitors, and resistors driven by electromotive forces. The examples of two-dimensional coupled oscillators include the Figures 8.1a, c; 8.2a, b, c; and 8.3a, b.

two masses. In the absence of these forces (8.99a) there are free oscillations, which are analyzed next (subsection 8.3.1) [subsequently (section 8.4)] in the absence (8.99b) [presence] of damping. The oscillators are decoupled if the middle spring is non-existent (8.99c):

$$F_1 = F_2 = \mu_1 = \mu_2 = \mu_3 = 0 = k_3: \quad \ddot{x}_{1,2} + \omega_{1,2}^2 \, x_{1,2} = 0, \quad \omega_{1,2} \equiv \frac{\sqrt{k_{1,2}}}{m_{1,2}}, \qquad (8.99\text{a–e})$$

in which case each mass oscillates independently (8.99d) with its own natural frequency (8.99e). The presence of the middle spring couples the oscillations of the two masses, for example, if only the mass m_1 is displaced, this deforms the spring k_3, which exerts a force on the mass m_2 and sets it in motion too. The coupled equations of motion (8.97a, b) $\equiv$ (8.98a, b) for the undamped motion (8.100a) can be written in matrix form (8.100b):

$$\mu_1 = \mu_2 = \mu_3 = 0: \quad \begin{bmatrix} \ddot{x}_1 \\ \\ \ddot{x}_2 \end{bmatrix} + \begin{bmatrix} \dfrac{k_1 + k_3}{m_1} & -\dfrac{k_3}{m_1} \\ \\ -\dfrac{k_3}{m_2} & \dfrac{k_2 + k_3}{m_2} \end{bmatrix} \begin{bmatrix} x_1 \\ \\ x_2 \end{bmatrix} = \begin{bmatrix} \dfrac{F_1(t)}{m_1} \\ \\ \dfrac{F_2(t)}{m_2} \end{bmatrix};$$

$$(8.100\text{a, b})$$

for a free (8.101a) undamped (8.101b) oscillator the modal frequencies are the roots of (8.101c):

$$F_1, F_2 = 0 = \mu_1 = \mu_2 = \mu_3: \quad \begin{vmatrix} \dfrac{k_1 + k_3}{m_1} - \omega^2 & -\dfrac{k_3}{m_1} \\ \\ -\dfrac{k_3}{m_2} & \dfrac{k_2 + k_3}{m_2} - \omega^2 \end{vmatrix} = 0,$$

$$(8.101\text{a–c})$$

that is, ω^2 are the eigenvalues (8.101c) of the matrix in (8.100).

The equation (8.101c) is a biquadratic (8.102) in ω:

$$0 = \left(k_1 + k_3 - m_1 \, \omega^2\right)\left(k_2 + k_3 - m_2 \, \omega^2\right) - k_3^2$$

$$= m_1 \, m_2 \, \omega^4 - \left[\left(k_1 + k_3\right)m_2 + \left(k_2 + k_3\right)m_1\right]\omega^2 + \left(k_1 + k_3\right)\left(k_2 + k_3\right) - k_3^2,$$

$$(8.102)$$

whose roots specify the modal frequencies:

$$2m_1 m_2 \omega_\pm^2 = (k_1 + k_3)m_2 + (k_2 + k_3)m_1 \pm \sqrt{\Omega}. \tag{8.103}$$

where the discriminant is given by (8.104a):

$$\Omega = \left[(k_1 + k_3)m_2 + (k_2 + k_3)m_1\right]^2 - 4(k_1 + k_3)(k_2 + k_3)m_1 m_2 + 4m_1 m_2 k_3^2$$

$$= \left[(k_1 + k_3)m_2 - (k_2 + k_3)m_1\right]^2 + 4\,m_1 m_2\,k_3^2$$

$$= \left[(k_1 + k_3)m_2 + (k_2 + k_3)m_1\right]^2 - 4m_1 m_2 (k_1 k_2 + k_1 k_3 + k_2 k_3).$$

$$\tag{8.104a–c}$$

From (8.104b) it follows (i) that the discriminant is positive Ω, and hence the modal frequencies are real and distinct $\omega_+^2 \neq \omega_-^2$ in (8.103); from (8.104c) it follows (ii) that $\sqrt{\Omega}$ is smaller than the term in square brackets in (8.102), and hence, (8.103) is positive. Thus (i) and (ii) imply that the modal frequencies $\omega_\pm$ are real and hence, the motion is an oscillation with constant amplitude. If the system is decoupled by removing the middle spring (8.105a):

$$k_3 = 0: \qquad \omega_\pm^2 = \frac{1}{2}\left[\left(\frac{k_1}{m_1} + \frac{k_2}{m_2}\right) \pm \left(\frac{k_1}{m_1} - \frac{k_2}{m_2}\right)\right] = \frac{k_{1,2}}{m_{1,2}} = \omega_\pm^2, \tag{8.105a–c}$$

the modal frequencies (8.103) simplify (8.105b) to the natural frequencies (8.105c) ≡ (8.99e). Thus, *(problem 445) the two-dimensional free (8.101a) oscillator consisting (Figure 8.1a) of two masses connected to each other and to two rigid walls by linear springs without dampers (8.101b) have (8.97a, b) ≡ (8.98a, b) the equations of motion (8.106a, b):*

$$m_1 \ddot{x}_1 + (k_1 + k_3)x_1 = k_3 x_2, \qquad m_2 \ddot{x}_2 + (k_2 + k_3)x_2 = k_3 x_1, \tag{8.106a, b}$$

leading to the coupled modal frequencies (8.103; 8.104a–c). In the absence of middle spring (8.107a) ≡ (8.105a) the decoupled (8.99d) natural frequencies are (8.99e) ≡ (8.105b) ≡ (8.107b):

$$k_3 = 0: \qquad \omega_\pm = \omega_{1,2} = \sqrt{\frac{k_{1,2}}{m_{1,2}}}; \qquad \omega_1 = \omega_2 \;\Leftrightarrow\; k_1 m_2 = k_1 m, \tag{8.107a–d}$$

which *coincide (8.107c) if the condition (8.103d) is met.* An electric analogue of this mechanical circuit is considered next (subsection 8.3.2).

8.3.2 Pair of Electrical Circuits with a Common Branch

In order to find the quasi-stationary electrical circuit analogous to the mechanical oscillator just described (subsection 8.2.1) the analogy between a mass m (self L), a spring k (capacitor $1/C$) and an external force $F(t)$ [electromotive force $E(t)$], is used (Figure 8.1b) leading to the pair of coupled electrical circuits (Figure 8.1c). The latter may be taken as the **analogue simulator** of the mechanical system. In the electromechanical analogy, the displacements x_1, x_2 correspond to electric charges q_1, q_2 and the velocities $\dot{x}_1, \dot{x}_2$ correspond to electric currents $\dot{q}_1, \dot{q}_2$. The equations of the coupled electrical circuits in Figure 8.1c are (8.108a, b):

$$L_1 \ddot{q}_1 + R_1 \dot{q}_1 - R_3 \left(\dot{q}_2 - \dot{q}_1 \right) + \frac{q_1}{C_1} - \frac{q_2 - q_1}{C_3} = E_1(t), \tag{8.108a}$$

$$L_2 \dot{q}_2 + R_3 \dot{q}_2 - R_3 \left(\dot{q}_1 - \dot{q}_3 \right) + \frac{q_2}{C_2} - \frac{q_1 - q_2}{C_3} = E_2(t), \tag{8.108b}$$

where the decoupled (coupled and forcing) terms on the l.h.s. (r.h.s.) of (8.109a, b) can be separated:

$$L_1 \ddot{q}_1 + (R_1 + R_3) \dot{q}_1 + \left(\frac{1}{C_1} + \frac{1}{C_3} \right) q_1 = E_1(t) + R_3 \dot{q}_2 + \frac{q_2}{C_3}, \tag{8.109a}$$

$$L_2 \ddot{q}_2 + (R_2 + R_3) \ddot{q}_1 + \left(\frac{1}{C_2} + \frac{1}{C_3} \right) q_2 = E_2(t) + R_3 \dot{q}_1 + \frac{q_1}{C_3}. \tag{8.109b}$$

In the absence of resistance (8.110b), the free oscillations (8.110a) of the two circuits are decoupled if the middle condenser C_3 is removed (8.110c):

$$E_1 = E_2 = R_1 = R_1 = R_3 = 0 = \frac{1}{C_3}: \quad \ddot{q}_1 + \omega_1^2 q_1 = 0 = \ddot{q}_2 + \omega_2^2 q_2, \quad \omega_{1,2} = \frac{1}{\sqrt{L_{1,2} C_{1,2}}},$$

$$\tag{8.110a–e}$$

in which case, each circuit oscillates independently (8.110d) at its own natural frequency (8.110e). In the coupled case, making the substitutions (8.111):

$$m_1, m_2, k_1, k_2, k_3 \quad \Leftrightarrow \quad L_1, L_2, \frac{1}{C_1}, \frac{1}{C_2}, \frac{1}{C_3}, \tag{8.111}$$

leads (8.103; 8.104b) to the modal frequencies (8.112a, b):

$$2 L_1 L_2 \, \omega_\pm^2 = L_2 \left(\frac{1}{C_1} + \frac{1}{C_3} \right) + L_1 \left(\frac{1}{C_2} + \frac{1}{C_3} \right) \pm \sqrt{\Omega} \, , \qquad (8.112a)$$

$$\Omega = \left[L_2 \left(\frac{1}{C_1} + \frac{1}{C_3} \right) - L_1 \left(\frac{1}{C_2} + \frac{1}{C_3} \right) \right]^2 + \frac{4 L_1 L_2}{C_3^2} . \qquad (8.112b)$$

In the decoupled case (8.113a):

$$C_3 = \infty: \quad \omega_\pm^2 = \frac{1}{2} \left[\left(\frac{1}{L_1 C_1} + \frac{1}{L_2 C_2} \right) \pm \frac{1}{L_1 C_1} - \frac{1}{L_2 C_2} \right] = \frac{1}{L_{1,2} \, C_{1,2}} = \omega_{1,2}^2 , \qquad (8.113a, b)$$

the modal frequencies (8.113b) coincide with the natural frequencies (8.110e). Thus, *(problem 446) the electrical simulator or analogue (Figure 8.1b) of the two-dimensional mechanical circuit in Figure 8.1a is the set of two electrical circuits in Figure 8.1c, each consisting of a self and a capacitor coupled by a common branch with a capacitor, excluding forcing (8.114a) and resistances (8.114b) in (8.114c, d):*

$$E_1 = E_2 = 0 = \mu_1 = \mu_2 = \mu_3: \quad L_1 \, \ddot{q}_1 + q_1 \left(\frac{1}{C_1} + \frac{1}{C_3} \right) = \frac{q_2}{C_3}, \; L_2 \, \ddot{q}_2 + \left(\frac{1}{C_2} + \frac{1}{C_3} \right) q_2 = \frac{q_1}{C_3} ,$$
$$(8.114a\text{–}d)$$

and has coupled natural frequencies (8.112a, b). In the absence of a middle capacitor (8.115a) ≡ (8.113a) the decoupled natural frequencies are (8.115b) ≡ (8.113b) ≡ (8.110e):

$$C_3 = \infty: \quad \omega_\pm = \omega_{1,2} = \frac{1}{\sqrt{L_{1,2} \, C_{1,2}}}; \quad \omega_1 = \omega_2 \;\Leftrightarrow\; L_1 \, C_1 = L_2 \, C_2 , \quad (8.115a\text{–}d)$$

which coincide (8.115c) if the condition (8.115d) is met. The same electrical circuit (Figure 8.1c) can simulate (subsection 8.3.4) distinct mechanical circuits (Figures 8.1a and 8.2a) through suitable choices of parameters (subsections 8.3.1 and 8.3.3).

8.3.3 Damped Suspension of a Two-Wheeled Vehicle

As a third example, consider a "plane" rigid body supported on two unequal springs and dampers, for example, to model the oscillations of a two-wheeled vehicle, like a motorcycle, consisting of: (i) heave, which is vertical displacement z; (ii) pitch, which is rotation θ. These are longitudinal motions, which are a simplification of a car (Figure 8.2a); in general,

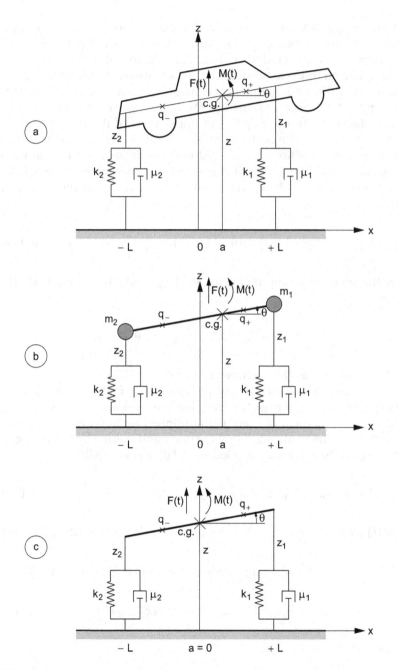

FIGURE 8.2
An example of two-dimensional oscillator is the motion in a plane consisting of coupled translation of (rotation around) the center of mass, and applies to: (a) a two-wheeled vehicle; (b) a diatomic molecule; (c) a homogeneous rod. In all cases the translational (rotational) forcing is by a force (moment).

for a four-wheeled vehicle there are also lateral, longitudinal, rolling, and yawing motions. In the case of a motorcycle, only the motion in the vertical plane is considered; excluded are lateral, longitudinal, rolling, and yawing motions. The methods to address these six-dimensional motions are similar to the two-dimensional motion considered next. Two motions, namely heave and pitch, serve to illustrate the coupling. The origin is placed at equal distance $\pm L$ from the point of application of the two springs k_1, k_2 and dampers μ_1, μ_2. The center of mass is located (Figure 8.2b) at the coordinate $x = a$, the position of the rigid body is determined by the vertical displacement z of the center of mass and the angular rotation θ relative to the horizontal, which determine the extensions $z_{1,2}$ of the two springs (8.116a):

$$\{z_1, z_2\} - z = \{L - a, L + a\} \tan \theta = \{L - a, L + a\} \theta + \left[1 + O(\theta^3)\right], \quad \text{(8.116a, b)}$$

where the small-angle approximation (8.116b) ≡ (8.117b, c) is made for linear oscillators:

$$-L \leq a \leq +L: \qquad z_1 = z + \theta(L - a), \qquad z_2 = z - \theta(L + a), \qquad \text{(8.117a–c)}$$

and the center of mass lies between the wheels (8.117a).

The equations of motion specify the balance of forces (8.118a) [moments (8.118b)] at the center of mass, by equating the inertia force (moment), equal to the mass m (moment of inertia I) multiplied by the linear $\ddot{z}$ (angular $\ddot{\theta}$) acceleration, to the total restoring force (moment) exerted by the springs and dampers plus the externally applied force $F(t)$ [moment $M(t)$]:

$$F(t) = m\ddot{z} + \mu_1 \dot{z}_1 + \mu_2 \dot{z}_2 + k_1 z_1 + \mu_2 z_2, \qquad \text{(8.118a)}$$

$$M(t) = I\ddot{\theta} + (L - a)\mu_1 \dot{z}_1 - (L + a)\mu_2 \dot{z}_2 + (L - a)k_1 z_1 - (L + a)k_2 z_2. \qquad \text{(8.118b)}$$

Substitution of (8.117b, c) in the restoring forces in (8.118a) leads to (8.119):

$$k_1 z_1 + k_2 z_2 = (k_1 + k_2)(z - a\theta) + (k_1 - k_2)\theta L, \qquad \text{(8.119)}$$

and implies (8.120a, b):

$$b \equiv (k_1 + k_2) a + (k_2 - k_1) L: \qquad k_1 z_1 + k_2 z_2 = (k_1 + k_2)z - b\theta, \qquad \text{(8.120a, b)}$$

$$c \equiv (\mu_1 + \mu_2) a + (\mu_2 - \mu_1) L: \qquad \mu_1 \dot{z}_1 + \mu_2 \dot{z}_2 = (\mu_1 + \mu_2)\dot{z} - c\,\dot{\theta}, \qquad \text{(8.121a, b)}$$

and likewise (8.121a, b) for the friction forces; substitution of (8.117b, c) in the moment of the restoring forces in (8.118b) leads to (8.122):

$$(L-a)\,k_1\,z_1 - (L+a)k_2\,z_2 = \left[(L-a)\,k_1 - (L+a)\,k_2\right]z + \left[(L-a)^2\,k_1 + (L+a)^2\,k_2\right]\theta,$$

$$(8.122)$$

and implies (8.123a, b):

$$\bar{b} = k_1(L-a)^2 + k_2(L+a)^2: \quad (L-a)\,k_1\,z_1 - (L+a)\,k_2\,z_2 = -bz + \bar{b}\,\theta, \quad (8.123a, b)$$

$$\bar{c} = (L-a)^2\,\mu_1 + (L+a)^2\,\mu_2: \quad (L-a)\,\mu_1\,\dot{z}_1 - (L+a)\,\mu_2\,\dot{z}_2 = -c\,\dot{z} + \bar{c}\,\dot{\theta},$$

$$(8.124a, b)$$

and likewise (8.124a, b) for the moments of the friction forces.

Substitution of (8.120b; 8.121b) [(8.123b; 8.124b)] in (8.118a) [(8.118b)] shows that *(problem 447) for a rigid body (car, motorcycle) with mass m and moment of inertia I relative to the center of mass at unequal distance from the two wheels with distinct sets of springs and dampers, the coupled translational (8.125a) [rotational (8.125b)] equations of motion:*

$$m\ddot{z} + (\mu_1 + \mu_2)\dot{z} + (k_1 + k_2)z = c\,\dot{\theta} + b\theta + F(t), \qquad (8.125a)$$

$$I\ddot{\theta} + \bar{c}\,\dot{\theta} + \bar{b}\,\theta = c\,\dot{z} + bz + M(t), \qquad (8.125b)$$

involve three sets of two constants: (i) for the free translational motion on the l.h.s. of (8.125a) the sum of the two frictions (resiliences) in the damping (restoring) forces; (ii) for the free rotation motion on the l.h.s. of (8.125b) the damping (restoring) moments involve the constants (8.124a) [(8.123a)] with the dimensions of square of length times friction coefficient (resilience); (iii) the terms coupling the translation and rotation motions on the r.h.s. of (8.125a, b) for the damping (restoring) forces in (8.125a) and moments in (8.125b) involve the constants (8.121a) [(8.120a)] with the dimensions of length multiplied by kinematic friction coefficient (spring resilience). The three two-dimensional oscillators (subsections 8.3.1–8.3.3) can be made equivalent by a suitable choice of parameters (subsection 8.3.4).

8.3.4 Three Analogue Mechanical and Electrical Circuits

The equations of motion (8.125a, b) can be written in matrix form (8.126):

$$\begin{bmatrix} m\ddot{z} \\ I\ddot{\theta} \end{bmatrix} + \begin{bmatrix} \mu_1 + \mu_2 & -c \\ -c & \bar{c} \end{bmatrix} \begin{bmatrix} \dot{z} \\ \dot{\theta} \end{bmatrix} + \begin{bmatrix} k_1 + k_2 & -b \\ -b & \bar{b} \end{bmatrix} \begin{bmatrix} z \\ \theta \end{bmatrix} = \begin{bmatrix} F(t) \\ M(t) \end{bmatrix};$$

$$(8.126)$$

the equations of the coupled electrical circuits (8.108a, b) can be put in matrix form (8.127):

$$
\begin{bmatrix} L_1 \ddot{q}_1 \\ L_2 \ddot{q}_2 \end{bmatrix} +
\begin{bmatrix} R_1 + R_3 & -R_3 \\ -R_3 & R_2 + R_3 \end{bmatrix}
\begin{bmatrix} q_1 \\ q_2 \end{bmatrix}
$$

$$
+ \begin{bmatrix} C_1^{-1} + C_3^{-1} & -C_3^{-1} \\ -C_3^{-1} & C_2^{-1} + C_3^{-1} \end{bmatrix}
= \begin{bmatrix} E_1(t) \\ E_2(t) \end{bmatrix} ;
\tag{8.127}
$$

the equations of motion (8.98a, b) take the matrix form (8.128):

$$
\begin{bmatrix} m_1 \ddot{x}_1 \\ m_2 \ddot{x}_2 \end{bmatrix} +
\begin{bmatrix} \mu_1 + \mu_3 & -\mu_3 \\ -\mu_3 & \mu_2 + \mu_3 \end{bmatrix}
\begin{bmatrix} \dot{x}_1 \\ \dot{x}_2 \end{bmatrix} +
\begin{bmatrix} k_1 + k_3 & -k_3 \\ -k_3 & k_2 + k_3 \end{bmatrix}
\begin{bmatrix} x_1 \\ x_2 \end{bmatrix}
$$

$$
= \begin{bmatrix} F_1(t) \\ F_2(t) \end{bmatrix} .
\tag{8.128}
$$

Thus, *the following three circuits are (problem 448) analogues: (i) the electrical (Figure 8.1c) and mechanical circuits [Figure 8.1a (8.2a)]; (ii) the currents correspond to linear (linear and angular displacements) in (8.129a, b):*

$$
q_1 \equiv \{x_1, z\}, \quad q_2 \equiv \{x_2, \theta\}; \quad E_1(t) \equiv \{F_1(t), F(t)\}, \quad E_2(t) = \{F(t), M(t)\},
\tag{8.129a–d}
$$

(iii) the electromotive forces correspond to forces (forces and moments) in (8.129c, d); (iv) the inductions correspond to masses and moment of inertia (8.130a, b):

$$
L_1 = \{m_1, m\}, \qquad L_2 = \{m_2, I\};
\tag{8.130a, b}
$$

(v) the resistances correspond to kinematic frictions (8.131a–c):

$$
R_3 = \{\mu_3, c\}: \quad R_1 = \{\mu_1 + \mu_3, \mu_1 + \mu_2\} - R_3 = \{\mu_1, \mu_1 + \mu_2 - c\},
\tag{8.131a, b}
$$

$$
R_2 = \{\mu_2 + \mu_3, \bar{c}\} - R_3 = \{\mu_2, \bar{c} - c\};
\tag{8.131c}
$$

(vi) the capacities correspond to resiliences (8.132a–c):

$$\frac{1}{C_3} = \left\{ k_3, b \right\}: \qquad \frac{1}{C_1} = \left\{ k_1 + k_3, k_1 + k_2 \right\} - \frac{1}{C_3} = \left\{ k_1, k_1 + k_2 - b \right\}, \qquad (8.132a-c)$$

$$\frac{1}{C_3} = \left\{ k_2 + k_3, \overline{b} \right\} - \frac{1}{C_3} = \left\{ k_2, \overline{b} - b \right\}. \qquad (8.132c)$$

The coupled equations of the electrical and mechanical circuits involve [subsection 8.3.4 (8.3.5)] the mass, friction, and resilience (damping and oscillation) matrices in the general form (8.28) [form with explicit accelerations (8.31a)].

8.3.5 Mass, Friction, and Resilience Matrices

The equivalent mechanical/electrical/bynamical (Figures 8.1a, 8.1c, 8.2a) linear two-dimensional circuits satisfy the same fundamental equations $(8.28) \equiv (8.126) \equiv (8.127) \equiv (8.128)$ involving: (i, ii) the physical coordinates (8.133a) and forcing vectors (8.133b):

$$\begin{bmatrix} x_1(t) \\ x_2(t) \end{bmatrix} = \begin{bmatrix} q_1(t) \\ q_2(t) \end{bmatrix} = \begin{bmatrix} z(t) \\ \theta(t) \end{bmatrix}, \qquad \begin{bmatrix} F_1(t) \\ F_2(t) \end{bmatrix} = \begin{bmatrix} E_1(t) \\ E_2(t) \end{bmatrix} = \begin{bmatrix} F(t) \\ M(t) \end{bmatrix};$$

$$(8.133a, b)$$

(iii) diagonal mass matrices:

$$m_{rs} = \begin{bmatrix} m_1 & 0 \\ 0 & m_2 \end{bmatrix} = \begin{bmatrix} L_2 & 0 \\ 0 & L_2 \end{bmatrix} = \begin{bmatrix} m & 0 \\ 0 & I \end{bmatrix}; \qquad (8.134a-c)$$

(iv) non-diagonal friction matrices:

$$\mu_{rs} = \begin{bmatrix} \mu_1 + \mu_3 & -\mu_3 \\ -\mu_3 & \mu_2 + \mu_3 \end{bmatrix} = \begin{bmatrix} R_1 + R_3 & -R_3 \\ -R_3 & R_2 + R_3 \end{bmatrix} = \begin{bmatrix} \mu_1 + \mu_2 & -c \\ -c & \overline{c} \end{bmatrix},$$

$$(8.135a-c)$$

the latter (8.135c) involving (8.121a; 8.124a); (v) the non-diagonal resilience matrices:

$$
k_{rs} = \begin{bmatrix} k_1 + k_3 & -k_3 \\ -k_3 & k_2 + k_3 \end{bmatrix} = \begin{bmatrix} C_1^{-1} + C_3^{-1} & -C_3^{-1} \\ -C_3^{-1} & C_2^{-1} + C_3^{-1} \end{bmatrix} = \begin{bmatrix} k_1 + k_2 & -b \\ -b & b \end{bmatrix},
$$

$$(8.136a\text{–}c)$$

the latter (8.136c) involving (8.120a; 8.123a).

The three terms of (problem 449) the modal matrix (8.81c), namely mass (8.134a–c), friction (8.135a–c), and resilience (8.136a–c) matrices, may be replaced in the reduced fundamental equations (8.31a) with explicit accelerations by the two terms in the dispersion matrix (8.35a), namely: (a) the (8.31b) damping matrix (8.137a–c):

$$
2\lambda_{rs} = \begin{bmatrix} \dfrac{\mu_1 + \mu_3}{m_1} & -\dfrac{\mu_3}{m_1} \\[2ex] -\dfrac{\mu_3}{m_2} & \dfrac{\mu_2 + \mu_3}{m_2} \end{bmatrix} = \begin{bmatrix} \dfrac{R_2 + R_3}{L_1} & -\dfrac{R_3}{L_1} \\[2ex] -\dfrac{R_3}{L_2} & \dfrac{R_2 + R_3}{L_2} \end{bmatrix} = \begin{bmatrix} \dfrac{\mu_1 + \mu_2}{m} & -\dfrac{c}{m} \\[2ex] -\dfrac{c}{I} & \dfrac{\overline{c}}{I} \end{bmatrix};
$$

$$(8.137a\text{–}c)$$

(b) the (8.31c) oscillation matrix (8.138a–c):

$$
\omega_{rs}^2 = \begin{bmatrix} \dfrac{k_1 + k_3}{m_1} & -\dfrac{k_3}{m_1} \\[2ex] -\dfrac{k_3}{m_2} & \dfrac{k_2 + k_3}{m_2} \end{bmatrix} = \begin{bmatrix} \dfrac{1}{L_2}\left(\dfrac{1}{C_1} + \dfrac{1}{C_3}\right) & -\dfrac{1}{L_1 C_3} \\[2ex] -\dfrac{1}{L_2 C_3} & \dfrac{1}{L_2}\left(\dfrac{1}{C_2} + \dfrac{1}{C_3}\right) \end{bmatrix}
$$

$$(8.138a\text{–}c)$$

$$
= \begin{bmatrix} \dfrac{k_1 + k_2}{m} & -\dfrac{b}{m} \\[2ex] -\dfrac{b}{I} & \dfrac{\overline{b}}{I} \end{bmatrix};
$$

(c) the reduced forcing vectors (8.139a–c):

$$
f_{1,2} = \dfrac{F_{1,2}}{m_{1,2}} = \dfrac{E_{1,2}}{L_{1,2}} = \left\{ \dfrac{F}{m}, \dfrac{M}{I} \right\},
$$

$$(8.139a\text{–}c)$$

appear in the presence of forcing. Since the three circuits are equivalent, any of them can be chosen for further analysis, for example, the two-dimensional oscillator (Figures 8.2a–c) in the case of free (forced) oscillations [section 8.4 (8.5)] without or with damping.

8.4 Coupled Natural Frequencies and Dampings

The two-dimensional (section 8.3) free oscillations (section 8.4) are considered first for the undamped motion of a rod supported on springs at the two ends (Figure 8.2a) in the coupled (uncoupled) cases when the forces exerted by the two springs are unequal (equal) so that the modal frequencies do not (do) coincide with the frequencies of translation and rotation. In general, the mass and moment of inertia of the rod are arbitrary as for a two-axle or two-wheeled vehicle, and the particular cases include: (i) two masses at the ends of a rod with negligible mass and moment of inertia (subsection 8.4.3), corresponding to the plane at oscillations of a diatomic molecule with the two atoms at a fixed distance (subsection 8.4.2); (ii)(iii) an inhomogeneous rod with center of mass in the middle (subsection 8.4.4), which includes as a further particular case the homogenous rod (subsection 8.4.5). Case (iii) serves to illustrate: (a) the relation between the modal and the physical coordinates satisfying the compatibility conditions (subsection 8.4.6); (b) the determination of the amplitudes and phases of the two modal coordinates from the initial positions and velocities (subsections 8.4.7–8.4.8). The modal frequencies and dampings are considered for free oscillations with dissipation (subsection 8.4.9) in the general coupled case (subsection 8.4.11) for an arbitrary rod, and in particular, (α) in the decoupled case with strong damping (subsection 8.4.10), and (β) in the coupled case with weak damping for the homogeneous rod (subsection 8.4.12).

8.4.1 Translational/Rotational Oscillations of a Rod

In the case of translational and rotational oscillations of a rod supported at the two ends by springs and dampers (Figure 8.2a), the equations of motion (8.118a, b; 8.117b, c) $\equiv$ (8.126; 8.120a, 8.121a, 8.123a, 8.124a) are written explicitly (8.140):

$$
\begin{bmatrix} m\,\ddot{z} \\ I\,\ddot{\theta} \end{bmatrix} + \begin{bmatrix} \mu_1 + \mu_2 & \mu_1(L-a) - \mu_2(L+a) \\ \mu_1(L-a) - \mu_2(L+a) & \mu_1(L-a)^2 + \mu_2(L+a)^2 \end{bmatrix} \begin{bmatrix} \dot{z} \\ \dot{\theta} \end{bmatrix}
$$

$$
+ \begin{bmatrix} k_1 + k_2 & k_1(L-a) - k_2(L+a) \\ k_1(L-a) - k_2(L+a) & k_1(L-a)^2 + k_2(L+a)^2 \end{bmatrix} \begin{bmatrix} z \\ \theta \end{bmatrix} = \begin{bmatrix} F(t) \\ M(t) \end{bmatrix}.
$$

$$(8.140)$$

In the case of unforced (8.141a) undamped (8.141b) oscillations, the natural frequencies are the roots of (8.141c):

$$F = M = 0 = \mu_1 = \mu_2: \quad \begin{vmatrix} k_1 + k_2 - m\omega^2 & k_1(L-a) - k_2(L+a) \\ k_1(L-a) - k_2(L+a) & k_1(L-a)^2 + k_2(L+a)^2 - I\omega^2 \end{vmatrix} = 0.$$

$$(8.141\text{a–c})$$

If the forces exerted by the two springs are equal (8.142a), then the translational (8.142b) [rotational (8.142c)] oscillations are decoupled:

$$k_1(L-a) = k_2(L+a): \qquad \ddot{z} + \omega_t^2 z = 0 = \ddot{\theta} + \omega_r^2 \theta; \qquad (8.142\text{a–c})$$

in this case, the translation ω_t (rotation ω_r) frequencies are given (8.143a–c) [(8.144a–c)] by:

$$\omega_t = \left| \frac{k_1 + k_2}{m} \right|^{1/2} = \left| \frac{2k_1 L}{m(L+a)} \right|^{1/2} = \left| \frac{2k_2 L}{m(L-a)} \right|^{1/2}, \qquad (8.143\text{a, b})$$

$$\omega_r = \left| \frac{k_1(L-a)^2 + k_2(L-a)^2}{I} \right|^{1/2} = \left| \frac{2k_1 L(L-a)}{I} \right|^{1/2} = \left| \frac{2k_2 L(L+a)}{I} \right|^{1/2}, \qquad (8.144\text{a–c})$$

where (8.142a) implies (8.145a–c) [(8.146a–c)], which were used in (8.143b, c) [(8.144b, c)]:

$$k_1 + k_2 = k_1 \left(1 + \frac{L-a}{L+a} \right) = \frac{2k_1 L}{L+a} = \frac{2k_2 L}{L-a}, \qquad (8.145\text{a–c})$$

$$k_1(L-a)^2 + k_2(L+a)^2 = 2k_1 L(L-a) = 2k_2 L(L+a). \qquad (8.146\text{a–c})$$

The ratio of the rotational (8.144c) to the translational (8.143c) frequencies is (8.147b):

$$I = mR^2: \qquad \frac{\omega_r}{\omega_t} = \left| \frac{m(L^2 - a^2)}{I} \right|^{1/2} = \left| \frac{L^2 - a^2}{R^2} \right|^{1/2}, \qquad (8.147\text{a–c})$$

where the **radius of gyration** was introduced in (8.147c), defined in (8.147a) as the distance from the center of mass where all the mass would be concentrated to produce the same moment of inertia. The decoupling condition (8.142a) implies that the two springs act in parallel, that is, in the case of a vertical displacement, the two springs exert an equal restoring force, implying that they produce no turning moment, so that rotation is not excited; (ii) also, if the decoupling condition (8.134a) is met, a rotation causes equal and opposite forces that cancel, so no translation is excited. Conversely if the decoupling condition is not met, a translation of the center of mass will cause a rotation, and vice-versa. Thus *(problem 450) the decoupling condition (8.142a) implies the relation (8.147a–c) between the frequencies of translation (8.143a–c) and rotation (8.144a–c) in the case of a rod (8.140) mounted on springs (Figure 8.2a) in the absence of forcing (8.141a) and damping (8.141b). In general, if the decoupling condition (8.142a) is not met, the coupled natural frequencies (8.148a, b):*

$$2mR^2\omega_\pm^2 = (k_1 + k_2)R^2 + k_1(L-a)^2 + k_2(L-a)^2$$

$$\pm \left| \left[(k_1 + k_2)R^2 + k_1(L-a)^2 + k_2(L-a) \right]^2 - 16k_1 k_2 L^2 R^2 \right|^{1/2},$$

$$(8.148a, b)$$

are the roots (8.141c) of the biquadraic (8.148c):

$$mI\omega^4 - \left\{ (k_1 + k_2)I + m\left[k_1(L-a)^2 + k_2(L-a)^2 \right] \right\}\omega^2 + 4k_1 k_2 L^2 = 0, \quad (8.148c)$$

using the gyration radius (8.147a). In the passage from (8.141c) to (8.148c) was made this simplification:

$$(k_1 + k_2)\left[k_1(L-a)^2 + k_2(L+a)^2 \right] - \left[k_1(L-a) - k_2(L+a) \right]^2$$

$$= k_1 k_2 \left[(L-a)^2 + (L+a)^2 + 2(L-a)(L+a) \right] = 4k_1 k_2 L^2.$$

$$(8.149a, b)$$

A further idealization of the two-wheeled vehicle (Figure 8.2a) is the two-point masses converted by a rod of negligible mass and inertia (Figure 8.2b), which also models the plane oscillations of a diatomic molecule with two atoms at a fixed distance (subsection 8.4.2).

8.4.2 Plane Oscillations of Two Atoms at a Fixed Distance

A further idealization of the two-wheeled vehicle (Figure 8.2b) is the two-point masses m_1, m_2, supported on the springs (k_1, k_2) and dampers (μ_2, μ_2), and connected by a rigid bar of negligible mass; this is also a physical model of the plane oscillations of a diatomic molecule. Both cases lead to the same equations of motion (8.150a, b):

$$(m_1 + m_2)\,\ddot{z} + \mu_1\,\dot{z}_1 + \mu_2\,\dot{z}_2 + k_1\,z_1 + k_2\,z_2 = F_1(t) + F_2(t), \qquad (8.150a)$$

$$\left[m_1(L-a)^2 + m_2(L+a)^2 \right]\ddot{\theta} + (\mu_1\,\dot{z}_1 + k_1\,z_1)(L-a)$$

$$- (\mu_2\,\dot{z}_2 + k_2\,z_2)(L+a) = (L-a)\,F_1(t) - (L+a)\,F_2(t). \qquad (8.150b)$$

Substitution of (8.117b, c) in (8.150a, b) leads to (8.151):

$$
\begin{bmatrix} m_1 + m_2 & \\ m_1(L-a)^2 + m_2(L+a)^2 & \end{bmatrix}
\begin{bmatrix} \ddot{z} \\ \ddot{\theta} \end{bmatrix}
+
\begin{bmatrix} \mu_1 + \mu_2 & \mu_1(L-a) - \mu_2(L+a) \\ \mu_1(L-a) - \mu_2(L+a) & \mu_1(L-a)^2 + \mu_2(L+a)^2 \end{bmatrix}
\begin{bmatrix} \dot{z} \\ \dot{\theta} \end{bmatrix}
$$

$$
\begin{bmatrix} k_1 + k_2 & k_1(L-a) - k_2(L+a) \\ k_1(L-a) - k_2(L+a) & k_1(L-a)^2 + k_2(L+a)^2 \end{bmatrix}
\begin{bmatrix} z \\ \theta \end{bmatrix}
=
\begin{bmatrix} F_1(t) + F_2(t) \\ (L-a)F_1(t) - (L+a)F_2(t) \end{bmatrix}
$$

$$(8.151)$$

as the equation of motion in terms of translation and rotations. In the unforced (8.152a) undamped (8.152b) case, the natural frequencies are the roots of (8.152c):

$$F_1 = F_2 = 0 = \mu_1 = \mu_2: \qquad (8.152a, b)$$

$$
\begin{vmatrix} k_1 + k_2 - (m_1 + m_2)\,\omega^2 & k_1(L-a) - k_2(L+a) \\ k_1(L-a) - k_2(L+a) & k_1(L-a)^2 + k_2(L+a)^2 - \omega^2\left[m_1(L-a)^2 + m_2(L+a)^2 \right] \end{vmatrix} = 0.
$$

$$(8.152c)$$

The decoupled case is (8.142a) ≡ (8.153a), and the natural frequencies of translation (8.143a–c) [rotation (8.144a–c)] are given by (8.153b) [(8.153c)]:

$$k_1(L-a) = k_2(L+a): \quad \omega_t = \left| \frac{k_1 + k_2}{m_1 + m_2} \right|^2, \quad \omega_r = \left| \frac{k_1(L-a)^2 + k_2(L-a)^2}{m_1(L-a)^2 + m_2(L+a)^2} \right|^{1/2},$$

$$(8.153a–c)$$

for (problem 451) the plane oscillator (8.150a, b) ≡ (8.151) with the two masses at fixed distance (Figure 8.2b) in the absence of forcing (8.152a) and damping (8.152b). The oscillator in the Figure 8.2b is a particular case of that in Figure 8.2a, as shown by the next comparison (subsection 8.3.3), which includes both decoupled and coupled translational and rotational frequencies.

8.4.3 Decoupled Rotational and Translational Natural Frequencies

The diatomic-molecule oscillator (Figure 8.2b) is the particular case of the rod oscillator (Figure 8.2a) with (8.140) ≡ (8.151): (i) the force is equal to the sum of forces (8.154a) and the moment of forces relative to the center of mass (8.154b):

$$F(t) = F_1(t) + F_2(t), \qquad\qquad M(t) = (L-a)F_1(t) - (L+a)F_2(t); \quad \text{(8.154a, b)}$$

$$m = m_1 + m_2, \qquad\qquad I = m_1(L-a)^2 + m_2(L+a)^2, \qquad \text{(8.155a, b)}$$

(ii) the total mass (8.155a) and the moment of inertia (8.155b). In the case of an inhomogeneous rod, the center of mass may lie anywhere within its length (8.117a), whereas for two-point masses it is given by (8.156a) leading to (8.156b):

$$a = \frac{m_1 - m_2}{m_1 + m_2}L, \qquad L \mp a = L\left(1 \mp \frac{m_1 - m_2}{m_1 + m_2}\right) = 2L\frac{\{m_2, m_1\}}{m_1 + m_2}. \qquad \text{(8.156a, b)}$$

Thus, the center of mass is at the origin for equal masses (8.157b) and shifts to the side of the larger mass if they are unequal (8.157a, c):

$$a \begin{cases} > 0 & \text{if} \quad m_1 > m_2, \\ = 0 & \text{if} \quad m_1 = m_2, \\ < 0 & \text{if} \quad m_1 < m_2; \end{cases} \qquad a = \begin{cases} L & \text{if} \quad m_1 \neq 0 = m_2 \\ -L & \text{if} \quad m_1 = 0 \neq m_2, \end{cases} \qquad \text{(8.157a–e)}$$

the extreme case is coincident with one of the masses if the other is zero (8.157d, e). From (8.155b) follows (8.156a), the moment of inertia (8.158a, b) and radius of gyration (8.158c, d):

$$I = 4L^2\frac{m_1 m_2^2 + m_2 m_1^2}{(m_1 + m_2)^2} = 4L^2\frac{m_1 m_2}{m_1 + m_2}, \qquad R = \sqrt{\frac{I}{m_1 + m_2}} = 2L\frac{\sqrt{m_1 m_2}}{m_1 + m_2}.$$

$$\text{(8.158a–d)}$$

The decoupled case (8.142a) ≡ (8.153a) corresponds (8.156b) to (8.159a), and the decoupled frequencies of translation (8.153b) ≡ (8.159b) [rotation (8.153c) ≡ (8.159c)] coincide (8.159d):

$$m_2 k_1 = m_1 k_2: \quad \omega_t = \left| \frac{k_1 + k_2}{m_1 + m_2} \right|^{1/2} = \left| \frac{k_1}{m_1} \frac{1 + k_2/k_1}{1 + m_2/m_1} \right|^{1/2} = \left| \frac{k_1}{m_1} \right|^{1/2} = \omega_1, \qquad (8.159a, b)$$

$$\omega_r = \left| \frac{k_1 (L-a)^2 + k_2 (L+a)^2}{m_1 (L-a)^2 + m_2 (L+a)^2} \right|^{1/2} = \left| \frac{k_1 + k_2 (k_1/k_2)^2}{m_1 + m_2 (m_1/m_2)^2} \right|^{1/2}$$

$$(8.159c, d)$$

$$= \left| \frac{k_1}{k_2} \frac{k_1 + k_2}{m_1 + m_2} \frac{m_2}{m_1} \right|^{1/2} = \left| \frac{k_1 + k_2}{m_1 + m_2} \right|^{1/2} = \omega_2 = \omega_1.$$

In the coupled case (8.160a), the natural frequencies are (8.152c; 8.156a, b) the roots (8.152c) of (8.160b):

$$m_2 k_1 \neq m_1 k_2: \quad \begin{vmatrix} k_1 + k_2 - m\omega^2 & (k_1 m_2 - m_2 k_1)\dfrac{2L}{m} \\[2ex] (k_1 m_2 - k_2 m_1)\dfrac{2L}{m} & \left[k_1 m_2^2 + k_2 m_1^2 - m_1 m_2 m \omega^2 \right]\dfrac{4L^2}{m^2} \end{vmatrix} = 0,$$

$$(8.160a, b)$$

which is a biquadratic equation for the frequency:

$$m_1 m_2 m^2 \omega^4 - \left[k_1 m_2^2 + k_2 m_1^2 + m_1 m_2 (k_1 + k_2) \right] m \omega^2$$

$$+ (k_1 + k_2)(k_1 m_2^2 + k_2 m_1^2) - (k_1 m_2 - k_2 m_1)^2 = 0,$$

$$(8.161a)$$

which simplifies to:

$$m_1 m_2 \omega^4 - (k_1 m_2 + k_2 m_1)\omega^2 + k_1 k_2 = 0. \qquad (8.161b)$$

The modal frequencies (8.162a, b) are the roots of (8.161b):

$$\omega_\pm = \left| \frac{k_1}{m_1} \right|^{1/2}, \left| \frac{k_2}{m_2} \right|^{1/2} = \omega_1, \omega_2; \quad m_2 k_1 = m_1 k_2: \quad \omega_\pm = \omega_1 = \omega_2; \qquad (8.162a–d)$$

and in the decoupled case (8.159a) ≡ (8.162c) coincide (8.159d) ≡ (8.162d). It has been shown that (*problem 452*) *two distinct masses at a fixed distance*

(Figure 8.2b) have total mass (8.155a), center of mass (8.156a; 8.157a–e) moment of inertia (8.158a, b), and radius of gyration (8.158c, d). When supported on unequal springs (8.151) in the absence of forcing (8.152a) and damping (8.152b), the natural frequencies: (i) are those of separate oscillators (8.162a, b) because the mass and moment of inertia of the connecting rod have been neglected; (ii) in the decoupled case (8.162c) the frequencies of translation and rotation coincide (8.162d). Thus, it is the mass and/or inertia of the rod (Figure 8.2a) that cou- ples the two natural frequencies in (8.152a–c), which will be simplified for an inhomogeneous (homogeneous) rod with center of mass at the middle of the rod (subsection 8.4.4).

8.4.4 Coupled Free Undamped Oscillations of a Rod

A particular case of a rigid body supported on unequal springs and dampers is a rod, homogeneous or not (Figure 8.2c) for which the center of mass is in the middle (8.163a). In this case, the translations and rotations are decoupled (8.142a) if the resiliences of the springs are equal (8.163b):

$$a = 0; \quad k_1 = k_2 \equiv k: \qquad \omega_t = \left|\frac{2k}{m}\right|^{1/2}, \qquad \omega_r = \left|\frac{2kL^2}{I}\right|^{1/2} = \frac{L}{R}\left|\frac{2k}{m}\right|^{1/2} = \frac{L}{R}\omega_t,$$

$$(8.163a\text{–}f)$$

and the modal frequencies of translation (8.153b) $\equiv$ (8.163c) and rotation (8.153c) $\equiv$ (8.163d, e) are related by (8.163f), the ratio of half-length to gyration radius. In the coupled case, of unequal springs (8.164a), the natural frequencies are the roots of (8.141a; 8.163a) $\equiv$ (8.164b):

$$k_1 \neq k_2: \qquad \begin{vmatrix} k_1 + k_2 - m\omega^2 & (k_1 - k_2)L \\ (k_1 - k_2)L & (k_1 + k_2)L^2 - mR^2\omega^2 \end{vmatrix} = 0, \qquad (8.164a, b)$$

which is a biquadratic equation:

$$m^2 R^2 \omega^4 - m(k_1 + k_2)(L^2 + R^2)\omega^2 + 4k_1 k_2 L^2 = 0. \qquad (8.165)$$

The roots of (8.165) are:

$$2mR^2 \omega_\pm^2 - (k_1 + k_2)(L^2 + R^2) = \left|(k_1 + k_2)^2(L^2 + R^2)^2 - 16k_1 k_2 L^2 R^2\right|^{1/2}, \qquad (8.166)$$

and specify *(problem 453) the modal frequencies (8.166) of a rod (Figure 8.2c) with center of the mass at the middle (8.163a), supported on springs at the two ends, without forcing (8.141a) or damping (8.141b). In the case of equal springs (8.163b),* the translational (8.163c) and rotational (8.163d) oscillations are decoupled; their ratio (8.163e) equals the ratio of the half-length of the rod to the gyration radius (8.163e) ≡ (8.167a):

$$\omega_r R = \omega_t L: \qquad\qquad R \leq L \quad\Rightarrow\quad \omega_r \geq \omega_t, \qquad\qquad (8.167\text{a–c})$$

since the radius of gyration cannot exceed the half-length of the rod (8.167b) the frequency of translation cannot exceed the frequency of rotation (8.167c). The equality in (8.167c) of the frequencies of rotation and translation is possible only if: (i) the gyration radius equals the half-length of the rod (8.167b); (ii) hence there are two equal masses concentrated at the ends (Figure 8.2b) with equal springs (8.163b), implying that (8.163f) is met; (iii) then (8.163c, d) confirm that the frequencies of rotation and translation are equal. A further simplification is a homogeneous rod (subsection 8.4.5) for which the radius of gyration is a fixed fraction of the length of the rod.

8.4.5 Coupled and Decoupled Natural Frequencies of a Homogeneous Rod

A homogeneous rod has a constant mass density or mass per unit length (8.168a, b), leading to; (i) the total mass (8.168c, d); (ii) center of mass (8.168e) at the origin (8.168f); (iii) moment of inertia (8.168g) ≡ (8.168h) and the radius of gyration (8.168i):

$$\sigma \equiv \frac{dm}{dx} = const: \quad m \equiv \int_{-L}^{+L} \sigma\, dx = 2\sigma L, \quad a \equiv \frac{1}{m}\int_{-L}^{+L}\sigma x\, dx = 0,$$

$$I \equiv \int_{-L}^{+L}\sigma x^2 dx = \frac{2\sigma L^3}{3} = \frac{mL^2}{3},\ R = \frac{L}{\sqrt{3}}. \qquad (8.168\text{a–i})$$

In the case of equal springs (8.163b) ≡ (8.169a), the frequency of rotation (8.163e) ≡ (8.169c) is larger than that of translation (8.163c) ≡ (8.169b) by a factor (8.163f) ≡ (8.169d):

$$k_1 = k_2 \equiv k: \qquad \omega_t = \left|\frac{2k}{m}\right|^{1/2}, \qquad \omega_t = \left|\frac{6k}{m}\right|^{1/2} = \omega_t\sqrt{3}. \qquad (8.169\text{a–d})$$

In the coupled case of distinct springs, the modal frequencies are the roots (8.164b) of (8.170c):

$$\omega_{1,2} = \left|\frac{\omega_{1,2}}{m}\right|: \qquad \begin{vmatrix} \omega_1^2 + \omega_2^2 - \omega^2 & \omega_1^2 - \omega_2^2 \\ 3\left(\omega_1^2 - \omega_2^2\right) & 3\left(\omega_1^2 + \omega_2^2\right) - \omega^2 \end{vmatrix} = 0, \qquad (8.170\text{a–c})$$

where appear the natural frequencies of translation of the rod supported on the spring $k_1(k_2)$ alone (8.170a) [(8.170b)]. The equation (8.170c) ≡ (8.171) is a biquadratic in ω:

$$0 = \omega^4 - 4\left(\omega_1^2 + \omega_2^2\right)\omega^2 + 12\,\omega_1^2\,\omega_2^2 = \left(\omega^2 - \omega_+^2\right)\left(\omega^2 - \omega_-^2\right) \equiv P_4(i\omega), \qquad (8.171)$$

with roots (8.172a):

$$P_4(\omega_\pm) = 0: \qquad \frac{1}{2}\omega_\pm^2 = \omega_1^2 + \omega_2^2 \pm \left|\left(\omega_1^2 + \omega_2^2\right)^2 - 3\omega_1^2\,\omega_2^2\right|^{1/2}$$

$$= \omega_1^2 + \omega_2^2 \pm \left|\omega_1^4 + \omega_2^4 - \omega_1^2\,\omega_2^2\right|^{1/2} \qquad (8.172a\text{–}d)$$

$$= \omega_1^2 + \omega_2^2 \pm \left|\left(\omega_1^2 - \omega_2^2\right)^2 + \omega_1^2\,\omega_2^2\right|^{1/2},$$

which show that: (i) $\omega_\pm^2$ is real (8.172d) and positive (8.172b); (ii) hence $\omega_\pm$ are real and the motion is oscillatory with constant amplitude. In the decoupled case (8.169a) ≡ (8.173a):

$$\omega_1 = \omega_2 = \sqrt{\frac{k}{m}} \equiv \omega_0: \qquad \omega_\pm^2 = 2(2 \pm 1)\omega_0^2 = \{2, 6\}\omega_0^2 = \{\omega_t^2, \omega_r^2\}, \qquad (8.173a\text{–}c)$$

the modal frequencies (8.173b, c) coincide with the translation and rotation frequencies (8.169b, c). Thus, *a homogeneous rod (8.168a–i) supported at the two ends by unequal springs (Figure 8.2c), in the absence of forcing (8.152a) and damping (8.152b) has (problem 454) the natural frequencies (8.171; 8.170a, b) ≡ (8.172a–d), which simplify (8.173a–c) to the translation (8.169b) and the rotation (8.169c) frequencies in the decoupled case (8.169d) of equal springs (8.169a).* The modal frequencies correspond to the modal coordinates, whose linear combination specifies the physical coordinates meeting the compatibility conditions (subsection 8.4.6).

8.4.6 Compatibility Relations between Modal and Physical Coordinates

In the coupled case, the modal coordinates (8.174a):

$$q_\pm(t) = C_\pm \cos\left(\omega_\pm t - \alpha_\pm\right), \qquad \ddot{q}_\pm + \omega_\pm^2\,q_\pm = 0, \qquad (8.174a, b)$$

each oscillate at one modal frequency (8.174b), with its own amplitude $C_\pm$ and phase $\alpha_\pm$. The modal coordinates $q_\pm$ are decoupled, unlike physical the translation z and rotation θ coordinates, which appear coupled in the equations of motion $(8.140) \equiv (8.175d, e)$:

$$F = M = 0 = \mu_1 = \mu_2, \sigma = \frac{dm}{dx} = const: \qquad (8.175a\text{--}c)$$

$$\ddot{z} + \left(\omega_1^2 + \omega_2^2\right)z + \left(\omega_1^2 - \omega_2^2\right)L\theta = 0, \qquad (8.175d)$$

$$L\ddot{\theta} + 3\left(\omega_1^2 - \omega_2^2\right)z + 3\left(\omega_1^2 + \omega_2^2\right)L\theta = 0, \qquad (8.175e)$$

where: (i) forcing (8.175a) and friction (8.175b) were neglected, leading to free undamped oscillations; (ii) the rod was assumed to be homogeneous $(8.175c) \equiv (8.168a)$ implying (8.168b–i). The angle of rotation θ is replaced as a dependent variable in (8.175d, e) by $L\theta$, which has the same dimensions as the translation z.

The translation is a superposition of modal coordinates (8.176a), including the amplitudes $C_\pm$ and phases $\alpha_\pm$ in the modal coordinates (8.174a, b):

$$z(t) = q_+(t) + q_-(t): \qquad \left(\omega_1^2 - \omega_2^2\right)L\theta = -\ddot{z} - \left(\omega_1^2 + \omega_2^2\right)z$$

$$= -\ddot{q}_+ - \ddot{q}_- - \left(\omega_1^2 + \omega_2^2\right)\left(q_+ + q_-\right)$$

$$= \left(\omega_+^2 - \omega_1^2 - \omega_2^2\right)q_+ + \left(\omega_-^2 - \omega_1^2 - \omega_2^2\right)q_-$$

$$(8.176a\text{--}d)$$

and the rotation (8.176b) is also a superposition of modal coordinates with other coefficients that are not independent of the former, since the equation of motion (8.175d) specifies the compatibility relation (8.176c, d). The relation $(8.176a, d) \equiv (8.177b)$ between the physical coordinates, which is the translation z and the rotation θ, and the normal coordinates $q_\pm$ involves the parameters (8.177a):

$$a_\pm \equiv \frac{\omega_\pm^2 - \omega_1^2 - \omega_2^2}{\omega_1^2 - \omega_2^2}: \qquad \begin{bmatrix} z(t) \\ L\theta(t) \end{bmatrix} = \begin{bmatrix} 1 & 1 \\ a_+ & a_- \end{bmatrix} \begin{bmatrix} q_+(t) \\ q_-(t) \end{bmatrix}. \qquad (8.177a, b)$$

The inverse of (8.177b) is (8.178b), which involves the inverse of the determinant (8.178a):

$$a_0 \equiv \frac{1}{a_- - a_+} = \frac{\omega_1^2 - \omega_2^2}{\omega_-^2 - \omega_+^2}: \qquad \begin{bmatrix} q_+(t) \\ q_-(t) \end{bmatrix} = a_0 \begin{bmatrix} a_- & -1 \\ -a_+ & 1 \end{bmatrix} \begin{bmatrix} z(t) \\ L\theta(t) \end{bmatrix}. \qquad (8.178a, b)$$

Thus, (8.178b) implies that:

$$\left(\omega_{\mp}^2 - \omega_{\pm}^2\right)q_{\pm}(t) = \left(\omega_{\mp}^2 - \omega_1^2 - \omega_2^2\right)z(t) - \left(\omega_1^2 - \omega_2^2\right)L\theta(t), \qquad (8.179a, b)$$

the modal coordinates (8.179a, b) specify (problem 455) the only two points (8.174a, b) on the rod that oscillate only at one modal frequency $\omega_{\pm}$. *The ampli-* tudes $C_{\pm}$ and phases $\alpha_{\pm}$ in the modal (8.174a) or physical (8.175a, b) coordi- nates are determined by four independent and compatible initial conditions (subsection 8.4.7).

8.4.7 Amplitudes, Phases, and Initial Conditions

Since the system of differential equations (8.175d, e) is of fourth-order, four initial conditions can be imposed, for example, the initial translation (8.180a), rotation (8.180c), linear (8.180b), and angular (8.180d) velocities:

$$z(0) = z_0, \qquad \dot{z}(0) = \dot{z}_0, \qquad \theta(0) = \theta_0, \qquad \dot{\theta}(0) = \dot{\theta}_0; \qquad (8.180a\text{--}d)$$

these determine the amplitudes $C_{\pm}$ and phases $\alpha_{\pm}$ of the modal coordinates by substitution in (8.174a), leading to (8.181a, b):

$$\begin{bmatrix} C_+ \cos\alpha_+ \\ C_- \cos\alpha_- \end{bmatrix} = \begin{bmatrix} q_+(0) \\ q_-(0) \end{bmatrix} = a_0 \begin{bmatrix} a_- & -1 \\ -a_+ & 1 \end{bmatrix} \begin{bmatrix} z_0 \\ L\theta_0 \end{bmatrix} = a_0 \begin{bmatrix} a_- z_0 - L\theta_0 \\ -a_+ z_0 + L\theta_0 \end{bmatrix},$$

$$(8.181a)$$

$$\begin{bmatrix} C_+ \omega_+ \sin\alpha_+ \\ C_- \omega_- \sin\alpha_- \end{bmatrix} = \begin{bmatrix} \dot{q}_+(0) \\ \dot{q}_-(0) \end{bmatrix} = a_0 \begin{bmatrix} a_- & -1 \\ -a_+ & 1 \end{bmatrix} \begin{bmatrix} \dot{z}_0 \\ L\dot{\theta}_0 \end{bmatrix} = a_0 \begin{bmatrix} a_- \dot{z}_0 - L\dot{\theta}_0 \\ -a_+ \dot{z}_0 + L\dot{\theta}_0 \end{bmatrix},$$

$$(8.181b)$$

where (8.178b) was used. Using (8.182a) [(8.182b)]:

$$\left(C_{\pm}\right)^2 = \left(C_{\pm}\cos\alpha_{\pm}\right)^2 + \left(C_{\pm}\sin\alpha_{\pm}\right)^2, \qquad \cot\alpha_{\pm} = \frac{C_{\pm}\cos\alpha_{\pm}}{C_{\pm}\sin\alpha_{\pm}}, \qquad (8.182a, b)$$

leads to the solution of (8.181a, b) for the amplitudes (phases) in (8.183a) [(8.183b)]:

$$C_{\pm} = a_0 \left| \left(a_{\mp} z_0 - L\theta_0\right)^2 + \left(\frac{a_{\mp} \dot{z}_0 - L\dot{\theta}_0}{\omega_{\pm}}\right)^2 \right|^{1/2}, \qquad \cot\alpha_{\pm} = \omega_{\pm} \frac{a_{\mp} z_0 - L\theta_0}{a_{\mp} \dot{z}_0 - L\dot{\theta}_0}.$$

$$(8.183a, b)$$

Thus, *the initial linear and angular positions and velocities (8.180a–d), specify (problem 456) the phases (8.183b) and amplitudes (8.183a) of the modal (8.174a) and physical (8.177b) coordinates of the free (8.175a) undamped (8.175b) oscillations of a homogeneous (8.175c) rod (8.175d, e) supported on springs (Figure 8.2c) involving the modal frequencies (8.172b–d; 8.170a, b) in the coefficients (8.177a; 8.178a).* The initial conditions (8.180a–d) can be applied in an alternative way (subsection 8.4.8).

8.4.8 Displacement, Rotation, and Linear and Angular Velocities

The modal coordinates can be rewritten (8.174a) ≡ (8.184c) in terms of four arbitrary constants (8.184a, b) alternative to the amplitudes and the phases:

$$\{A_\pm, B_\pm\} = C_\pm \{\cos\alpha_\pm, \sin\alpha_\pm\}: \qquad q_\pm(t) = A_\pm \cos(\omega_\pm t) + B_\pm \sin(\omega_\pm t).$$
$$(8.184\text{a–c})$$

Substitution of (8.184c) in (8.176a) [(8.176d)] specifies the physical coordinates, namely the translation of (8.185a) [rotation around (8.185b)] the center of mass at the middle of the homogeneous rod:

$$z(t) = A_+ \cos(\omega_+ t) + B_+ \sin(\omega_+ t) + A_- \cos(\omega_- t) + B_- \sin(\omega_- t), \qquad (8.185\text{a})$$

$$\left(\omega_2^2 - \omega_1^2\right) L\theta(t) = \left(\omega_+^2 - \omega_1^2 - \omega_2^2\right)\left[A_+ \cos(\omega_+ t) + B_+ \sin(\omega_+ t)\right]$$
$$+ \left(\omega_-^2 - \omega_1^2 - \omega_2^2\right)\left[A_- \cos(\omega_- t) + B_- \sin(\omega_- t)\right], \qquad (8.185\text{b})$$

The corresponding linear (angular) velocities are (8.184a) [(8.184b)]:

$$\dot{z}(t) = B_+\omega_+ \cos(\omega_+ t) - A_+\omega_+ \sin(\omega_+ t) + B_-\omega_- \cos(\omega_- t) - A_-\omega_- \sin(\omega_- t), \qquad (8.186\text{a})$$

$$\left(\omega_2^2 - \omega_1^2\right) L\dot{\theta}(t) = \left(\omega_+^2 - \omega_1^2 - \omega_2^2\right)\left[B_+\omega_+ \cos(\omega_+ t) - A_+\omega_+ \sin(\omega_+ t)\right]$$
$$+ \left(\omega_-^2 - \omega_1^2 - \omega_2^2\right)\left[B_-\omega_- \cos(\omega_- t) - A_-\omega_- \sin(\omega_- t)\right]. \qquad (8.186\text{b})$$

Substituting (8.185a, b) [(8.186a, b)] in the initial conditions (8.180a–d) leads to (8.187a, b) [(8.187c, d)]:

$$z_0 = A_+ + A_-, \quad \left(\omega_2^2 - \omega_1^2\right) L\theta_0 = \left(\omega_+^2 - \omega_1^2 - \omega_2^2\right)A_+ + \left(\omega_-^2 - \omega_1^2 - \omega_2^2\right)A_-,$$
$$(8.187\text{a, b})$$

$$\dot{z}_0 = \omega_+ B_+ + \omega_- B_-, \quad \left(\omega_2^2 - \omega_1^2\right) L\dot{\theta}_0 = \left(\omega_+^2 - \omega_1^2 - \omega_2^2\right)\omega_+ B_+ + \left(\omega_-^2 - \omega_1^2 - \omega_2^2\right)\omega_- B_-,$$
$$(8.187\text{c, d})$$

which can be solved for the arbitrary constants (8.188a) [(8.188b)]:

$$\left(\omega_\pm^2 - \omega_\mp^2\right) A_\mp = \left(\omega_\pm^2 - \omega_1^2 - \omega_2^2\right) z_0 - \left(\omega_2^2 - \omega_1^2\right) L\theta_0,$$ (8.188a)

$$\left(\omega_\pm^2 - \omega_\mp^2\right) \omega_\mp B_\mp = \left(\omega_\pm^2 - \omega_1^2 - \omega_2^2\right) \dot{z}_0 - \left(\omega_2^2 - \omega_1^2\right) L\dot{\theta}_0.$$ (8.188b)

Thus, *the free (8.175a) undamped (8.175b) oscillations of a homogeneous (8.175c) rod supported on springs (Figure 8.2c) are specified (problem 457) for the initial conditions (8.180a–d) by the modal (physical) coordinates in terms of: (i) amplitudes (8.183a) and phases (8.183b) in (8.174a) [(8.176a, d)]; (ii) alternative (8.184a, b) constants (8.188a, b) in (8.184c) [(8.185a, b)]; (iii) the translation (8.185a) [rotation (8.185b)], linear (8.186a) [angular (8.186b)] velocities involve the pairs of constants (8.188a, b) and initial conditions (8.180a–d) that satisfy similar relations with the interchanges (8.189a, b):*

$$A_\pm \quad \leftrightarrow \quad \omega_\pm B_\pm, \qquad \left\{z_0, L\theta_0\right\} \quad \leftrightarrow \quad \left\{\dot{z}_0, L\dot{\theta}_0\right\}.$$ (8.189a, b)

The inclusion of friction forces associated with dissipation leads to modal dampings (subsection 8.4.9) in addition to the oscillation frequencies.

8.4.9 Linear Free Oscillations with Dissipation

In the case of damped oscillation, the solutions of (8.140) without forcing (8.190a, b) are sought in the form (8.190c, d):

$$F(t) = 0 = M(t): \quad \left\{z(t), L\theta(t)\right\} = e^{\xi t}\left\{z_0, L\theta_0\right\}, \quad \left\{z_0, \theta_0\right\} \neq \{0, 0\}, \quad (8.190a–e)$$

leading to a linear homogeneous system of equations. which has non-trivial solutions (8.190e) if the determinant of coefficients is zero (8.191):

$$0 = \begin{vmatrix} m\xi^2 + (\mu_1 + \mu_2)\xi + k_1 + k_2 & (\mu_1\xi + k_1)(L-a) - (\mu_2 + k_2\xi)(L+a) \\ (\mu_1\xi + k_1)(L-a) - (\mu_2\xi + k_2)(L+a) & I\xi^2 + \left[\mu_1(L-a)^2 - \mu_2(L+a)^2\right]\xi + k_1(L-a)^2 + k_2(L+a)^2 \end{vmatrix}$$ (8.191)

$$\equiv P_4(\xi).$$

The vanishing of the modal-damping determinant (8.191) that has real coefficients leads to real roots for monotonic motion or complex conjugate pairs:

$$P_4(\xi) = m I(\xi - \xi_+)(\xi - \xi_+^*)(\xi - \xi_-)(\xi - \xi_-^*),\qquad(8.192)$$

for damped oscillatory motion. Denoting by (8.193a) the pair of complex roots and by (8.193b) their conjugates follow (8.193c):

$$\xi_\pm = -\lambda_\pm + i\omega_\pm,\ \xi_\pm^* = -\lambda_\pm - i\omega_\pm :\qquad(8.193a, b)$$

$$(\xi - \xi_\pm)(\xi - \xi_\pm^*) = (\xi + \lambda_\pm - i\omega_\pm)(\xi + \lambda_\pm + i\omega_\pm) = (\xi + \lambda_\pm)^2 + \omega_\pm^2,\qquad(8.193c)$$

showing that the quartic polynomial (8.192) can be rewritten (8.194):

$$0 = P_4(\xi) = \left[(\xi + \lambda_+)^2 + \omega_+^2\right]\left[(\xi + \lambda_-)^2 + \omega_-^2\right];\qquad(8.194)$$

each complex conjugate pair of roots corresponds to one modal coordinate (8.195b) with (8.54a) oscillation frequency (8.195a):

$$\bar{\omega}_\pm = \left|(\omega_\pm)^2 + (\lambda_\pm)^2\right|^{1/2} :\qquad q_\pm(t) = C_\pm \exp(-\lambda_\pm t)\cos(\bar{\omega}_\pm t - \alpha_\pm).\qquad(8.195a, b)$$

Thus, *the strong subcritically damped (subsection 2.4.1) free (8.1a, b) oscillations of a rod (8.140) supported by unequal springs and dampers at the two ends (Figure 8.2a) leads (problem 458) to the modal coordinates (8.195b) with the: (i) modal frequencies $\omega_\pm$ and dampings $\lambda_\pm$ specified by the pair of complex conjugate (8.193a–c) roots (8.192) of the modal damping determinant (8.191); (ii) oscillation frequencies (8.195a); (iii) the amplitudes $C_\pm$ and the phases $\alpha_\pm$ are determined by four compatible and independent initial conditions,* as in the subsections 8.4.7– 8.4.8. The roots of the quartic polynomial (8.191) ≡ (8.192) ≡ (8.194), specifying the modal frequencies and dampings, can be determined explicitly in two cases: (i) strong damping of decoupled oscillations (subsection 8.4.10) when it factorizes into the product of two quadratic polynomials; (ii) weak damping of coupled oscillations (subsection 8.4.12) that leads to a polynomial of first degree. Both are particular cases of strong damping of coupled oscillations (subsection 8.4.11).

8.4.10 Strong Damping of Decoupled Free Oscillations

The decoupled case corresponds to the vanishing of the off-diagonal terms in (8.191) leading to (8.142a) ≡ (8.196a) for the resilience and (8.196b) for the friction implying (8.196c, d):

$$k_1(L-a) = k_2(L+a), \quad \mu_1(L-a) = \mu_2(L+a): \tag{8.196a, b}$$

$$k_1(L-a)^2 + k_2(L+a)^2 = 2k_1 L(L-a), \tag{8.196c}$$

$$\mu_1(L-a)^2 + \mu_2(L+a)^2 = 2\mu_1 L(L-a). \tag{8.196d}$$

The quartic polynomial (8.191) splits into two factors that vanish separately:

$$m\xi^2 + (\mu_1+\mu_2)\xi + k_1 + k_2 = 0 = mR^2\xi^2 + 2L\left(\mu_1\xi + k_1\right)(L-a), \tag{8.197a, b}$$

for the motion of translation (8.197a) [rotation (8.197b)]. The roots of (8.197a) specify (8.198a, b):

$$2m\xi_{\pm t} = -\mu_1 - \mu_2 \pm \left|(\mu_1+\mu_2)^2 - 4m(k_1+k_2)\right|^{1/2} = 2m\left(-\lambda_t \pm i\omega_t\right), \tag{8.198a, b}$$

the modal translational damping (8.199a) and oscillation frequency (8.199b):

$$\lambda_t = \frac{\mu_1+\mu_2}{2m}, \qquad \bar{\omega}_t = \left|\frac{k_1+k_2}{m} - \left(\frac{\mu_1+\mu_2}{2m}\right)^2\right|^{1/2}, \tag{8.199a, b}$$

and the roots of (8.197b) specify (8.200a, b):

$$mR^2\xi_{\pm r} = \mu_1 L(L-a) \pm \left|\left[\mu_1 L(L-a)\right]^2 - 2mR^2 k_1 L(L-a)\right|^{1/2} = mR^2\left(-\lambda_r \pm i\omega_r\right), \tag{8.200a, b}$$

the modal rotational damping (8.201a) and oscillation frequency (8.201b):

$$\lambda_r = \frac{\mu_1 L(L-a)}{mR^2}, \qquad \bar{\omega}_r = \left|\frac{2k_1 L(L-a)}{mR^2} - \left[\frac{\mu_1 L(L-a)}{mR^2}\right]^2\right|^{1/2}. \tag{8.201a, b}$$

Thus, *the free (8.190a, b) oscillations of a bar (8.140) supported on unequal springs and dampers at the two ends (Figure 8.2a) in the decoupled case*

(8.196a–d) leads (problem 459) to the physical coordinates of translation (8.202a) [(8.202b)]:

$$z(t) = C_t \exp(-\lambda_t t)\cos(\bar{\omega}_t t - \alpha_t), \quad L\theta(t) = C_r \exp(-\lambda_r t)\cos(\bar{\omega}_r t - \alpha_r),$$

$$(8.202a, b)$$

with: (i) modal dampings (8.199a) [(8.201a)] and oscillation frequencies (8.199b) [(8.201b)]; (ii) the oscillation frequencies are affected by strong damping (8.199a, b) [(8.201a, b)] but not by weak damping (8.203a) [(8.203c)] when they simplify to the modal frequencies (8.203b) [(8.203c)]:

$$\omega_t^2 \gg \lambda_t^2: \quad \bar{\omega}_t = \sqrt{\frac{2k}{m}} = \omega_r, \quad \omega_r^2 \gg \lambda_r^2: \quad \bar{\omega}_r = \sqrt{\frac{2k_1 L(L-a)}{mR^2}} = \omega_r. \quad (8.203a–d)$$

The latter property can be used to determine the weak damping of coupled oscillations (subsection 8.4.12) as a particular case of the strong damping of coupled oscillators (subsection 8.4.11), which is considered for the homogeneous rod (Figure 8.2c).

8.4.11 Strong Damping of Coupled Oscillators

In the case of a homogeneous rod (8.168a–i), the unforced (8.204a, b) oscillations (8.140) are specified by (8.204c):

$$F(t) = 0 = M(t): \quad \begin{bmatrix} m\ddot{z} \\ mL\ddot{\theta} \end{bmatrix} + \begin{bmatrix} \mu_1 + \mu_2 & \mu_1 - \mu_2 \\ 3(\mu_1 - \mu_2) & 3(\mu_1 + \mu_2) \end{bmatrix} \begin{bmatrix} \dot{z} \\ \dot{\theta} \end{bmatrix}$$

$$+ \begin{bmatrix} k_1 + k_2 & k_1 - k_2 \\ 3(k_1 - k_2) & 3(k_1 + k_2) \end{bmatrix} \begin{bmatrix} z \\ L\theta \end{bmatrix} = 0.$$

$$(8.204a–c)$$

Since (8.204c) is a coupled system of linear ordinary differential equations with constant coefficients, it has solutions as exponentials of time (8.190c, d) that are non-trivial if (8.190e) determinant (8.205) vanishes:

$$0 = \begin{vmatrix} \xi^2 + \dfrac{\mu_1 + \mu_2}{m}\xi + \dfrac{k_1 + k_2}{m} & \dfrac{\mu_1 - \mu_2}{m}\xi + \dfrac{k_1 - k_2}{m} \\ 3\dfrac{\mu_1 - \mu_2}{m}\xi + 3\dfrac{k_1 - k_2}{m} & \xi^2 + 3\dfrac{\mu_1 + \mu_2}{m}\xi + 3\dfrac{k_1 + k_2}{m} \end{vmatrix} \equiv P_4(\xi).$$

$$(8.205)$$

Using the natural frequencies (8.170a, b) [dampings (8.206a, b)] of the rod supported on the springs $k_{1,2}$ (dampers μ_1, μ_2) alone, the dispersion relation (8.205) becomes (8.206c):

$$\lambda_{1,2} = \frac{\mu_{1,2}}{2m}: \quad 3\left[2(\lambda_1 - \lambda_2)\xi + \omega_1^2 - \omega_2^2\right]^2 = \left[\xi^2 + 2(\lambda_1 + \lambda_2)\xi + \omega_1^2 + \omega_2^2\right]$$

$$\times \left[\xi^2 + 6(\lambda_1 + \lambda_2)\xi + 3(\omega_1^2 + \omega_2^2)\right].$$
(8.206a–c)

The dispersion relation (8.206c) ≡ (8.207) is:

$$0 = \xi^4 + 8(\lambda_1 + \lambda_2)\xi^3 + 4\left[\omega_1^2 + \omega_2^2 - 3(\lambda_1 - \lambda_2)\right]\xi^2$$
$$+ 24(\lambda_1 \omega_2^2 + \lambda_2 \omega_1^2)\xi + 12\omega_1^2 \omega_2^2 \equiv P_4(\xi),$$
(8.207)

a polynomial of fourth-degree.

The dispersion relation (8.207) must coincide with (8.194) ≡ (8.208a) in terms of (8.208b) modal dampings and oscillation frequencies (8.195a):

$$0 = P_4(\xi) \equiv (\xi^2 + 2\lambda_+ \xi + \bar{\omega}_+^2)(\xi^2 + 2\lambda_- \xi + \bar{\omega}_-^2),$$
(8.208a)

$$= \xi^4 + 2(\lambda_+ + \lambda_-)\xi^3 + (\bar{\omega}_+^2 + \bar{\omega}_-^2 + 4\lambda_- \lambda_+)\xi^2 + 2(\lambda_+ \bar{\omega}_-^2 + \lambda_- \bar{\omega}_+^2)\xi + \bar{\omega}_+^2 \bar{\omega}_-^2.$$
(8.208b)

The coincidence of the coefficients of the polynomials (8.207) ≡ (8.208b) leads to four relations (8.209a–d):

$$\lambda_+ + \lambda_- = 4(\lambda_1 + \lambda_2), \qquad \bar{\omega}_+^2 + \bar{\omega}_-^2 + 4\lambda_- \lambda_+ = 4\left[\omega_1^2 + \omega_2^2 - 3(\lambda_1 - \lambda_2)\right],$$
(8.209a, b)

$$\lambda_- \bar{\omega}_+^2 + \lambda_+ \bar{\omega}_-^2 = 12(\lambda_1 \omega_2^2 + \lambda_2 \omega_1^2), \qquad \bar{\omega}_+^2 \bar{\omega}_-^2 = 12\omega_1^2 \omega_2^2,$$
(8.209c, d)

Thus, *the free (8.204a, b) damped oscillations (8.204c) of a homogeneous rod (8.168a–i) supported on springs and dampers (Figure 8.2c) are specified by the modal coordinates (8.195b) with modal dampings and oscillation frequencies satisfying (problem 460) (8.209a–d) where appear the natural frequencies (8.170a, b) [dampings (8.206a, b)] for each spring (damper) in isolation.* Two particular cases are considered: (i) no damping (subsection 8.4.4); (ii) weak damping of coupled oscillations (subsection 8.4.12).

8.4.12 Weak Damping of Coupled Oscillations

In the absence of damping (8.210a, b), only two relations (8.209a–d) are non-trivial (8.209b, d) $\equiv$ (8.210d, e):

$$\lambda_{1,2} = 0 = \lambda_\pm: \quad \bar{\omega}_\pm = \omega_\pm: \quad \omega_+^2 + \omega_-^2 = 4\left(\omega_1^2 + \omega_2^2\right), \quad \omega_+^2\,\omega_-^2 = 12\,\omega_1^2\omega_2^2, \quad (8.210\text{a–e})$$

and (8.195a) the oscillation and modal frequencies coincide (8.210c). The modal frequencies (8.210c) satisfying (8.210d, e) are the roots of (8.211a–c):

$$0 = \left(\omega^2 - \omega_+^2\right)\left(\omega^2 - \omega_-^2\right) = \omega^4 - \left(\omega_+^2 + \omega_-^2\right)\omega^2 + \omega_+^2\,\omega_-^2$$
$$= \omega^4 - 4\left(\omega_1^2 + \omega_2^2\right)\omega^2 + 12\,\omega_1^2\,\omega_2^2, \tag{8.211a–c}$$

which coincides with (8.211c) $\equiv$ (8.171), obtained before (subsection 8.4.4). In the case of weak damping, when the square or product of dampings is small compared with the square of frequencies (8.212a, b):

$$\left(\lambda_{1,2}\right)^2, \lambda_1\lambda_2 << \left(\omega_{1,2}\right)^2 \sim \left(\bar{\omega}_{1,2}\right)^2, \quad \left(\lambda_\pm\right)^2, \lambda_+\lambda_- << \left(\omega_\pm\right)^2 \sim \left(\bar{\omega}_\pm\right)^2: \tag{8.212a, b}$$

$$\lambda_\mp\left(\omega_\pm^2 - \omega_\mp^2\right) = 4\left[\lambda_1\left(3\omega_2^2 - \omega_\mp^2\right) + \lambda_2\left(3\omega_1^2 - \omega_\mp^2\right)\right], \tag{8.212c, d}$$

then: (i) the modal frequencies are unchanged since (8.209b, d) simplify to (8.210d, e) as before (8.211a–c) $\equiv$ (8.171); (ii) the modal dampings satisfy (8.209a, c), whose solution for $\lambda_\pm$ is (8.212c, d). Thus, *(problem 461) the weakly damped (8.212a; 8.170a, b; 8.206a, b) linear unforced (8.204a, b) oscillations (8.204c) of a homogeneous rod (8.168a–i), supported on springs and dampers (Figure 8.2c) have modal coordinates (8.195b) with oscillation frequencies equal (8.210c) to the modal frequencies (8.172b–d) and weak modal dampings (8.212c, d).* Following the free oscillations (subsections 8.4.10–8.4.12) next (section 8.5) the forced oscillations of the homogeneous rod are considered.

8.5 Forced Oscillations, Beats, and Resonance

The forced coupled oscillations are considered first without damping in the non-resonant (resonant) cases [subsection 8.5.1 (8.5.2)]. The modal coordinates and forces (subsection 8.5.3) provide the simplest representation of undamped resonant and non-resonant oscillations, as well as the intermediate case of beats (subsection 8.5.4). The case of damped forcing leads (subsection 8.5.5), as usual, to constant amplitude and a phase shift such that the work of the applied forces is balanced by dissipation.

8.5.1 Undamped Non-Resonant Forcing

Consider (8.140) the undamped (8.213c) oscillations of a rod with center of mass at the middle (8.213a) supported on springs and forced (8.213b) [(8.213d)] by a force (moment) of amplitude F_0 (M_0) and applied frequency ω_a:

$$a = 0: \qquad m\ddot{z} + (k_1 + k_2)z + (k_1 - k_2)L\theta = F(t) = F_0\cos(\omega_a t), \qquad (8.213a, b)$$

$$\mu_1 = 0 = \mu_2: \quad I\ddot{\theta} + (k_1 - k_2)Lz + (k_1 + k_2)L^2\,\theta = M(t) = M_0\cos(\omega_a t); \quad (8.213c, d)$$

in the case of the homogeneous rod (8.168a–i), the equations of motion take the form:

$$\begin{bmatrix} \ddot{z} \\ L\ddot{\theta} \end{bmatrix} + \begin{bmatrix} \omega_1^2 + \omega_2^2 & \omega_1^2 - \omega_2^2 \\ 3(\omega_1^2 - \omega_2^2) & 3(\omega_1^2 + \omega_2^2) \end{bmatrix} \begin{bmatrix} z \\ L\theta \end{bmatrix} = \begin{bmatrix} F_0 L \\ 3 M_0 \end{bmatrix} \frac{\cos(\omega_a t)}{mL},$$

$$(8.214)$$

involving (8.170a, b) the oscillation matrix (8.31c) for the applied frequency. The particular integral of (8.214) is sought as an oscillation at the same applied frequency (8.215a, b):

$$z_a(t) = A\cos(\omega_a t) = A\,\mathrm{Re}\left(e^{i\omega_a t}\right), \qquad L\theta_a(t) = B\cos(\omega_a t) = B\,\mathrm{Re}\left(e^{i\omega_a t}\right),$$

$$(8.215a, b)$$

with amplitudes A, B satisfying:

$$mL \begin{bmatrix} \omega_1^2 + \omega_2^2 - \omega_a^2 & \omega_1^2 - \omega_2^2 \\ 3(\omega_1^2 - \omega_2^2) & 3(\omega_1^2 + \omega_2^2) - \omega_a^2 \end{bmatrix} \begin{bmatrix} A \\ B \end{bmatrix} = \begin{bmatrix} F_0 L \\ 3 M_0 \end{bmatrix}. \qquad (8.216)$$

Inverting the system (8.216) and substituting in (8.215a, b), specifies the forced oscillation (8.217b):

$$\omega_a \neq \omega_\pm: \qquad \begin{bmatrix} z_a(t) \\ L\theta_a(t) \end{bmatrix} = \frac{\cos(\omega_a t)}{mL\,P_4(i\omega_a)} \begin{bmatrix} 3(\omega_1^2 + \omega_2^2) - \omega_a^2 & \omega_2^2 - \omega_1^2 \\ 3(\omega_2^2 - \omega_1^2) & \omega_1^2 + \omega_2^2 - \omega_a^2 \end{bmatrix} \begin{bmatrix} F_0 L \\ 3 M_0 \end{bmatrix},$$

$$(8.217a, b)$$

where $P(i\omega_a)$ is the dispersion polynomial (8.171) calculated at the applied frequency ω_a, which is assumed to be distinct from the natural frequencies (8.217a), so that it does not vanish in non-resonant conditions $P(\omega_a) \neq 0$. Thus, *(problem 462) the uniform (8.168a–i) rod supported on springs (Figure 8.2c) forced by sinusoidal forces and moments (8.213a, b) ≡ (8.214) at an applied frequency distinct (8.217a) from the modal frequencies (8.172a–d) has oscillations (8.217b) with constant amplitude and in phase with the forcing, corresponding to the non-resonant case without damping.* The resonant case without damping is considered next (subsection 8.5.2).

8.5.2 Undamped Resonant Forcing

If the applied frequency ω_a coincides with one of the modal frequencies $\omega_\pm$, then (8.217a, b) fails and the resonant response is obtained (subsection 8.2.13) by applying l'Hôspital rule (I.19.35), which is differentiating the numerator and denominator with regards to ω_a and letting $\omega_a \to \omega_\pm$:

$$
\begin{bmatrix} z_a(t) \\ L\theta_a(t) \end{bmatrix} = \lim_{\omega_a \to \omega_\pm} \left(\frac{\partial P_4(i\omega_a)}{\partial \omega_a} \right)^{-1}
$$

$$
\times \frac{\partial}{\partial \omega_a} \left\{ \frac{\cos(\omega_a t)}{mL} \begin{bmatrix} 3(\omega_1^2 + \omega_2^2) - \omega_a^2 & 3(\omega_2^2 - \omega_1^2) \\ \omega_2^2 - \omega_1^2 & \omega_1^2 + \omega_2^2 - \omega_a^2 \end{bmatrix} \begin{bmatrix} F_0 L \\ 3 M_0 \end{bmatrix} \right\}.
$$

(8.218)

In (8.218), three sets of derivatives with regards to the applied frequency appear, namely: (i) the derivatives of the numerator (8.219a, b):

$$
\frac{\partial}{\partial \omega_a} \left[\cos(\omega_a t) \right] = -t \sin(\omega_a t),
$$

(8.219a)

$$
\frac{\partial}{\partial \omega_a} \begin{bmatrix} 3(\omega_1^2 + \omega_2^2) - \omega_a^2 & 3(\omega_2^2 - \omega_1^2) \\ \omega_2^2 - \omega_1^2 & \omega_1^2 + \omega_2^2 - \omega_a^2 \end{bmatrix} = \begin{bmatrix} -2\omega_a & 0 \\ 0 & -2\omega_a \end{bmatrix};
$$

(8.219b)

(ii) the derivative of the denominator (8.220b), which is the dispersion polynomial (8.171) without damping at the applied frequency (8.220a):

$$
P_4(i\omega_a) = (\omega_a^2 - \omega_+^2)(\omega_a^2 - \omega_-^2), \qquad \frac{\partial P_4(i\omega_a)}{\partial \omega_a} = 2\omega_a (2\omega_a^2 - \omega_+^2 - \omega_-^2).
$$

(8.220a, b)

Substitution of (8.219a, b; 8.220b) in (8.218) specifies the translation and rotation (8.221b) in the resonant case (8.221a):

$$\omega_a = \omega_\pm: \quad 2mL\omega_\pm\left(\omega_\pm^2 - \omega_\mp^2\right)\begin{bmatrix} z_a(t) \\ L\theta_a(t) \end{bmatrix}$$

$$= \begin{bmatrix} -2\omega_\pm & 0 \\ 0 & -2\omega_\pm \end{bmatrix}\begin{bmatrix} F_0 L \\ 3M_0 \end{bmatrix}\cos(\omega_\pm t) \qquad \text{(8.221a, b)}$$

$$- \begin{bmatrix} 3\left(\omega_1^2 + \omega_2^2\right) - \omega_\pm^2 & 3\left(\omega_2^2 - \omega_1^2\right) \\ \omega_2^2 - \omega_1^2 & \omega_1^2 + \omega_2^2 - \omega_\pm^2 \end{bmatrix}\begin{bmatrix} F_0 L \\ 3M_0 \end{bmatrix}t\sin(\omega_\pm t),$$

Thus, *the undamped (8.213c) resonant forcing (8.213a, b) ≡ (8.214) of a homogeneous (8.168a–i) rod supported on springs (Figure 8.2c) at an applied frequency coincident (8.221a) with one of the natural frequencies (8.172a–d) leads (problem 463) to oscillations (8.221b) including a term out-of-phase with amplitude increasing linearly with time.* Both the non-resonant (resonant) forcing [subsection 8.5.1 (8.5.2)] in terms of physical coordinates, forces, and moments become decoupled in terms of modal coordinates and forces (subsection 8.5.3).

8.5.3 Forcing in Terms of Modal Coordinates and Forces

The power or activity of forces, or rate of change of the work with time, can be expressed both in terms of applied force $F(t)$, [moment $M(t)$], and translation $\dot{z}$ (rotation $\dot{\theta}$), velocity (8.222a):

$$\left[F(t)M(t)\right]\begin{bmatrix} \dot{z}(t) \\ \dot{\theta}(t) \end{bmatrix} = \dot{E} = \left[Q_+(t)\,Q_-(t)\right]\begin{bmatrix} \dot{q}_+(t) \\ \dot{q}_-(t) \end{bmatrix}, \qquad \text{(8.222a, b)}$$

or in terms (8.222b) of modal velocities $\dot{q}_\pm$ and forces $Q_\pm$ as in (8.67a, b). Substituting (8.177b) in (8.222a) leads to (8.223):

$$\left[F(t)\quad M(t)\right]\begin{bmatrix} 1 & 1 \\ a_+/L & a_-/L \end{bmatrix}\begin{bmatrix} \dot{q}_+(t) \\ \dot{q}_-(t) \end{bmatrix} = \dot{E}, \qquad \text{(8.223)}$$

comparison of (8.223) with (8.222b), specifies the normal forces:

$$\begin{bmatrix} Q_+(t) & Q_-(t) \end{bmatrix} = \begin{bmatrix} F(t) & M(t) \end{bmatrix} \begin{bmatrix} 1 & 1 \\ a_+/L & a_-/L \end{bmatrix}$$

$$= \begin{bmatrix} F(t)+(a_+/L)\,M(t) & F(t)+(a_-/L)\,M(t) \end{bmatrix},$$

(8.224a, b)

where (8.177a) can be substituted leading to (8.255a, b):

$$\left(\omega_1^2 - \omega_2^2\right)Q_\pm(t) = \left(\omega_1^2 - \omega_2^2\right)F(t) + \left(\omega_\pm^2 - \omega_1^2 - \omega_2^2\right)\frac{M(t)}{L}. \qquad (8.225)$$

The equations of forced motion (8.226a) are decoupled (subsection 8.2.11) in terms of modal coordinates and forces (8.226a), so that the forced oscillations are given, respectively, by (8.226b) [(8.226c)] in the non-resonant (resonant) case:

$$\ddot{q}_\pm + \omega_\pm^2\, q_\pm(t) = Q_\pm(t) \equiv Q_0^\pm \cos(\omega_a t): \quad q_\pm(t) = \begin{cases} \dfrac{Q_0^\pm}{\omega_\pm^2 - \omega_a^2}\cos(\omega_a t) & \text{if } \omega_a \neq \omega_a, \\[4mm] -\dfrac{Q_0^\pm\, t}{2\omega_\pm}\sin(\omega_\pm t) & \text{if } \omega_a \neq \omega_\pm. \end{cases}$$

(8.226a–c)

It has been shown that [problem 464 (465)] *both the non-resonant (8.217a, b) [resonant (8.221a, b)] undamped forced oscillations of a homogeneous rod (8.168a–i) supported on springs (Figure 8.2c) and forced at an applied frequency (8.213a, b) can be decoupled (8.226a) in terms of modal coordinates (8.177a, b) and forces (8.225) leading to simple non-resonant (8.226b) [resonant (8.226c)] oscillations.* The intermediate case between non-resonant and resonant oscillations is beats at an applied frequency close to, but not coincident with, a natural frequency, which are considered next in terms of the modal coordinates (subsection 8.5.4).

8.5.4 Beats at One of the Normal Coordinates

If the applied frequency ω_a is close to but not equal to a natural frequency $\omega_\pm$, there is a phenomenon of beats that applies to one dimensional oscillators (section 2.7) as well as to multidimensional oscillators (section 8.5) with closer analogy using modal coordinates in the latter case. As an example, consider a forced oscillation (8.226b) at the applied frequency ω_a, contaminated by free oscillation at the natural frequency $\omega_\pm$, both with the same amplitude $Q_0^\pm$:

$$q_\pm(t) = \frac{Q_0^\pm}{\omega_\pm^2 - \omega_a^2}\left[\cos(\omega_a t) - \cos(\omega_\pm t)\right], \tag{8.227a}$$

$$= -\frac{2Q_0^\pm}{\omega_\pm^2 - \omega_a^2}\left[\sin\left(\frac{\omega_a - \omega_\pm}{2}t\right)\sin\left(\frac{\omega_a + \omega_\pm}{2}t\right)\right], \tag{8.227b}$$

leading to (8.227b) by (II.5.88b).

Assuming that the difference between applied and natural frequency is small (8.228a, b) compared with the sums (8.228a, b):

$$4\varepsilon_\pm^2 \equiv (\omega_\pm - \omega_a)^2 \ll (\omega_\pm + \omega_a)^2: \qquad \omega_\pm^2 - \omega_a^2 = (\omega_\pm - \omega_a)(\omega_\pm + \omega_a) \sim 4\omega_\pm \varepsilon_\pm,$$

$$\tag{8.228a, b}$$

there are beats (8.229):

$$q_\pm(t) = -\frac{Q_0^\pm}{2\omega_\pm \varepsilon_\pm}\sin(\varepsilon_\pm t)\sin(\omega_\pm t), \tag{8.229}$$

which are oscillations at a "fast" frequency $\omega_\pm$ with amplitude modulation at a "slow" frequency $\varepsilon_\pm$. In the limit of coincidence (8.230a) $\equiv$ (II.7.13b) of the applied and natural frequencies:

$$\lim_{b \to 0}\frac{\sin b}{b} = 1: \qquad \lim_{\varepsilon_\pm \to 0} q_\pm(t) = -\frac{Q_0^\pm}{2\omega_\pm}t\sin(\omega_\pm t), \tag{8.230a,b}$$

the beats (8.229) lead to resonance (8.230b) $\equiv$ (8.226c). *The beats (8.229) [resonance (8.230b) $\equiv$ (8.226c)] correspond [problem 466 (465)] to oscillations at the natural frequency $\omega_\pm$, with an amplitude that is sinusoidal (linearly growing) with time [Figure 2.22c (b)]. These phenomena apply only to one modal coordinate $q_\pm$ (or q_-), namely, that which corresponds to the coincidence frequency $\omega_a \to \omega_+$ (or $\omega_a \to \omega_-$). For example, in the case (8.231a) there are beats (8.229) [no beats (8.227a)] in the* modal coordinate $q_+(t)[q_-(t)]$, and both affect both translation and rotation in (8.177a, b) leading to (8.231b):

$$\omega_a = \omega_+ + \varepsilon_+: \quad \left(\omega_1^2 + \omega_2^2\right)\begin{bmatrix} x_a(t) \\ L\theta_a(t) \end{bmatrix}$$

$$= \begin{bmatrix} 1 & 1 \\ \omega_a^2 - \omega_1^2 - \omega_2^2 & \omega_-^2 - \omega_1^2 - \omega_2^2 \end{bmatrix} \times \begin{bmatrix} \dfrac{Q_0^+}{2\varepsilon_+\omega_+}\sin(\varepsilon_+t)\sin(\omega_+t) \\ \dfrac{Q_0^-}{\omega_-^2 - \omega_a^2}\left[\cos(\omega_a t) - \cos(\omega_- t)\right] \end{bmatrix}.$$

$$(8.231a, b)$$

The beats are not possible at more than modal frequency because they are distinct, and the applied frequency cannot excite both; for the same reason, there is in this case no double resonance, that is, an amplitude growing in the square of time when the applied frequency coincides with a double modal frequency. The presence of damping changes fundamentally the forced oscillations due to the ability to dissipate the work of the applied forces (subsection 8.5.5).

8.5.5 Forced Damped Oscillations

The last case of forced damped oscillations is the solution of the complete system (8.140) for a possibly inhomogeneous rod with center of mass at the midposition with forcing (8.232a) at an applied frequency ω_a:

$$m\ddot{z}+(\mu_1+\mu_2)\dot{z}+(\mu_1-\mu_2)L\dot{\theta}+(k_1+k_2)z+(k_1-k_2)L\theta = F_0\exp(i\omega_a t),$$
$$(8.232a)$$

$$I\ddot{\theta}+(\mu_1-\mu_2)L\dot{z}+(\mu_1+\mu_2)L^2\dot{\theta}+(k_1-k_2)Lz+(k_1+k_2)L^2\theta = M_0\exp(i\omega_a t).$$
$$(8.232b)$$

Seeking as a solution an oscillation at the same applied frequency (8.215a, b) leads to the system (8.233):

$$\begin{bmatrix} \omega_1^2 + \omega_2^2 + 2i\omega_a(\lambda_1+\lambda_2)-\omega_a^2 & \omega_1^2 - \omega_2^2 + i\omega_a(\lambda_1-\lambda_2) \\ 3(\omega_1^2-\omega_2^2)+6i\omega_a(\lambda_1-\lambda_2) & 3(\omega_1^2+\omega_2^2)+6i\omega_a(\lambda_1+\lambda_2)-\omega_a^2 \end{bmatrix}\begin{bmatrix} A \\ B \end{bmatrix} = 0,$$

$$(8.233)$$

for the case (8.168a–i) of a homogeneous rod. The determinant of the matrix in (8.233) is not zero because in the presence of damping the free oscillations cannot have constant amplitude. Thus, the system (8.233) can be solved for $\{A, B\}$ to specify the forced oscillations (8.215a, b). The same method would apply to an inhomogeneous rod with center of mass at the middle (8.233) or not (8.140; 8.232a, b). Thus, *the oscillations (8.215a, b) of the homogeneous (8.168a–i) rod supported (Figure 8.2c) on springs and dampers in the presence of sinusoidal forcing (8.232a, b) have constant amplitudes and phases specified (problem 467) by the complex constants (A, B) as solutions of (8.233). The matrix in (8.233) simplifies at resonance $\omega_a = \omega_+$ or $\omega_a = \omega_-$, and becomes diagonal in the decoupled case; in all cases, the amplitude is constant and there is a phase shift between the response (8.233) and the forcing (8.215a, b) so that dissipation balances the work of the applied forces and the amplitude of the oscillations is constant.* A particular case of coupled oscillator is the vibration absorber (section 8.6), which uses an undamped secondary circuit to absorb the three vibrations of a damped primary circuit.

8.6 Principle of the Vibration Absorber

A two-dimensional coupled oscillator of special interest is the vibration absorber, whose principle of operation can be explained as follows: (i) consider a primary second-order damped system forced at an applied frequency ω_a; (ii) a second-order undamped system is coupled (subsection 8.6.1) with natural frequency tuned to be equal to the applied frequency $\omega_2 = \omega_a$; (iii) it follows that the forced oscillation in the first system is suppressed, and is transferred to the second system (subsection 8.6.2); (iv) the free oscillations of both systems decay on account of the damping (subsection 8.6.3); (v) the vibration absorption does not apply to an undamped system (subsection 8.6.4), but a weak damping is sufficient (subsection 8.6.5) for it to become effective after a sufficiently long time. Thus, in the vibration absorption mode both circuits have transient oscillations, but only the secondary circuit, and not the primary circuit, has forced oscillations (subsection 8.6.6).

8.6.1 Primary Damped Forced System with Auxiliary Undamped Unforced Circuit

Consider a primary second-order damped system performing forced oscillations with applied frequency ω_a in $(2.22) \equiv (8.234)$:

$$\ddot{x} + 2\lambda_1 \dot{x} + \omega_1^2 x = f \cos(\omega_a t) = \mathrm{Re}\{f \exp(i\omega_a t)\}, \qquad (8.234)$$

such as a mechanical (electrical) circuit (Figure 8.1b) with a mass m_1 (self L_1), damper μ_1(resistor R_1), spring k_1 (capacitor C_1), and an applied F (electromotive E) force in (2.23a–c) ≡ (8.235a–c):

$$\lambda_1 \equiv \left\{ \frac{\mu_1}{2m_1}, \frac{R_1}{2L_1} \right\}, \qquad \omega_1 \equiv \left\{ \sqrt{\frac{k_1}{m_1}} , \frac{1}{\sqrt{L_1 C_1}} \right\}, \qquad f \equiv \left\{ \frac{F(t)}{m_1}, \frac{E(t)}{L_1} \right\}.$$

(8.235a–c)

The response:

$$\bar{\omega}_1 \equiv \sqrt{\omega_1^2 - \lambda_1^2}; \quad \lambda_1 < \omega_1: \quad x_0(t) = C \exp(-\lambda_1 t) \cos(\bar{\omega}_1 t - \alpha)$$

$$+ \operatorname{Re} \left\{ f \left(\omega_1^2 - \omega_a^2 + 2i\lambda_1 \omega_a \right)^{-1} \exp(i\omega_a t) \right\},$$

(8.236a–c)

consists (8.236c) of: (i) a free oscillation (2.106b) with subcritical damping (2.106a) ≡ (8.236b) and oscillation frequency (2.105c) ≡ (8.54a) ≡ (8.236a), and amplitude C and phase α determined by initial conditions, which decays due to damping; (ii) a forced oscillation with constant amplitude (2.194), which is the only one remaining after a sufficiently long time. In order to suppress the latter oscillation: (i) a secondary system (8.237b) is coupled, undamped, and unforced, having only [Figure 8.3a (b)] mass m_2 (self L_2), and spring k_2 (capacitor C_2), leading to the natural frequency (8.237a):

$$\omega_2 \equiv \left\{ \sqrt{\frac{k_2}{m_2}}, \frac{1}{\sqrt{L_2 C_2}} \right\}: \qquad \ddot{x}_2 + \omega_2^2 (x_2 - x_1) = 0, \qquad (8.237a, b)$$

$$\omega_{12}^2 \equiv \left\{ \sqrt{\frac{k_2}{m_1}}, \frac{1}{\sqrt{L_1 C_2}} \right\}: \quad \ddot{x}_1 + 2\lambda_1 \dot{x}_1 + \omega_1^2 x_1 - \omega_{12}^2 (x_2 - x_1) = \operatorname{Re} \left\{ \left[f \exp(i\omega_a t) \right] \right\},$$

(8.237c, d)

(ii) instead of (8.234), there is a coupled system (8.237b, d) with parameters (8.235a–c; 8.237a, c). Thus: (i) only the primary system (8.237d) is forced and involves the cross-frequency (8.237c); (ii) the secondary system (8.237b) is unforced, undamped, and coupled only through a mass-spring (self-capacitor) in the mechanical (electrical) case. Thus, *the mechanical (electrical)* **vibration absorber** *in Figure 8.3a(b) consists (problem 468) of a forced, damped primary system (8.237c, d; 8.235a–c) to which an undamped, unforced secondary system (8.237a, b) is coupled.* Since only the forced solution does not decay with

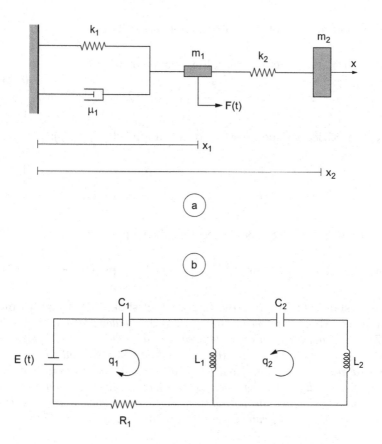

FIGURE 8.3
The mechanical (a) [electrical (b)] vibration absorber adds to a primary damped and forced circuit another undamped, unforced secondary circuit whose natural frequency equals the applied frequency; apart from transient oscillations that decay with time the permanent forced oscillations are transferred from the primary to the secondary circuit.

time, only the particular integral of the forced system (8.237b, d) is considered next (subsection 8.6.2) as a first instance.

8.6.2 Suppression of Forced Oscillations in the Primary System

The particular integral of the forced system (8.237b, d) is sought in the form of an oscillation at the applied frequency (8.238a, b) where the amplitudes satisfy (8.238c):

$$x_{1,2}(t) = A_{1,2}\exp(i\omega_a t): \quad \begin{bmatrix} \omega_1^2 + \omega_{12}^2 + 2i\lambda_1\omega_a - \omega_a^2 & -\omega_{12}^2 \\ -\omega_2^2 & \omega_2^2 - \omega_a^2 \end{bmatrix}\begin{bmatrix} A_1 \\ A_2 \end{bmatrix} = \begin{bmatrix} f \\ 0 \end{bmatrix}.$$

$$(8.238a\text{--}c)$$

Since the determinant of the matrix is not zero (8.239a, b):

$$P_4(i\omega_a) = \left(\omega_1^2 + \omega_{12}^2 - \omega_a^2 + 2i\lambda_1\omega_a\right)\left(\omega_2^2 - \omega_a^2\right) - \omega_2^2\,\omega_{12}^2$$

$$= \omega_a^4 - 2i\lambda_1\omega_a^3 - \left(\omega_1^2 + \omega_{12}^2 + \omega_2^2\right)\omega_a^2 + 2i\lambda_1\omega_2^2\,\omega_a + \omega_1^2\,\omega_2^2, \qquad (8.239\text{a, b})$$

the system (8.238c) can be inverted for the amplitudes (A_1, A_2):

$$P_4(i\omega_a)\begin{bmatrix} A_1 \\ A_2 \end{bmatrix} = \begin{bmatrix} \omega_2^2 - \omega_a^2 & \omega_{12}^2 \\ \omega_2^2 & \omega_1^2 + \omega_{12}^2 - 2i\lambda_1\omega_a - \omega_a^2 \end{bmatrix}\begin{bmatrix} f \\ 0 \end{bmatrix}. \qquad (8.240)$$

Substituting (8.240) in (8.238a, b) specifies the responses:

$$\{x_1(t), x_2(t)\} = f\{\omega_2^2 - \omega_a^2, \omega_2^2\}\,\mathrm{Re}\left\{\left[P_4(i\omega_a)\right]^{-1}\exp(i\omega_a t)\right\} + \dots \qquad (8.241\text{a, b})$$

where ... stands for the free oscillations that should decay with time due to damping. Thus: *if (problem 469) a secondary undamped, unforced oscillator (8.237a, b) is coupled to a primary damped, forced mechanical (electrical) oscillator (8.234; 8.235a–c) then [Figure 8.3a(b)] the coupled (8.237c, d) oscillators are forced at the applied frequency (8.241a, b) and: (i) the forced oscillation is always transferred to the auxiliary circuit (8.241b)* ≡ *(8.242c); (ii) the forced oscillation is suppressed in the primary circuit (8.242b) if the natural frequency of the secondary circuit is chosen to coincide with the applied frequency of forcing of the first circuit (8.242a):*

$$\omega_2 = \omega_a: \qquad x_1(t) = \dots = x_2(t) - f\omega_a^2\,\mathrm{Re}\left\{\left[P(i\omega_a)\right]^{-1}\exp(i\omega_a t)\right\}, \qquad (8.242\text{a–c})$$

where ... stands for the free oscillations that decay with time is shown in next (subsection 8.6.3).

8.6.3 Transfer of Forced Vibrations to the Secondary System

Both the suppression (transfer) of vibrations in (to) the primary (8.242b) [secondary (8.242c)] system occur as the free oscillations decay with time due to damping. Although only (not) the primary (secondary) system has dissipation, their coupling implies that the free oscillations decay in both. This is proved next by showing that the eigenvalues of the unforced system [(8.237b, d) with $f = 0$] have negative real parts. The solution is sought in the form (8.243a, b) leading to the system (8.243c):

$$x_{1,2}(t) = B_{1,2}\,e^{\xi t}: \qquad \begin{bmatrix} \xi^2 + 2\lambda_1\xi + \omega_1^2 + \omega_{12}^2 & -\omega_{12}^2 \\ -\omega_2^2 & \xi^2 + \omega_2^2 \end{bmatrix}\begin{bmatrix} B_1 \\ B_2 \end{bmatrix} = 0. \qquad (8.243\text{a–c})$$

The solution (8.243a, b) is the same as (8.238a, b) with $\xi = i\omega_a$, and thus, the system (8.243c) has the same matrix as (8.238c); since the system (8.243c) is unforced, the eigenvalues are roots of (8.239b) ≡ (8.244b):

$$-\lambda \equiv \text{Re}(\xi) < 0: \quad 0 = P_4(\xi) = \xi^4 + 2\lambda_1 \xi^3 + \left(\omega_1^2 + \omega_{12}^2 + \omega_2^2\right)\xi^2 + 2\lambda_1 \omega_2^2 \xi + \omega_1^2 \omega_2^2 ;$$

$$(8.244\text{a, b})$$

the free oscillations are damped, provided that all eigenvalues ξ have negative real parts (8.244a). Instead of finding the roots of the quartic dispersion polynomial (8.244b) a quadratic polynomial is formed from (8.243c) by multiplying the equations (8.243c) for the complex amplitudes (B_1, B_2) by the conjugates (B_1^*, B_2^*), leading to (8.245a):

$$0 = \left[\left(\xi^2 + 2\lambda_1 \xi + \omega_1^2 + \omega_{12}^2\right)B_1 - \omega_{12}^2 B_2\right]B_1^* + \left[\left(\xi^2 + \omega_2^2\right)B_2 - \omega_2^2 B_1\right]B_2^*$$

$$(8.245\text{a–c})$$

$$= H_2 \xi^2 + 2H_1 \xi + H_0 = H_2 (\xi - \xi_+)(\xi - \xi_-),$$

which is (8.245b, c), a binomial in ξ with positive real coefficients (8.246a–c):

$$H_2 = B_1 B_1^* + B_2 B_2^* = |B_1|^2 + |B_2|^2 > 0, \quad H_1 = \lambda_1 B_1 B_1^* = \lambda_1 |B_1|^2 > 0, \quad (8.246\text{a, b})$$

$$H_0 = \left(\omega_1^2 + \omega_{12}^2\right)B_1 B_1^* - \omega_{12}^2 B_2 B_1^* + \omega_2^2 B_2 B_2^* - \omega_2^2 B_1 B_2^*. \quad (8.246\text{c})$$

In the case (8.247a) implying (8.247b), the third coefficient (8.246c) is positive (8.247c) like the other two (8.246a, b):

$$\{m_1, L_1\} = \{m_2, L_2\}; \quad \omega_{12}^2 = \omega_2^2: \quad (8.247\text{a, b})$$

$$H_0 = \omega_1^2 B_1 B_1^* + \omega_2^2 (B_1 - B_2)(B_1^* - B_2^*) = \omega_1^2 |B_1|^2 + \omega_2^2 |B_2 - B_1|^2 > 0. \quad (8.247\text{c})$$

The roots of (8.245b, c) are (8.248a):

$$H_2 \xi_\pm = -H_1 \pm \sqrt{H_1^2 - H_0 H_2}, \quad \text{Re}(\xi_\pm) < 0, \quad (8.248\text{a, b})$$

and satisfy (8.248b) ≡ (8.244a) in all cases:

$$H \equiv \left|H_1^2 - H_0 H_2\right|^{1/2}: \quad \xi_\pm = \begin{cases} -\dfrac{H_1}{H_2} < 0 & \text{if} \quad H_0 H_2 = H_1^2, & (8.249\text{b, c}) \\[2ex] -\dfrac{H_1 \mp iH}{H_2} & \text{if} \quad H_0 H_2 > H_1^2, & (8.249\text{d, e}) \\[2ex] -\dfrac{H_1 \mp H}{H_2} < 0 & \text{if} \quad H_0 H_1 < H_1^2, & (8.249\text{f, g}) \end{cases}$$

because: (i) in the case (8.249c) there is a real negative double root (8.249b); (ii) in the case (8.249e) the complex conjugate roots have (8.249d) negative real parts not involving (8.249a); (iii) in the case (8.249g) the real roots (8.249f) are both negative since $H < H_1$ in (8.249a). *Quod erat demonstrandum.* It has been shown that *(problem 470) for a primary damped (secondary undamped) system (8.237a–d; 8.235a–c) with the same (8.247a) mass/induction in the case of mechanical/electrical circuits, all free oscillations are damped (8.244a).* The vibration absorption: (a) depends on the decay of free oscillations and does not occur in the absence of damping (subsection 8.6.4); (b) the decaying free oscillations are transient both in the primary and secondary systems (subsection 8.6.5). The preceding method applies for strong damping and has by-passed the calculation of the modal frequencies and dampings, which is considered next (subsections 8.6.4).

8.6.4 Modal Frequencies and Dampings of the Vibration Absorber

The vibration absorption does not apply to an undamped system because the free oscillations do not decay in the primary nor in the secondary system; the natural frequencies are unchanged by weak damping, and thus, coincide with the modal frequencies that are calculated next. The modal frequencies (8.250a) in the absence of damping (8.250b) are the roots of the dispersion polynomial (8.244b) ≡ (8.250c):

$$\xi = i\omega, \qquad \lambda_1 = 0: \qquad 0 = P_4(i\omega) = \omega^4 - \left(\omega_1^2 + \omega_{12}^2 + \omega_2^2\right)\omega^2 + \omega_1^2\,\omega_2^2 ,$$

$$(8.250\text{a–c})$$

The dispersion polynomial is biquadratic (8.250c) and has roots (8.251a):

$$2\omega_\pm^2 = \omega_1^2 + \omega_{12}^2 + \omega_2^2 \pm \sqrt{\Omega}: \quad \Omega = \left(\omega_1^2 + \omega_{12}^2 + \omega_2^2\right)^2 - 4\omega_1^2\,\omega_2^2$$

$$= \left(\omega_1^2 + \omega_2^2\right)^2 - 4\omega_1^2\,\omega_2^2 + \omega_2^4 + 2\omega_2^2\left(\omega_1^2 + \omega_{12}^2\right)$$

$$= \left(\omega_2^2 - \omega_2^2\right)^2 + \omega_2^2\left(2\omega_1^2 + 2\omega_{12}^2 + \omega_2^2\right),$$

$$(8.251\text{a–d})$$

where: (i) Ω is positive by (8.251d) and hence $\omega_\pm^2$ is real; (ii) from (8.251a, b) it follows that $\omega_\pm^2$ is positive. Thus, *(8.251a–d) are (problem 471) the natural frequencies of the undamped free motion (8.250b) ≡ (8.252a) of the coupled oscillator (8.252b, c):*

$$\lambda_1 = 0: \qquad x_1 + \omega_1^2\,x_1 + \omega_{12}^2\,x_2 = 0 = x_2 + \omega_2^2\left(x_2 - x_1\right), \qquad (8.252\text{a–c})$$

that have constant amplitude.

In the case of weak damping (8.253a), substitution of (8.253b, c) in the dispersion polynomial (8.244b) leads to (8.253d):

$$\lambda^2 \ll \omega^2: \qquad \xi = -\lambda \pm i\omega, \qquad \xi^2 = -\omega^2 \mp 2i\lambda\omega:$$

$$0 = \omega^4 \pm 4i\lambda\omega^3 \mp 2i\lambda_1\omega^3 + \left(\omega_1^2 + \omega_{12}^2 + \omega_2^2\right)\left(-\omega^2 \mp 2i\lambda\omega\right) \tag{8.253a–d}$$

$$\pm 2i\lambda_1\omega_2^2\omega + \omega_1^2\omega_2^2 + 0\left(\lambda^2, \lambda_1^2, \lambda_1\lambda\right),$$

where: (i) the vanishing of the real part leads to (8.250c), showing that the modal frequencies coincide with the natural frequencies (8.251a–d), which is unchanged by weak damping (8.253a) ≡ (8.254a); (ii) the vanishing of the imaginary part specifies the modal dampings (8.254b):

$$\lambda^2 \equiv \lambda_\pm^2 \ll \omega_\pm^2 \equiv \omega^2: \qquad \lambda_\pm = \lambda_1 \frac{\omega_\pm^2 - \omega_2^2}{2\omega_\pm^2 - \omega_1^2 - \omega_{12}^2 - \omega_2^2}, \tag{8.254a, b}$$

for weak damping. Thus, *the two-dimensional coupled mechanical (electrical) oscillator [Figure 8.3a(b)], corresponding to the unforced vibration absorber (8.237a–d; 8.235a–c) in the case of weak damping (8.253a–c) ≡ (8.254a) has (problem 472): (i) modal frequencies (8.251a–d) unaffected by damping; (ii) modal dampings specified by (8.254b).* These specify the transient oscillations in the primary and secondary circuits (subsection 8.6.5), in addition to the forced oscillations (subsection 8.6.2).

8.6.5 Transient and Forced Oscillatory Components

In the case of subcritical damping (8.255a), the oscillations of the secondary circuit (8.255c) consist of: (i) free oscillations, which are a superposition of two modal oscillations (8.243a; 8.253b) with dampings (8.254b) and oscillation frequencies (8.251a–d) leading to the oscillation frequencies (8.255b); (ii) the forced oscillation (8.241b):

$$\lambda_\pm^2 < \omega_\pm^2, \quad \bar{\omega}_\pm = \left|(\omega_\pm)^2 - (\lambda_\pm)^2\right|^{1/2}: \tag{8.255a, b}$$

$$x_2(t) = C_+ \exp(-\lambda_+ t)\cos(\bar{\omega}_+ t - \alpha_+) + C_- \exp(-\lambda_- t)\cos(\bar{\omega}_- t - \alpha_-)$$

$$+ f\omega_2^2 \operatorname{Re}\left\{\left[P_4(i\omega_a)\right]^{-1}\exp(i\omega_a t)\right\}. \tag{8.255c}$$

The amplitudes $C_\pm$ and phases $\alpha_\pm$ are determined from four compatible and independent initial conditions. Thus, (8.255c) completes (8.241b) by specifying explicitly the transient oscillations, formerly symbolized by dots. For the primary circuit, the free oscillations are obtained from (8.237b) ≡ (8.256a) by applying the corresponding operator (8.256b) to the first two terms on the r.h.s. of (8.255c):

$$x_1(t) = x_2(t) + \omega_2^{-2}\ddot{x}_2(t) = \left\{1 + \omega_2^{-2}\frac{d^2}{dt^2}\right\}$$

$$\left\{C_+\exp(-\lambda_+ t)\cos(\overline{\omega}_+ t - \alpha_+) + C_-\exp(-\lambda_- t)\cos(\overline{\omega}_- t - \phi_-)\right\}.$$

(8.256a, b)

Evaluating (8.256b) for strong damping (8.255b) and adding the forced part (8.241a), specifies the total oscillation in the primary circuit:

$$\omega_2^2 x_1(t) = C_+\exp(-\lambda_+ t)\left[(\omega_2^2 - \overline{\omega}_+^2 + \lambda_+^2)\cos(\overline{\omega}_+ t - \alpha_+) + 2\lambda_+\overline{\omega}_+\sin(\overline{\omega}_+ t - \alpha_+)\right]$$

$$+ C_-\exp(-\lambda_- t)\left[(\omega_2^2 - \overline{\omega}_-^2 + \lambda_-^2)\cos(\overline{\omega}_- t - \alpha_-) + 2\lambda_-\overline{\omega}_-\sin(\overline{\omega}_- t - \alpha_-)\right]$$

$$+ f(\omega_2^2 - \omega_a^2)\mathrm{Re}\left\{\left[P_4(i\omega_a)\right]^{-1}\exp(i\omega_a t)\right\}.$$

(8.257)

The total oscillation in the primary (8.257) [secondary (8.255c)] circuit includes the free oscillations that were omitted in (8.241a) [(8.241b)] and represented by ...; this completes the solution of the problem of the vibration absorber, which is summarized next (subsection 8.6.6).

8.6.6 Total Oscillations in the Primary and Secondary Circuits

It has been shown that: *a mechanical (electrical) damped and forced primary circuit (8.234; 8.235a–c) to which is coupled [Figure 8.3a(b)] a mechanical (electrical) undamped, unforced secondary circuit (8.237a–d), performs (problem 473) oscillations (8.255c; 8.257) consisting of: (i) free oscillations at the oscillation frequencies (8.255b) in the case of subcritical damping (8.255a), which is transient oscillations, for any initial conditions, specifying the amplitudes and phases; (ii) after the transient oscillations have decayed, only the forced oscillations (8.241a, b) remain as t → ∞; (iii) the forced oscillations can be suppressed (8.242b) in the primary circuit x → 0 as t → ∞ by tuning the natural frequency of the secondary circuit to coincide with the applied frequency in the primary circuit (8.242a); (iv) in this case, the forced oscillation remain only in the secondary circuit, that is, as t → ∞ then x_2 tends to (8.242c). The roots of (8.244b; 8.253b) specify the modal frequencies ω_± and dampings λ_±, in general; in the particular case of weak damping (8.254a) the oscillation frequencies (8.255b) simplify to the modal frequencies (8.251a–d) and are independent of the weak dampings (8.254b). The amplitudes C_± and phases α_± are specified by four non-redundant and compatible initial conditions, for example, the initial displacement (8.258a) [(8.258c)] and velocity (8.258b) [(8.258d)] of the secondary (primary) circuit:*

$$x_{20} \equiv x(0) = C_+ \cos\alpha_+ + C_- \cos\alpha_- + f\,\omega_2^2 \operatorname{Re}\left\{ \left[P_4\left(i\,\omega_a\right) \right]^{-1} \right\}, \quad (8.258a)$$

$$\dot{x}_{20} \equiv \dot{x}(0) = C_+\left(\bar{\omega}_+ \sin\alpha_+ - \lambda_+ \cos\alpha_+\right) + C_-\left(\bar{\omega}_- \sin\alpha_- - \lambda_- \cos\alpha_-\right)$$
$$+ f\,\omega_2^2 \operatorname{Re}\left\{ i\,\omega_a \left[P_4\left(i\,\omega_a\right) \right]^{-1} \right\}, \quad (8.258b)$$

$$\omega_2^2\, x_{10} \equiv \omega_2^2\, x_1(0) = C_+\left[\left(\omega_2^2 - \bar{\omega}_+^2 + \lambda_+^2\right)\cos\alpha_+ - 2\,\lambda_+\bar{\omega}_+ \sin\alpha_+\right]$$
$$+ C_-\left[\left(\omega_2^2 - \omega_-^2 + \lambda_-^2\right)\cos\alpha_- - 2\,\lambda_-\bar{\omega}_- \sin\alpha_-\right] \quad (8.258c)$$
$$+ f\left(\omega_2^2 - \omega_a^2\right)\operatorname{Re}\left\{ \left[P_4\left(i\,\omega_a\right) \right]^{-1} \right\},$$

$$\omega_2^2\, \dot{x}_{10} \equiv \omega_2^2\, \dot{x}_1(0) = C_+\left[\lambda_+\left(3\bar{\omega}_+^2 - \omega_2^2 - \lambda_+^2\right)\cos\alpha_+ + \bar{\omega}_+\left(2\lambda_+^2 + \omega_2^2 - \omega_+^2\right)\sin\alpha_+\right]$$
$$+ C_-\left[\lambda_-\left(3\bar{\omega}_-^2 - \omega_2^2 - \lambda_-^2\right)\cos\alpha_- + \bar{\omega}_-\left(2\lambda_-^2 + \omega_2^2 - \omega_-^2\right)\sin\alpha_-\right]$$
$$+ f\left(\omega_2^2 - \omega_a^2\right)\operatorname{Re}\left\{ i\,\omega_a \left[P_4\left(i\,\omega_a\right) \right]^{-1} \right\}. \quad (8.258d)$$

The N-dimensional linear oscillator (sections 8.1–8.2) is illustrated most simply in the two-dimensional case considered first (sections 8.3–8.6) followed by any finite (infinite) dimension [section 8.8 (8.9)]. As a preliminary N-dimensional simultaneous system is considered a radioactive disintegration chain (section 8.7).

8.7 A Markov Chain: Radioactive Disintegration

The general theory of linear damped and forced oscillators with N degrees of freedom (sections 8.1–8.2) was illustrated by detailed examples with two degrees-of-freedom (sections 8.3–8.6). Proceeding to an arbitrary finite number of degrees-of-freedom, a particular case is **Markov chains,** in which each degree-of-freedom depends only on itself and the one preceding. The examples of Markov chains with N degrees-of-freedom of order one include (section 8.7), a radioactive disintegration chain. A radioactive disintegration chain consists of N elements, each decaying to the following (subsection 8.7.1).

The solution of the Markov chain of first-order ordinary differential equations (subsection 8.7.2) can be obtained iteratively (subsection 8.7.4) starting with the first element and: (i) the second element has a non-resonant (resonant) case if (subsection 8.7.3) the first two decay rates are distinct (coincide); (iii) the third element has non-resonant/singly/doubly resonant solutions (subsection 8.7.5, 8.7.6, 8.7.7) if the three decay rates are distinct/two/three coincide. The non-resonant and resonant cases can be combined at higher order (subsection 8.7.8) between the non-resonant and all resonant extremes. The constants of integration are determined by the initial masses of all elements (subsection 8.7.8). The total mass is conserved (subsection 8.7.1) and asymptotically for a long time is concentrated in the last element of the radioactive disintegration chain.

8.7.1 Sequence of N Elements and $N - 1$ Distintegration Rates

Consider (Figure 8.4a) a sequence of N elements, each disintegrating into the next at a constant rate:

$$\dot{M}_1 = -v_1 M_1, \quad \dot{M}_N = v_{N-1} M_{N-1}; \quad n = 2,...,N-1: \quad \dot{M}_n = v_{n-1} M_{n-1} - v_n M_n,$$
$$(8.259a\text{–}d)$$

so that: (i) the mass of the first element decays (8.259a) due to its disintegration at a rate v_1; (ii) the mass of the last element accumulates (8.259b) due to the disintegration of the penultimate element at a rate v_{N-1}; (iii) for every intermediate element (8.259c) its mass (8.259d) increases by disintegration of the preceding element like (ii) and decreases by its own disintegration like (i). Adding all of the intermediate equations (8.259c, d) and also using the first (8.259a) and last (8.259b) leads to (8.260a):

$$\sum_{n=2}^{N-1} \dot{M}_n = \sum_{n=2}^{N-1} \left(v_{n-1} M_{n-1} - v_n M_n \right) = v_1 M_1 - v_{N-1} M_{N-1} = -\dot{M}_1 - \dot{M}_N, \quad (8.260a)$$

implying that *(problem 474) for a radioactive disintegration chain (8.259a–d), the total mass is conserved at all times (8.260b):*

$$const = \sum_{n=1}^{N} M_n(t) = \sum_{n=1}^{N} M_n(0) = M_N(\infty); \quad n = 1,...,N-1: \quad M_n(\infty) = 0.$$
$$(8.260b\text{–}f)$$

and hence equals: (i) the sum of initial masses of all elements (8.260b); (ii) the asymptotic mass of the last element at infinite time (8.260d), because all others will have decayed (8.260e–f). The last statement is proved next for the second element of the radioactive disintegration chain in the non-resonant (resonant) case [subsections 8.7.2(8.7.3)], when the two decay rates are (are not) distinct.

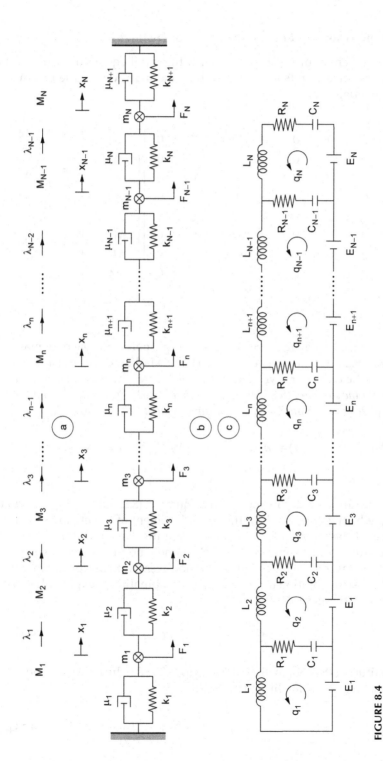

FIGURE 8.4

A radioactive disintegration chain (a) with N elements can be compared with an N-dimensional mechanical (b) [electrical (c)] oscillator consisting of circuits in series. The former (latter) is described by a system of N first- (second-)order differential equations. Each element is affected only by the preceding (both by the preceding and following) element.

8.7.2 Non-Resonant Radioactive Decay at Distinct Rates

The Markov chain of linear first-order differential equations with constant coefficients corresponds to a **banded diagonal matrix** with one line in addition to the diagonal:

$$
\begin{bmatrix}
-v_1 & 0 & 0 & 0 & \cdots & 0 & 0 & 0 \\
v_1 & -v_2 & 0 & 0 & \cdots & 0 & 0 & 0 \\
0 & v_2 & -v_3 & 0 & \cdots & 0 & 0 & 0 \\
0 & 0 & v_3 & -v_4 & \cdots & 0 & 0 & 0 \\
\vdots & \vdots & \vdots & \vdots & \ddots & \vdots & 0 & \vdots \\
0 & 0 & 0 & 0 & & v_{N-1} & -v_{N-1} & 0 \\
0 & 0 & 0 & 0 & \cdots & v_{N-1} & 0 & 0 \\
0 & 0 & 0 & 0 & \cdots & 0 & v_{N-1} & 0
\end{bmatrix}
\begin{bmatrix}
M_1 \\ M_2 \\ M_3 \\ M_4 \\ \vdots \\ M_{N-2} \\ M_{N-1} \\ M_N
\end{bmatrix}
\begin{matrix}
= \\ = \\ = \\ = \\ = \\ \\ = \\ = \\ =
\end{matrix}
\begin{bmatrix}
\dot{M}_1 \\ \dot{M}_2 \\ \dot{M}_3 \\ \dot{M}_4 \\ \vdots \\ \dot{M}_{N-2} \\ \dot{M}_{N-1} \\ \dot{M}_N
\end{bmatrix} ;
$$

$$(8.261)$$

the form of the matrix in (8.261) suggests the property (8.259a–d) of mass conservation (8.260a–f). To prove (8.260e, f), the Markov chain must be solved, which can be done iteratively: (i) in the *case I of (problem 475) the first element of the chain the equation (8.259a) has a solution (8.262b) where the constant of integration (8.262a) is the initial mass of the first element:*

$$M_{10} \equiv M_1(0): \qquad M_1(t) = M_{10}\, e^{-v_1 t}; \qquad \dot{M}_2 + v_2\, M_2 = v_1\, M_1 = v_1\, M_{10}\, e^{-v_1 t},$$

$$(8.262\text{a–d})$$

(ii) substituting (8.262b) in the second equation (8.259d) with $n = 2$ leads to (8.262c), which is the case II of the second element of the chain (8.262d); (iii) the mass of the second element of the chain involves in (8.262d) two decay rates, leading to two subcases IIA (IIB), namely non-resonant (resonant) for distinct (equal) decay rates; (iv) in the non-resonant case of distinct decay rates (8.263a) the solution must be a linear combination of exponential decays with time with rates (8.263b):

$$v_2 \neq v_1: \qquad M_{2A}(t) = C_{21}\, e^{-v_1 t} + C_{22}\, e^{-v_2 t}; \qquad (8.263\text{a, b})$$

(v) substituting (8.263b) in (8.262d) leads to (8.264a), which specifies one of the constants in (8.263b) leading to (8.264b):

$$(v_2 - v_1)C_{21} = v_1\, M_{10}: \qquad M_{2A}(t) = C_{22}\, e^{-v_2 t} + \frac{v_1}{v_2 - v_1}\, M_{10}\, e^{-v_1 t}; \qquad (8.264\text{a, b})$$

(vi) the initial mass of the second element of the chain (8.265a) specifies the remaining constant in (8.264b):

$$M_{20} = C_{22} + \frac{v_1}{v_2 - v_1} M_{10} : \qquad M_{2A}(t) = M_{20} e^{-v_2 t} + \frac{v_1}{v_2 - v_1} M_{10}\left(e^{-v_1 t} - e^{-v_2 t}\right),$$

$$(8.265a, b)$$

and *(problem 476) determines (8.263b) the mass of the second element for all time (8.265b) in the non-resonant subcase IIA of distinct (8.263a) disintegration rates.*

8.7.3 Single Resonance Due to the Coincidence of the Two Disintegration Rates

Proceeding to (vii) the subcase IIB of resonant forcing, when the two decay rates coincide (8.266a), the mass of the second element of the chain (8.265b) is obtained from the limit (8.266b):

$$v_2 = v_1 : \qquad M_{2B}(t) = \lim_{v_2 \to v_1} \frac{(v_2 - v_1) M_{20} e^{-v_2 t} + v_1 M_{10}\left(e^{-v_1 t} - e^{-v_2 t}\right)}{v_2 - v_1} ; \quad (8.266a, b)$$

(viii) the indetermination of type 0:0 in (8.266b) can be resolved by the L'Hospital rule (I.19.35) by differentiating separately the number and denominator with regards to v_2 before taking the limit, leading to (8.267):

$$M_{2B}(t) = \lim_{v_2 \to v_1} \frac{\partial}{\partial v_2}\left[(v_2 - v_1) M_{20} e^{-v_2 t} + v_1 M_{10}\left(e^{-v_1 t} - e^{-v_2 t}\right)\right], \quad (8.267)$$

since the derivative of the denominator is unity; (ix) from (8.267) follows (8.268a):

$$M_{2B}(t) = \lim_{v_2 \to v_1}\left(M_{20} e^{-v_2 t} + v_1 M_{10} t e^{-v_2 t}\right) = \left(M_{20} + v_1 M_{10} t\right) e^{-v_1 t}, \quad (8.268a, b)$$

as the mass of the second element of the chain (8.268b) in the resonant (8.266a) subcase IIB; (x) the same result can be obtained noting that the coincidence of decay rates (8.266a) $\equiv$ (8.269a) implies that the solution must be (8.269b), an exponential decay multiplied by a polynomial of degree one in time:

$$v_2 = v_1 : \qquad M_{2B}(t) = \left(C_{11} + C_{12} t\right) e^{-v_1 t} ; \qquad (8.269a, b)$$

(xi) substitution of (8.269b) in (8.262d) leads to (8.270a), which together with (8.270b) specifies (8.270c) $\equiv$ (8.268b):

$$C_{12} = v_1 M_{10}, \quad M_{20} = M_{2B}(0) = C_{11} : \qquad M_{2B}(t) = \left(M_{20} + v_1 M_{10} t\right) e^{-v_1 t} ;$$

$$(8.270a\text{--}c)$$

234   *Simultaneous Differential Equations and Multi-Dimensional Vibrations*

(xii) thus *(problem 477) the mass of the second element for all time (8.269a)* ≡ *(8.266a) in the resonant subcase IIB coincides (8.270c)* ≡ *(8.268b), as specified by the two equivalent methods.* Thus, considering (Figure 8.4a) the radioactive disintegration chain (8.259a–d) ≡ (8.261): (a) the case I of the first element (8.259a) has an exponential decay (8.262b) from the initial mass (8.262a); (b) the case II of the second element of the chain (8.262d) in the non-resonant (resonant) subcase IIA (IIB) of distinct (8.263a) [equal (8.266a)] decay rates the mass as function of time (8.265b) [(8.270c)] is a linear combination of negative exponentials (a negative exponential multiplied by a linear function) of time. Concerning the case III of the third element, its mass is determined proceeding with the solution of the sequence of differential equations (subsection 8.7.4), which describes the radioactive disintegration chain.

8.7.4 Sequential Solution of a Chain of Ordinary Differential Equations

In the case III of (xiii), the third element of the chain, the differential equation (8.259d) is linear, providing a method of solution (section 3.3 that could have been applied before to the subcases IIA, B as an alternative to the derivation from (8.263a, b) to (8.270a–c), and is applied next to some of the five cases, IIIA, B, C, D, E, in Diagram 8.2; (xiv) the differential equation (8.259d) with $n = 3$ for the mass of the third element of the chain (8.271a):

$$\dot{M}_3 + v_3 M_3 = v_2 M_2: \qquad P = -v_3, \qquad Q = v_2 M_2, \qquad (8.271a\text{–}c)$$

RADIOACTIVE DESINTEGRATION CHAIN

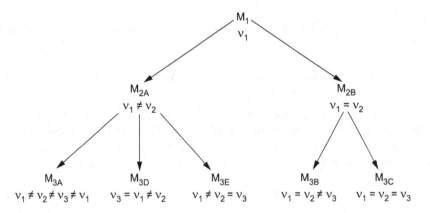

DIAGRAM 8.2
Considering a radioactive disintegration chain (Figure 8.4a) the non-resonant (resonant) cases correspond to distinct (coincident) disintegration rates, leading to two cases 2A–B for the first disintegration. The second disintegration has five cases 3A–E, of which one non-resonant, three singly resonant and one doubly resonant. The N-th disintegration has $N!/(N-k)!$ distinct k-times resonant cases, including one non-resonant case $k = 0$ and one N-times resonant case $k = N$.

is linear (3.27) with coefficients (8.271b, c); (xv) the solution involves (3.20a) ≡ (8.272a) and (3.31a) ≡ (8.272b) in (3.31b) ≡ (8.272c):

$$X(t) = e^{-v_3 t}, \quad Y(t) = v_2 \int^t e^{v_3 \tau} M_2(\tau) \, d\tau: \quad M_3(t) = e^{-v_3 t} \left[C_3 + Y(t) \right],$$

$$(8.272a\text{–}c)$$

where C_3 is an arbitrary constant determined from the initial mass. The first sub-case IIIA is three distinct decay rates that is totally non-resonant (sub-section 8.7.5).

8.7.5 Totally Non-Resonant Case for Three Distinct Decay Rates

In (xvi), the subcases IIIA, B apply if the first two decay rates do not coincide (8.263a) ≡ (8.273a) leading (8.265b; 8.272b) to (8.273b):

$$v_1 \neq v_2: \quad Y(t) = v_2 M_{20} \int^t e^{(v_3 - v_2)\tau} \, d\tau + \frac{v_1 v_2}{v_2 - v_1} M_{10} \int^t \left[e^{(v_3 - v_1)\tau} - e^{(v_3 - v_2)\tau} \right] d\tau;$$

$$(8.273a, b)$$

In (xvii), *(problem 478) the **totally non-resonant** subcase IIIA, where the three decay rates are all distinct (8.274a), substitution of (8.273b) in (8.272c) yields (8.274c) for the mass of the third element of the chain as a function of time:*

$$v_1 \neq v_2 \neq v_3 \neq v_1: \qquad M_{30} \equiv M_{3A}(0) = C_{3A} + \frac{v_2 M_{20}}{v_2 - v_1} - \frac{v_1 v_2 M_{10}}{(v_3 - v_1)(v_3 - v_2)},$$

$$(8.274a, b)$$

$$M_{3A}(t) = C_{3A} e^{-v_3 t} + \frac{v_2}{v_3 - v_2} M_{20} e^{-v_2 t} + \frac{v_1 v_2}{v_2 - v_1} M_{10} \left(\frac{e^{-v_1 t}}{v_3 - v_1} - \frac{e^{-v_2 t}}{v_3 - v_2} \right), \quad (8.274c)$$

where the constant C_{3A} is determined from the initial mass (8.274b); (xviii), the coincidence of the first two decay rates (8.266a) ≡ (8.275a) leads (8.270c; 8.272c) to (8.275b):

$$v_1 = v_2: \qquad Y(t) = v_2 \int^t \left(M_{20} + v_1 M_{10} \tau \right) e^{(v_3 - v_1)\tau} \, d\tau. \qquad (8.275a, b)$$

The subcases IIID/E/B correspond (Diagram 8.2) to a single resonance due to the coincidence of two decay rates $v_1 = v_3 \neq v_2/v_1 \neq v_2 = v_3/$ and $v_1 = v_2 \neq v_3$, and the last is considered next (subsection 8.7.6).

8.7.6 Coincidence of Two Out of Three Decay Rates

In (xix), *(problem 479) subcase IIIB of a third decay rate distinct from the first two* (8.276a), *there is a single resonance leading* (8.275b; 8.272c) *to* (8.276c):

$$v_1 = v_2 \neq v_3: \qquad M_{30} = C_{3B} + \frac{v_1}{v_3 - v_1}\left(M_{20} - M_{10}\frac{v_1}{v_3 - v_1} \right), \qquad \text{(8.276a, b)}$$

$$M_{3B}(t) = C_{3B}\, e^{-v_3 t} + \frac{v_1}{v_3 - v_1}\left[M_{20} + v_1 M_{10}\left(t - \frac{1}{v_3 - v_1} \right) \right], \qquad \text{(8.276c)}$$

where: (a) the remaining constant of integration is determined by the initial mass (8.276b); (b) the last term in (8.276c) results from the evaluation of the second term in (8.275b) in the integral (8.277a).

$$e^{-v_3 t}\, v_1 M_{10} \int^t \tau e^{(v_3 - v_1)\tau}\, d\tau = e^{-v_3 t}\, v_1 M_{10}\, \frac{\partial}{\partial(v_3 - v_1)} \int^t e^{(v_3 - v_1)\tau}\, d\tau$$

$$\text{(8.277a–d)}$$

$$= e^{-v_3 t}\, v_1 M_{10}\, \frac{\partial}{\partial(v_3 - v_1)}\left[\frac{e^{(v_3 - v_1)\tau}}{v_3 - v_1} \right] = \frac{v_1}{v_3 - v_1}\, e^{-v_1 t} M_{10}\left(t - \frac{1}{v_3 - v_1} \right),$$

using parametric differentiation (8.277b) to reduce to a simple primitive (8.277c), leading to the final result (8.277d). Of the five cases III (Diagram 8.2) for the mass of the third element of the radioactive disintegration chain, one IIIA is non-resonant (subsection 8.7.5) and three, IIIB, D, E (one IIIC) is singly (doubly) resonant [subsection 8.7.6 (8.7.7)].

8.7.7 Double Resonance for the Coincidence of Three Decay Rates

In (xx), the subcase IIIC of coincidence of the first three decay rates (8.278a) there is a double resonance for the third element of the chain with (8.275b) leading to (8.278b):

$$v_1 = v_3: \qquad Y(t) = v_1 \int^t \left(M_{20} + v_1 M_{10}\, \tau \right) d\tau; \qquad \text{(8.278a, b)}$$

Hence, (xxi) (8.275a; 8.278a) ≡ (8.279a) *leads to* (8.272c; 8.278b) *in the cases IIIC of* *(problem 480) three coincident disintegration rates to the mass of the third element of* *the radioactive disintegration chain as a function of time* (8.279c):

$$v_1 = v_2 = v_3 \equiv v; \qquad M_{30} = M_{3C}(0) = C_{3C}: \qquad \text{(8.279a, b)}$$

$$M_{3C}(t) = e^{-vt}\left[C_{3C} + v M_{20}\, t + \frac{v^2}{2} M_{10}\, t^2 \right], \qquad \text{(8.279c)}$$

with the constant determined by the initial mass (8.279b). Thus, concerning the case III of the third element (8.271a) of the (Figure 8.4a) radioactive disintegration chain (8.259a–d) ≡ (8.261), there are (Diagram 8.2) five (problem 481) subcases: (c-1) the totally non-resonant subcase IIIA of distinct (8.274a) decay rates leading a mass that is a linear combination of negative exponentials (8.274b, c); (c-2) the subcase IIIB of single resonance by coincidence of the first two decay rates (8.276a) leading to a linear combination of two negative exponentials, one with a factor linear in time (8.276b, c); (c-3) the doubly resonant subcase IIIC of coincidence of the first three decay rates (8.279a), leading to a mass that is the product of a negative exponential by a quadratic function of time (8.279b, c); (c-4/5) there are two more subcases IIID (IIIE) with a single resonance distinct from (8.276a) due to the coincidence of the third decay rate with the first $v_1 = v_3 \neq v_2$ (second $v_1 \neq v_2 = v_3$). Similar methods apply to elements further down the radioactive chain (subsection 8.7.8) up to the last.

8.7.8 Higher-Order Resonances along the Disintegration Chain

Concerning (xxii), the k-th element (8.280a) of the radioactive disintegration chain (8.259a–d) ≡ (8.261) the possible cases are: (xxiii) the (*problem 482*) *non-resonant extreme* of all decay rates distinct (8.280b), leading to a mass that is a linear combination of negative exponentials (8.280c):

$$1 \leq k \leq N-1; \quad (v_1,...,v_k)\,distinct: \quad M_k(t) = \sum_{\ell=1}^{k} C_{K,\ell} \exp(-v_k t); \quad (8.280a\text{–}c)$$

(*xxiv*) the opposite extreme (*problem 483*) of a (*problem 484*) **maximum resonance** with all decay rates equal (8.280a) leading to a negative exponential multiplied by a polynomial of degree $k-1$ of time (8.281b):

$$v_1 = v_2 = ... = v_k \equiv v: \quad M_k(t) = e^{-vt} \sum_{\ell=1}^{k} C_{k,\ell}\, t^{\ell-1}; \quad (8.281a,\, b)$$

(*xxv*) the intermediate cases of (*problem 484*) **multiple resonances**, for example, s coincident decay rates (8.282a) and $k - s$ distinct (8.282b) leading to $k-s+1$ negative exponentials with a polynomial of time of degree $s-1$ multiplying one of them (8.282c):

$$v_1 = v_2 = ... = v_s = v; \quad (v, v_{s+1},...,v_k)\,distinct:$$

$$M_k(t) = e^{-vt} \sum_{\ell=1}^{s} C_{k,\ell}\, t^{\ell-1} + \sum_{\ell=s+1}^{k} C_{k,\ell}\, e^{-\lambda_e t}. \quad (8.282a\text{–}c)$$

The last element (problem 485) of the radioactive disintegration chain (8.258b) ≡ (8.283a) simply accumulates (8.283b) from the decay of the preceding one:

$$\dot{M}_N = \nu_{N-1} M_{N-1}: \qquad M_N(t) = M_{N0} + \nu_{N-1} \int_0^t M_{N-1}(\tau)\,d\tau. \qquad \text{(8.283a, b)}$$

The constants (problem 486) in all cases (8.280a–c; 8.281a, b; 8.282a–c) depend (8.284b) on the decay rates [initial masses (8.284a)] of all elements up to and including the k-th elements:

$$M_{k0} = M_k(0): \qquad C_{k,\ell} = C_{k,\ell}\left(\nu_1, \ldots, \nu_k; M_{10}, \ldots, M_{k0}\right). \qquad \text{(8.284a, b)}$$

The radioactive disintegration chain (chain of linked damped and forced oscillators) lead [Figure 8.4a(b, c)] to a sequence of ordinary differential equations [section 8.7 (8.8)] of the first (second) order.

8.8 Sequence of Damped and Forced Oscillators

Considering a sequence of second-order systems, for example, the mechanical (electrical) circuits in Figure 8.4b(c), this is not a Markov chain because each intermediate element depends both on the preceding and following (subsection 8.8.1). In the case of three masses and four springs, if one of the intermediate elements has a very different mass from all the others (subsection 8.8.3) then: (i) it splits the chain into two if its mass is much larger; (ii) if its mass is much smaller, it can be omitted reducing the number of degrees-of-freedom by one (subsection 8.8.2). The analogy between mechanical (electrical) circuits [subsection 8.8.4)] applies with any number of circuits. In the general case of the damped free oscillations of a chain of N circuits, the: (i) modal dampings (frequencies) are specified (subsection 8.8.5) by the real (imaginary) parts of the complex conjugate roots of the modal polynomial of degree 2N; (ii) the time dependence of each oscillator is (subsection 8.8.6) a superposition of modal coordinates with complex coefficients. The method of solution for a chain of oscillators (subsections 8.8.5–8.8.6) is illustrated explicitly (subsection 8.8.7) in the simplest cases of triple or quadruple oscillators.

8.8.1 Sequence of Coupled Mechanical or Electrical Circuits

Considering the sequence of N damped and forced mechanical oscillators in Figure 8.4b with masses m_n, springs k_n, dampers μ_n, and applied forces F_n, the displacements x_n are specified by: (i) for the first mass (8.285):

$$m_1 \ddot{x}_1 + \mu_1 \dot{x}_1 - \mu_2 (\dot{x}_2 - \dot{x}_1) + k_1 x_1 - k_2 (x_2 - x_1) = F_1(t); \qquad \text{(8.285)}$$

$$m_N \ddot{x}_N + \mu_N (\dot{x}_N - \dot{x}_{N-1}) + \mu_{N+1} \dot{x}_N + k_N (x_N - x_{N-1}) + k_{N+1} x_N = F_N(t). \qquad \text{(8.286)}$$

(ii) for the last mass by (8.286); (vii) for the $(N-2)$ remaining masses (8.287a) by (8.287b):

$$n = 2, ..., N-1: \qquad m_n \ddot{x}_n + \mu_n \left(\dot{x}_n - \dot{x}_{n-1} \right) - \mu_{n+1} \left(\dot{x}_{n+1} - \dot{x}_n \right)$$
$$+ k_n \left(x_n - x_{n-1} \right) - k_{n+1} \left(x_{n+1} - x_n \right) = F_n(t). \qquad (8.287a, b)$$

Due to the different notation for the sequence of three mechanical (electrical) circuits (1,3,2) in Figure 8.1a(c) and (1,2,3) in Figure 8.4b(a) with $N = 2$ the correspondence: (i) between (8.97a) and (8.285) involves the changes $\{\mu_3, k_3\}$ and $\{\mu_2, k_2\}$; (ii) between (8.97b) and (8.286) appear the same changes with $N = 2$. The coupling of the system is similar for the dampers and springs, so it is sufficient to consider the latter:

$$
\begin{bmatrix} m_1 \ddot{x}_1 \\ m_2 \ddot{x}_2 \\ m_3 \ddot{x}_3 \\ \vdots \\ m_{N-1} \ddot{x}_{N-1} \\ m_N \ddot{x}_{N-1} \end{bmatrix}
+
\begin{bmatrix}
k_1 + k_2 & -k_2 & 0 & \cdots & 0 & 0 \\
-k_2 & k_2 + k_3 & -k_3 & \cdots & 0 & 0 \\
0 & -k_3 & k_3 + k_4 & \cdots & 0 & 0 \\
\vdots & \vdots & \vdots & \ddots & \vdots & \vdots \\
0 & 0 & 0 & \cdots & k_{N-1} + k_N & -k_N \\
0 & 0 & 0 & \cdots & -k_N & k_N + k_{N+1}
\end{bmatrix}
\begin{bmatrix} x_1 \\ x_2 \\ x_3 \\ \vdots \\ x_{N-1} \\ x_N \end{bmatrix}
$$

$$
= \begin{bmatrix} F_1(t) \\ F_2(t) \\ F_3(t) \\ \vdots \\ F_{N-1}(t) \\ F_N(t) \end{bmatrix}. \qquad (8.288)
$$

*A chain of N first (8.259a–d) [second (8.285, 8.286; 8.287a, b)] order systems [problem 474 (487)] leads to a double (8.261) [triple (8.288)] banded matrix, because each element depends only on one (on both) of the two neighbors, so that a sequential solution involves a two (three)-term recurrence relation [subsections 8.7.3–8.7.8 (8.8.2–8.8.4)]. The sys-*tem simplifies if one of the masses is much larger or smaller than the others; this can be demonstrated with three masses and four springs (subsection 8.8.2), which is the next case after two masses and three springs (subsection 8.3.1).

8.8.2 Oscillations of Three Masses Coupled by Four Springs

In the unforced (8.289a), undamped (8.289b) case of three masses coupled by four springs, the system (8.285; 8.286; 287a, b) simplifies to (8.289c–e):

$$F_1(t) = F_2(t) = F_3(t) = 0 = \mu_1 = \mu_2 \mu_3: \qquad m \ddot{x}_1 + (k_1 + k_2) x_1 = k_2 x_2, \qquad (8.289a, b)$$

$$m_3 \ddot{x}_3 + (k_3 + k_4) x_3 = k_3 x_2, \qquad m_2 \ddot{x}_2 + (k_2 + k_3) x_2 = k_2 x_1 + k_3 x_3. \qquad (8.289d, e)$$

The solution of (8.289a–c) is sought as undamped free oscillations (8.290a) whose amplitudes satisfy (8.290b):

$$x_{1-3}(t) = A_{1-3}\, e^{i\omega t}: \quad \begin{bmatrix} k_1 + k_2 - m_1\omega^2 & -k_2 & 0 \\ -k_2 & k_2 + k_3 - m_2\omega^2 & -k_3 \\ 0 & -k_3 & k_3 + k_4 - m_3\omega^2 \end{bmatrix} \begin{bmatrix} A_1 \\ A_2 \\ A_3 \end{bmatrix} = 0;$$

$$(8.290a, b)$$

since not all amplitudes are zero (8.291a), the determinant must vanish (8.291b):

$$(A_1, A_2, A_3) \neq (0,0,0): \quad 0 = P_3(i\omega) = -(k_1 + k_2 - m_1\omega^2)k_3^2 - (k_3 + k_4 - m_3\omega)^2 k_2^2$$

$$+ (k_1 + k_2 - m_1\omega^2)(k_2 + k_3 - m_2\omega^2)(k_3 + k_4 - m_3\omega^2).$$

$$(8.291a, b)$$

Thus *(problem 488) an unforced undamped mechanical oscillator (Figure 8.4b) with N = 3 degrees-of-freedom (8.289a–e) has modal frequencies (8.290a) that are the roots of the cubic dispersion polynomial (8.291b) in* ω^2. The roots simplify if the middle mass is very different from the other two, which is either much larger or much smaller (subsection 8.8.3).

8.8.3 Limits of Middle Mass Much Larger/Smaller Than the Others

If the middle mass is much larger than the others (8.292a), only the terms multiplying m_2 in (8.291b) matter, leading to (8.292b):

$$m_2 \gg m_1, m_3: \qquad 0 = \omega^2 (k_1 + k_2 - m_1\,\omega^2)(k_3 + k_4 - m_3\,\omega^2); \qquad (8.292a, b)$$

the large mass does not oscillate (8.293a) and acts as an anchoring point for two decoupled oscillators with natural frequencies (8.293b, c):

$$\omega_2 = 0: \qquad \omega_1 = \left| \frac{k_1 + k_2}{m_1} \right|^{1/2}, \qquad \omega_3 = \left| \frac{k_3 + k_4}{m_3} \right|^{1/2}. \qquad (8.293a–c)$$

In the case opposite to (8.292a), when the middle mass is much smaller than the others (8.294a), only the terms in (8.291b) not multiplied by m_2 matter leading to (8.294b):

$$m_2 \ll m_1, m_3: \qquad 0 = \left(k_1 + k_2 - m_1\,\omega^2\right)k_3^2 - \left(k_3 + k_4 - m_3\,\omega^2\right)k_2^2$$
$$+ \left(k_2 + k_3\right)\left(k_1 + k_2 - m_1\,\omega^2\right)\left(k_3 + k_4 - m_3\,\omega^2\right),$$

(8.294a, b)

which is a biquadratic equation (8.294c) for the modal frequencies (8.294d):

$$0 = m_1 m_3\left(k_2 + k_3\right)\omega^4 - \left\{m_1\,k_3^2 + m_3 k_2^2 - \left(k_2 + k_3\right)\left[m_1\left(k_3 + k_4\right) + m_3\left(k_1 + k_2\right)\right]\right\}\omega^2$$

$$- \left(k_1 + k_2\right)k_3^2 - \left(k_3 + k_4\right)k_2^2 + \left(k_1 + k_2\right)\left(k_2 + k_3\right)\left(k_3 + k_4\right)$$

$$\equiv m_1 m_3\left(k_2 + k_3\right)\left(\omega^2 - \omega_+^2\right)\left(\omega^2 - \omega_-^2\right).$$

(8.294c, d)

Thus, *in a sequence of (problem 489) three masses and four springs, a large (8.292a) [small (8.294a)] middle mass decouples (8.292b) [couples (8.294c)] the outer masses and specifies the natural frequencies (8.293a–c) [(8.294c, d)].* The preceding results on sequences of mechanical oscillators (subsections 8.8.1–8.8.3) apply equally well (Figure 8.4a, b) to sequences of electrical circuits (subsection 8.8.4).

8.8.4 Comparison of Sequences of Mechanical and Electrical Circuits

Considering a sequence of N damped and forced electrical circuits in Figure 8.4c, with selfs L_n, resistors R_n, capacitors C_n, and electromotive forces E_n, the electric charges q_n are specified: (i, ii) for the first (last) circuit by (8.295) [(8.296)]:

$$L_1\,\ddot{q}_1 + R_1\,\dot{q}_1 - R_2\left(\dot{q}_2 - \dot{q}_1\right) + \frac{q_1}{C_1} - q_2\left(\frac{1}{C_2} - \frac{1}{C_1}\right) = E_1(t),$$

(8.295)

$$L_N\,\ddot{q}_N + R_N\left(\dot{q}_N - \dot{q}_{N-1}\right) + R_{N+1}\,\dot{q}_N + \frac{q_N - q_{N-1}}{C_N} + \frac{q_N}{C_{N+1}} = E_n(t);$$

(8.296)

(iii) for the (8.297a) intermediate circuits (8.297b):

$$2 \leq n \leq N - 1: \qquad L_n\ddot{q}_n + R_n\left(\dot{q}_n - \dot{q}_{n-1}\right) - R_{n+1}\left(\dot{q}_{n+1} - \dot{q}_n\right)$$

$$+ \frac{q_n - q_{n-1}}{C_n} - \frac{q_{n+1} - q_n}{C_{n+1}} = E_n(t).$$

(8.297a, b)

The dependence on the resistances R_n is similar to that on the inverse capacities $1/C_n$, so it is sufficient to consider only the former in the triple-banded matrix system:

$$
\begin{bmatrix}
L_1\ddot{q}_1 \\
L_1\ddot{q}_2 \\
L_1\ddot{q}_3 \\
\vdots \\
L_{N-1}\ddot{q}_{N-1} \\
L_N\ddot{q}_N
\end{bmatrix}
+
\begin{bmatrix}
R_1+R_2 & -R_2 & 0 & \cdots & 0 & 0 \\
-R_2 & R_2+R_3 & -R_3 & \cdots & 0 & 0 \\
0 & -R_3 & R_3+R_4 & \cdots & 0 & 0 \\
\vdots & \vdots & \vdots & \vdots & \vdots & \vdots \\
0 & 0 & 0 & \cdots & R_{N-1}+R_N & -R_N \\
0 & 0 & 0 & \cdots & -R_N & R_N+R_{N+1}
\end{bmatrix}
\begin{bmatrix}
\dot{q}_1 \\
\dot{q}_2 \\
\dot{q}_3 \\
\vdots \\
\dot{q}_{N-1} \\
\dot{q}_N
\end{bmatrix}
$$

$$
+
\begin{bmatrix}
\dfrac{1}{C_1}+\dfrac{1}{C_2} & -\dfrac{1}{C_2} & 0 & \cdots & 0 & 0 \\
-\dfrac{1}{C_2} & \dfrac{1}{C_2}+\dfrac{1}{C_3} & -\dfrac{1}{C_3} & \cdots & 0 & 0 \\
0 & -\dfrac{1}{C_3} & \dfrac{1}{C_3}+\dfrac{1}{C_4} & \cdots & 0 & 0 \\
\vdots & \vdots & \vdots & \vdots & \vdots \\
0 & 0 & 0 & \cdots & \dfrac{1}{C_{N-1}}+\dfrac{1}{C_N} & -\dfrac{1}{C_N} \\
0 & 0 & 0 & \cdots & -\dfrac{1}{C_N} & \dfrac{1}{C_N}+\dfrac{1}{C_{N+1}}
\end{bmatrix}
\begin{bmatrix}
\dot{q}_1 \\
\dot{q}_2 \\
\dot{q}_3 \\
\vdots \\
\dot{q}_{N-1} \\
\dot{q}_N
\end{bmatrix}
=
\begin{bmatrix}
E_1(t) \\
E_2(t) \\
E_3(t) \\
\vdots \\
E_{N-1}(t) \\
E_N(t)
\end{bmatrix}.
$$

$$\text{(8.298)}$$

The sequence of electrical (8.298) [mechanical (8.288)] circuits can be solved similarly, noting that a distinct choice of elements was made, namely resistors (springs) that are dissipative (not dissipative). *The chain of radioactive disintegration (8.259a–d) ≡ (8.261) in Figure 8.4a can be compared (problem 490) with the sequence of mechanical (8.285; 8.286; 8.287a, b) ≡ (8.288) [electrical (8.295; 8.296; 8.297a, b) ≡ (8.298)] circuits in Figure 8.4b(c) showing two notable differences between them. The radioactive chain (sequence of oscillators) is: (i) specified by a simultaneous system of N first (second)-order differential equations; (ii) each element depends only on its predecessor (both on its predecessor and successor) implying a two (three-banded) diagonal matrix that corresponds to a two (three)-term recurrence relation. The sequence of mechanical (8.285; 8.286; 8.287a, b) [electrical (8.255; 8.296; 8.297a, b; 8.298)] circuits [Figure 8.4b(c)] satisfies the analogy mass-self, damper-resistor, spring-capacitor (2.17a–c) and applied-electromotive force; in the triple-banded diagonal matrix system (8.288) [(8.298)] was considered the spring (resistor), which is analogous to the capacitor (damper), so the set of the two matrices applies to the general mechanical or electrical sequence of circuits.* Having considered subsection(s) [8.8.4 (8.8.1-8.1-8.8.3)] separately, damping (oscillations) next are considered both together (subsections 8.8.5–8.8.7).

8.8.5 Coupled Modal Frequencies and Dampings

The system of N coupled damped unforced (8.299a) oscillators has exponential solutions (8.299b) leading from the differential equations (8.285)/(8.286)/(8.287a, b) to the algebraic system (8.299c):

$$F_n(t) = 0: \qquad x_n(t) = e^{\xi t} A_n(\xi), \qquad \sum_{m=1}^{n} B_{m,n}(\xi) A_n(\xi) = 0, \qquad (8.299\text{a–c})$$

where the non-zero elements of the modal matrix are, respectively, (8.300a, b)/(8.301a, b)/(8.302a–d):

$$B_{1,1}(\xi) = m_1 \xi^2 + (\mu_1 + \mu_2)\xi + k_1 + k_2, \qquad B_{1,2}(\xi) = -\mu_2 \xi - k_2, \qquad (8.300\text{a, b})$$

$$B_{N,N}(\xi) = m_N \xi^2 + (\mu_N + \mu_{N+1})\xi + k_N + k_{N+1}, \quad B_{N,N-1}(\xi) = -\mu_N \xi - k_N, $$
$$(8.301\text{a, b})$$

$$n = 2,3,...,N-1: \qquad B_{n,n}(\xi) = m_n \xi^2 + (\mu_n + \mu_{n+1})\xi + k_n + k_{n+1},$$

$$B_{n,n-1}(\xi) = -\mu_n \xi - k_n, \quad B_{n,n+1}(\xi) = -\mu_{n+1} \xi - k_{n+1}.$$
$$(8.302\text{a–d})$$

A non-trivial solution requires that the amplitudes in (8.299b) be not all zero (8.303a) and thus, the determinant of the coefficients in (8.299c) is zero (8.303b):

$$\{A_1,...,A_N\} \neq \{0,...,0\}: \quad 0 = \text{Det}\left[B_{m,n}(\xi)\right] \equiv P_{2N}(\xi)$$

$$= m_1...m_N \prod_{\ell=1}^{N} (\xi + \lambda_\ell - i\bar{\omega}_\ell)(\xi + \lambda_\ell + i\bar{\omega}_\ell),$$

$$(8.303\text{a–d})$$

leading to the vanishing of the modal polynomial (8.303c) of degree $2N$, whose pairs of complex conjugate roots (8.303d) specify the modal frequencies and dampings. Thus, *the modal dampings (frequencies) of the unforced (8.299a) coupled damped oscillators (8.285; 8.286; 8.287a, b) are (problem 491) minus the real part (the modulus of the imaginary part) of the roots (8.303d) of the modal polynomial (8.303c), which is the determinant (8.303b) of the three-banded diagonal matrix with non-zero elements (8.300a, b; 8.301a, b; 8.302a–d).* The modal frequencies and dampings appear in the time dependence of the free damped oscillations (subsection 8.8.6).

8.8.6 Amplitudes and Phases of the Coupled Oscillations

The complex factors A_n in (8.299b) specify the amplitudes (phases) through their moduli (arguments) and are related by (8.299c), leading: (i)(ii) from (8.300a, b) [(8.301a, b)] to (8.304a) [(8.304b)] for the first (last) oscillator, which has only one neighbor:

$$\frac{A_2(\xi)}{A_1(\xi)} = -\frac{B_{1,1}(\xi)}{B_{1,2}(\xi)}, \qquad\qquad \frac{A_N(\xi)}{A_{N-1}(\xi)} = -\frac{B_{N,N-1}(\xi)}{B_{N,N}(\xi)}; \qquad (8.304\text{a, b})$$

(iii) the intermediate oscillators (8.302a) have two neighbors, leading to a three-term recurrence relation (8.303a):

$$0 = A_n\,B_{n,n}(\xi) + A_{n-1}\,B_{n,n-1}(\xi) + A_{n+1}\,B_{n,n+1}(\xi), \qquad\qquad (8.305\text{a})$$

which can be solved (subsection II.1.6.1) as a finite continued fraction:

$$\frac{A_{n+1}(\xi)}{A_n(\xi)} = -\frac{B_{n,n}(\xi)}{B_{n,n+1}(\xi)} - \frac{B_{n,n-1}(\xi)}{B_{n,n+1}(\xi)}\,\frac{1}{A_n(\xi)/A_{n-1}(\xi)}. \qquad\qquad (8.305\text{b})$$

Thus, *(problem 492) the damped oscillations of the first mass are a linear superposition (8.306a) of all modal coordinates (8.306b):*

$$x_1(t) = \sum_{\ell=1}^{N}\left[q_\ell^+(t) + q_\ell^-(t)\right]: \qquad\qquad q_\ell^\pm(t) = C_\ell^\pm\,e^{-\lambda_\ell t}\,e^{\pm i\bar\omega_\ell t}, \qquad (8.306\text{a, b})$$

with: (i) the modal frequencies and dampings (8.303b–d) obtained before (8.300a, b; 8.301a, b; 8.302a–d); (ii) 2N amplitudes $C_\ell^\pm$ that are determined by 2N independent and compatible initial conditions, such as the initial displacements and velocities of each oscillator. The damped oscillations of the remaining masses (8.307a) are a linear superposition (8.305b) of the same modal coordinates (8.306b):

$$m = 2,\ldots,N: \quad x_m(t) = \sum_{\ell=1}^{N}\left[A_m\left(-\lambda_\ell + i\bar\omega_\ell\right)q_\ell^+(t) + A_m\left(-\lambda_\ell - i\bar\omega_\ell\right)q_\ell^-(t)\right],$$

$$(8.307\text{a, b})$$

*with **modal amplitudes** $A_2,\ldots,A_N$ determined successively by (8.304a; 8.305b; 8.304b).* This method of determination of all interacting oscillations (subsections 8.8.5–8.8.6) applies to all orders; the simplest beyond the double oscillator is the triple oscillator (subsections 8.8.2–8.8.3) and quadruple oscillator (subsection 8.8.7).

8.8.7 Interactions in Triple/Quadruple Oscillators

In the case of three oscillators, $N = 3$, the three modal coordinates (8.306b) add to specify the motion of the first $m = 1$ oscillator (8.306a). The second $m = 2$ oscillator (8.307b) involves the complex factor (8.304a) with (8.308a) leading (8.300a, b) to the second modal amplitude (8.308b):

$$A_1 = 1: \qquad A_2(\xi) = \frac{m_1 \xi^2 + (\mu_1 + \mu_2)\xi + k_1 + k_2}{\mu_2 \xi + k_2}. \qquad (8.308a, b)$$

The last $m = 3$ triple (8.309a) oscillator (8.304b) involves (8.304b) the complex factor (8.309b, c), specifying the third modal amplitude:

$$N = 3: \qquad A_3(\xi) = -A_2(\xi) \frac{B_{3,2}(\xi)}{B_{3,3}(\xi)} = A_2(\xi) \frac{\mu_3 \xi + k_3}{m_3 \xi^2 + (\mu_3 + \mu_4)\xi + k_3 + k_4}.$$

$$(8.309a\text{–}c)$$

In the case (8.310a) of the quadruple oscillator, the first and second modal amplitudes (8.308a, b) still hold, but not the third modal amplitude (8.309a–c), which is replaced (8.305b) by (8.310b, c):

$$N = 4: \qquad A_3(\xi) = -A_2(\xi) \frac{B_{2,2}(\xi)}{B_{2,3}(\xi)} - \frac{B_{2,1}(\xi)}{B_{2,3}(\xi)}$$

$$(8.310a\text{–}c)$$

$$= A_2(\xi) \frac{m_2 \xi^2 + (\mu_2 + \mu_3)\xi + k_2 + k_3}{\mu_3 \xi + k_3} - \frac{\mu_2 \xi + k_2}{\mu_4 \xi + k_4}.$$

In addition to (8.308a, b; 8.310c) there is another (8.304b) complex factor (8.311b, c) in the case (8.311a) of the quadruple oscillator, specifying the fourth modal amplitude:

$$N = 4: \qquad A_4(\xi) = -A_3(\xi) \frac{B_{4,3}(\xi)}{B_{4,4}(\xi)} = A_3(\xi) \frac{\mu_4 \xi + k_4}{m_4 \xi^2 + (\mu_4 + \mu_5)\xi + k_4 + k_5}.$$

$$(8.311a\text{–}c)$$

It has been shown that *the triple (8.309a) [quadruple (8.310a) ≡ (8.311a)] chain of oscillators (8.285; 8.286; 8.287a, b) has (problem 493): (i) modal frequencies and dampings specified by the roots of (8.303b–d; 8.300a, b; 8.301a, b; 8.302a–d); (ii) displacements (8.306a; 8.307a,b) that are linear combinations of the modal coordinates (8.306b); (iii) the modal amplitudes $C_i^\ddagger$ of the modal coordinates are determined by initial conditions; (iv) the factors in the $N - 1 = 2(3)$ oscillators (8.307a,b) beyond the first (8.306a) are given by (8.308a, b; 8.309c) [(8.308a, b; 8.310c; 8.311c).*

The forced oscillations can be considered using the previous methods (sub-sections 8.2.9–8.2.16). After the oscillators in two (any finite number of) dimensions [sections 8.3–8.5 (8.1, 8.2, 8.6, 8.8)] is considered an infinite trans-mission line (section 8.9).

8.9 Passing Bandwidth of a Transmission Line

Proceeding with discrete circuits, from two (sections 8.3–8.7), to a finite number N (sections 8.1–8.2 and 8.8) to an infinite number $N \to \infty$ (section 8.9) leads to a transmission line (subsection 8.9.3) where each mechanical (electri-cal) circuit (subsection 8.9.1) can be represented by its impedance (subsection 8.9.2). For impedances consisting of capacitors and selfs (springs and masses) there is (subsection 8.9.4) either lossless transmission or decay by reflection (subsection 8.9.5). The lossless transmission is associated with a frequency bandpass and cut-off frequency (subsection 8.9.6) that lead to five regimes of signal transmission (subsection 8.9.7).

8.9.1 Signals and Spectra in Electrical and Mechanical Circuits

Consider an electrical (mechanical) circuit in the Figure 2.1 ≡ 8.5a (2.3 ≡ 8.5c) with a self L (mass m), resistor R (damper μ), and capacitor C (spring k) sub-ject to an electromotive $F_e \equiv E$ (applied mechanical $F_m = F$) force for which the electric charge q (displacement x) satisfies the linear second-order differen-tial equation (2.21) ≡ (8.312b) [(2.15) ≡ (8.314d)]:

$$I \equiv \dot{q}: \quad L\ddot{q} + R\dot{q} + \frac{q}{C} = E(t); \quad v \equiv \dot{x}: \quad m\ddot{x} + \mu\dot{x} + kx = F(t); \quad \text{(8.312a–c)}$$

the time derivative of the electric charge (displacement) is the electric current (8.312a) [velocity (8.312c)]. The Fourier transform (1.549a–d) relates a function of time to its spectrum, for example, the spectra of the electric current (8.313a) [velocity (8.313b)] and electromotive (8.313c) [mechanical (8.313d)] force:

$$\left\{ I(t), v(t), E(t), F(t) \right\} = \int_{-\infty}^{+\infty} e^{i\omega t} \left\{ \tilde{I}(\omega), \tilde{v}(\omega), \tilde{E}(\omega), \tilde{F}(\omega) \right\} d\omega. \quad \text{(8.313a–d)}$$

The time derivative applied to a function is equivalent (8.314a) to multiplica-tion by $i \equiv \sqrt{-1}$ times the frequency:

$$\frac{\partial}{\partial t} \to i\omega: \quad \tilde{I} = \tilde{\dot{q}} = i\omega\tilde{q}, \quad \tilde{v} = \tilde{\dot{x}} = i\omega\tilde{x}, \quad \tilde{\dot{q}} = i\omega\tilde{I}, \quad \tilde{\dot{x}} = \tilde{v} = i\omega\tilde{v}, \quad \text{(8.314a–e)}$$

and thus, the spectrum of the electric current $\tilde{I}$ (velocity $\tilde{v}$) is related to the spectra of the electric change (8.314b) [velocity (8.314c)] and the spectra of the second derivative of the electric charge (8.314d) [acceleration (8.314e)]. These results are used in next (subsection 8.9.3) to introduce the electrical (mechanical) impedances.

8.9.2 Impedances Due to Selfs/Masses, Resistors/ Dampers, and Capacitors/Springs

Substitution of the spectra (8.314b, d) [(8.314c, e)] in the linear second-order differential equation for the electrical (8.313b) [mechanical (8.313d)] circuit, *in the case of constant coefficients, shows that the spectrum of the electromotive (8.315a) [mechanical (8.315b)] force is [problem 494 (495)] proportional to the spectrum of the electric charge (velocity):*

$$\tilde{E}(\omega) = \left(i\omega L + R + \frac{1}{i\omega C} \right) \tilde{I}(\omega), \qquad \tilde{F}(\omega) = \left(i\omega m + \mu + \frac{k}{i\omega} \right) \tilde{v}(\omega), \qquad \text{(8.315a, b)}$$

*through (8.315a) ≡ (8.316b)] [(8.315b) ≡ (8.317a)] the **electrical mechanical impedance** (8.316b) [(8.317b)]:*

$$\tilde{E}(\omega) = Z_e(\omega)\, \tilde{I}(\omega); \qquad Z_e(\omega) = R + i\left(\omega L - \frac{1}{\omega C} \right) \equiv X_e + iY_e, \qquad \text{(8.316a, b)}$$

$$\tilde{F}(\omega) = Z_m(\omega)\, \tilde{v}(\omega); \qquad Z_m(\omega) = \mu + i\left(\omega m - \frac{k}{\omega} \right) \equiv X_m + iY_m, \qquad \text{(8.317a, b)}$$

*which is generally (problem 496) a complex function of the frequency, whose: (i) real part X_e (X_m) or **resistance** is the electrical resistance R (mechanical kinematic friction coefficient μ); (ii) imaginary part Y_e (Y_m) or **inductance** equals the induction L (mass m) multiplied by the frequency ω minus the inverse of the capacity C (resilience of the spring k) divided by the frequency. The **admittance** (8.318a) is the inverse of the impedance and is given by (8.318b) in terms of the resistance and the inductance:*

$$A \equiv \frac{1}{Z} = \frac{1}{X + iY} = \frac{X - iY}{X^2 + Y^2}. \qquad \text{(8.318a, b)}$$

The impedances may be used to represent associations of electric (mechanical) circuits (chapter I.4), for example, along an infinite transmission line (subsection 8.9.3).

8.9.3 Transmission Line with Impedances in Parallel and in Series

Consider an infinite **transmission line** (Figure 8.6) with impedances in parallel Z_a (series Z_b), so that the electric currents I_n in successive loops satisfy (8.319a):

$$0 = Z_b I_n + Z_a \left(I_n - I_{n+1} \right) + Z_a \left(I_n - I_{n-1} \right) = Z_b I_n + Z_a \left(2 I_n - I_{n-1} - I_{n+1} \right); \quad \text{(8.319a, b)}$$

the condition of lossless transmission is that the linear finite difference equation (8.319b) with constant coefficients has solutions $|I_n| = const$ independent of n. The feasibility of this condition and other possible cases can be assessed after (8.319b) is solved. The solution of the finite difference equation (8.319b) is sought in the form (1.444a) $\equiv$ (8.320a), which substituted in (8.319b) leads to (8.320b) involving (8.320c) a quadratic characteristic polynomial (8.320d):

$$I_n = \zeta^n: \quad 0 = \zeta^{n-1} \left[\left(Z_b + 2 Z_a \right) \zeta - Z_a \left(1 + \zeta^2 \right) \right]$$

$$= -Z_a \zeta^{n-1} \left[1 - \left(2 + \frac{Z_b}{Z_a} \right) \zeta + \zeta^2 \right] \equiv -Z_a \zeta^{n-1} P_2 \left(\zeta \right). \quad \text{(8.320a–d)}$$

The roots (8.321a) of the characteristic polynomial (8.320c, d) specify (8.321b) the general solution (8.321c):

$$P_2 \left(\zeta_{\pm} \right) = 0: \quad \zeta_{\pm} = 1 + \frac{Z_b}{2 Z_a} \pm \sqrt{\frac{Z_b}{Z_a} \left(1 + \frac{Z_b}{4 Z_a} \right)}, \quad I_n = C_+ \zeta_+^n + C_- \zeta_-^n, \quad \text{(8.321a–c)}$$

where $C_{\pm}$ are arbitrary constants determined from initial conditions, leading to five cases. In the case I (8.322a) [II (8.323a)] of a double root (8.322b) [(8.323b)]:

I: $Z_b = 0$: $\zeta_{\pm} = 1$, $I_n = C_+ + C_- n$,   (8.322a–c)

II: $Z_b = -4 Z_a$: $\zeta_{\pm} = -1$, $I_n = (-)^n \left[C_+ + C_- n \right]$,   (8.323a–c)

the currents (8.322c) [(8.323c)]: (i) in general (8.324a) diverge in both directions (8.324b):

$$C_- \neq 0: \quad \lim_{n \to \pm\infty} |I_n| = \infty; \quad C_- = 0: \quad |I_n| = |C_+|, \quad \text{(8.324a–d)}$$

(ii) in the particular case (8.324c) remain finite (8.324d). The cases I and II of a double real root separate the case(s) III (IV and V) of complex conjugate (real and distinct) roots that (subsection 8.9.4) lead to lossless transmission (decay by reflection).

8.9.4 Lossless Transmission or Decay by Reflection

In the case III of (8.325a, b) the roots (8.321b) are complex conjugate (8.325c):

$$\text{III:} \quad 0 > \frac{Z_b}{Z_a} > -4: \quad \zeta_\pm = 1 + \frac{Z_b}{2Z_a} \pm i \left| \frac{Z_b}{Z_a} - \left(\frac{Z_b}{2Z_a} \right)^2 \right|^{1/2}, \tag{8.325a–c}$$

implying that: (i) the modulus is unity (8.326a–c):

$$|\zeta_\pm|^2 = \left[\operatorname{Re}(\zeta_\pm) \right]^2 + \left[\operatorname{Im}(\zeta_\pm) \right]^2 = \left(1 + \frac{Z_b}{2Z_a} \right)^2 - \frac{Z_b}{Z_a} - \left(\frac{Z_b}{2Z_a} \right)^2 = 1; \tag{8.326a–c}$$

$$\zeta_\pm = e^{\pm i\phi}: \qquad \pm \tan\phi = \frac{\operatorname{Im}(\zeta_\pm)}{\operatorname{Re}(\zeta_\pm)} = \frac{\left| -Z_b(Z_b + 4Z_a) \right|^{1/2}}{Z_b + 2Z_a}, \tag{8.327a–c}$$

(ii) the phases (8.327a) are opposite (8.327b, c). The general solution (8.327a; 8.321c) ≡ (8.328a):

$$I_n = C_+ e^{in\phi} + C_- e^{-in\phi} = C \cos(n\phi - \alpha), \tag{8.328a, b}$$

has (8.328b): (i) constant amplitude C implying lossless transmission; (ii) phase jumps (8.327c) with a constant phase shift α. The remaining cases IV (8.329a) [V(8.329b)] exclude (8.322a, 8.323a) and (8.325a) and lead to real roots (8.321b), one larger (8.329c) and the other smaller (8.329d) than unity:

$$\text{IV or V:} \quad \frac{Z_b}{Z_a} > 0 \text{ or } \frac{Z_b}{Z_a} < -4: \quad \zeta_+ > 1 > \zeta_-; \quad C_\pm \neq 0: \quad \lim_{n \to \pm\infty} |I_n| = \infty, \tag{8.329a–f}$$

so that: (i) in general (8.329e), there is (8.321e) divergence in both directions (8.329f); (ii)(iii) in the particular case (8.330b) [(8.331b)] the signal decays (8.330c) [(8.331c)] in the direction of increasing (8.330a) [decreasing (8.330b)] n:

$$n \to \infty: \qquad C_+ = 0, \qquad I_n = C_-(\zeta_-)^n \to 0, \tag{8.330a–c}$$

$$n \to -\infty: \qquad C_- = 0, \qquad I_n = C_+(\zeta_+)^n \to 0. \tag{8.331a–c}$$

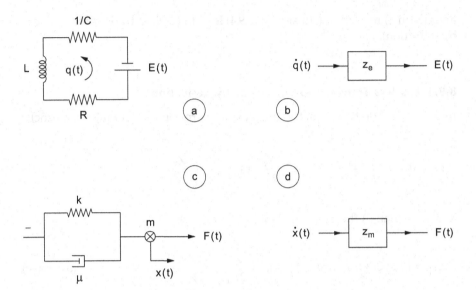

FIGURE 8.5
The representation of sinusoidal oscillations in an electrical (a) [mechanical (c)] circuit can be made via the electrical (b) [mechanical (d)] impedance, which is the ratio of the electromotive (mechanical) force to the electric current (velocity). The electrical (mechanical) impedance depends on the frequency, and does not vary with time, for constant self (mass), resistance (friction), and capacity (resilience).

Thus, *a transmission line (Figure 8.6) consisting of an infinite sequence of parallel Z_a and series Z_b impedances for mechanical (electrical) circuits [Figure 8.5a, b (c, d)] operates (problem 497) in five cases: (III) in the range (8.325a) there is lossless transmission (8.328a, b) with constant amplitude C, phase jumps (8.327c), and a constant phase shift α; (IV/V) above (8.329a) or below (8.329b) the range (8.325a) there is divergence in general (8.329e, f), and in particular cases (8.330a–c; 8.331a–c) there is decay of the signal due to successive reflections, even in the absence of dissipation;*

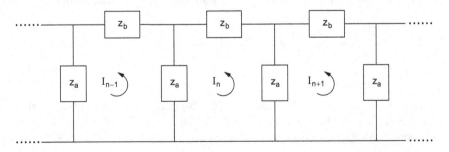

FIGURE 8.6
A transmission line is an infinite sequence of impedances in series Z_b and parallel Z_a, relating the electric currents I_n in successive loops from $n = -\infty$ to $n = +\infty$. Each impedance represents an electric (mechanical) circuit [Figures 8.5a, b (c, d)] leading to three possibilities in each case of one (two) elements(s) [Figures 8.7a–c (8.8a–c)] in the side branch.

(I/II) the boundary cases (8.322a; 8.323a) lead to divergence in general (8.324a, b) and lossless transmission in a particular case (8.324c, d). There is no dissipation in order that the ratio of impedances (8.316b) or (8.317b) be real. These results are applied next to the six cases of transmission lines with one or two elements in each impedance (subsection 8.9.5).

8.9.5 Six Transmission Lines including Two Lossless Cases

In (problem 498) there are six possible types of transmission lines in two sets of three, with self/resistance/capacitor in parallel (Figures 8.7a, 8.7b, 8.7c) [in series (Figures 8.8a, 8.8b, 8.8c] leading respectively to the six impedances (8.333a–f) in parallel and (8.333a–f) in series:

$$Z_{a,1-6} = \left\{ iL_a\omega, R_a, -\frac{i}{C_a\omega}, R_a - \frac{i}{C_a\omega}, iL_a\omega - \frac{i}{C_a\omega}, iL_a\omega + R_a \right\}, \quad (8.332\text{a–f})$$

$$Z_{b,1-6} = \left\{ R_b - \frac{i}{C_b\omega}, L_b - \frac{i}{C_b\omega}, iL_b\omega + R_b, iL_b\omega, R_b, -\frac{i}{C_b\omega} \right\}. \quad (8.333\text{a–f})$$

The conditions (8.325a, b) for a lossless passband require that the ratio of impedances to be real and this is possible (8.316b) only in two cases: (a) only resistance; (b) no resistance. The cases (a) when there are resistances (no selfs or capacitors) implies that the conditions (8.325a, b) are independent of frequency; also, the dissipative effect of the resistance excludes lossless transmission. Thus, if lossless transmission is possible it can only be the case (b), which is considered next (subsection 8.9.4).

8.9.6 Frequency Passband and Cut-off Frequency

For lossless transmission to be possible, dissipation must be absent, thus, (problem 499) excluding resistors (dampers) from the electrical (mechanical) circuits (8.332d, f) [(8.333d, f)] and leaving only (8.332e) [(8.333e)]:

$$Z_a = \left\{ iL_a\omega - \frac{i}{C_a\omega}, im_a\omega - \frac{ik_a}{\omega} \right\}, \qquad Z_b = \left\{ iL_b\omega - \frac{i}{C_b\omega}, im_b\omega - \frac{ik_b}{\omega} \right\}.$$

$$(8.334\text{a–d})$$

which have impedances (8.334a, c) [(8.334b, d)]. As an example, an electrical circuit (8.334a, c), substitution in (8.325a, b), specifies the **conditions for lossless transmission** (8.335a, b):

$$0 > \frac{L_b\omega - \dfrac{1}{C_b\omega}}{L_a\omega - \dfrac{1}{C_a\omega}} > -4: \quad \omega^2 > \frac{\dfrac{1}{C_b} + \dfrac{4}{C_a}}{L_b + 4L_a} = \frac{C_a + 4C_b}{L_b + 4L_a}\frac{1}{C_aC_b} \equiv \omega_*^2, a \quad (8.335\text{a–d})$$

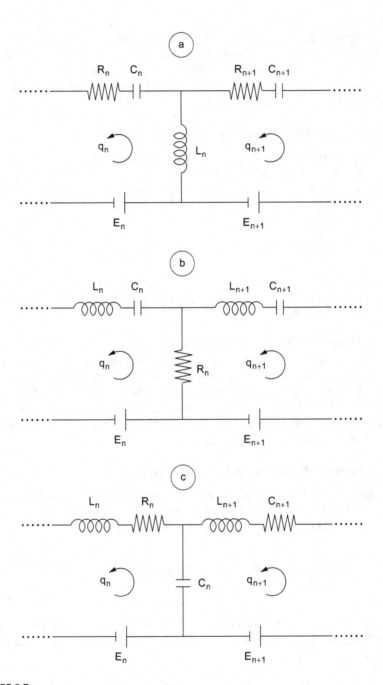

FIGURE 8.7
The three transmission lines with two elements in series and one in parallel in Figures 8.7a, b, c are the converses of Figures 8.8a, b, c. The most general case of a transmission line (Figure 8.6) with lossless signal transmission excludes resistances; the lossless transmission is possible only in the part of a frequency passband not affected by a cut-off frequency from below.

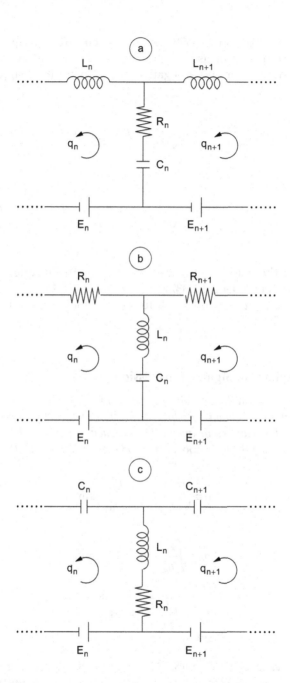

FIGURE 8.8
The transmission line (Figure 8.6) whose impedances consists only of one element in series, lead to three cases (a) self in series and resistances and capacitors in parallel; (b) resistances in series and selfs and capacitors in parallel; (c) capacitors in series and selfs and resistances in parallel. The converse three cases, exchanging the elements in series by those in parallel, appear in Figures 8.7a, b, c.

namely: (i) the condition (8.335b) leads to a **cut-off-frequency** (8.335c, d) below which transmission is not possible; (ii) the condition (8.335a) is met for a positive numerator and a negative denominator (8.336a) [or vice-versa (8.337a)]:

$$L_b\omega - \frac{1}{C_b\omega} > 0 > L_a\omega - \frac{1}{C_a\omega}: \quad \underline{\omega} \equiv \frac{1}{\sqrt{L_bC_b}} < \omega < \frac{1}{\sqrt{L_aC_a}} \equiv \bar{\omega} \quad \text{if} \quad L_bC_b > L_aC_a,$$

$$(8.336a\text{–}c)$$

$$L_b\omega - \frac{1}{C_b\omega} < 0 < L_a\omega - \frac{1}{C_a\omega}: \quad \underline{\omega} \equiv \frac{1}{\sqrt{L_aC_a}} < \omega < \frac{1}{\sqrt{L_bC_b}} \equiv \bar{\omega} \quad \text{if} \quad L_bC_b < L_aC_a,$$

$$(8.337a\text{–}c)$$

implying that there is lossless transmission in the **frequency passband** (8.336b) [(8.337b)] if (8.336c) [(8.337c)] holds. The cut-off frequency combined with the frequency passband leads to five regimes of signal transmission (subsection 8.9.7).

8.9.7 Five Regimes of Signal Transmission

Thus, *the transmission line (problem 500) consisting (Figure 8.6) of electrical (mechanical) circuits without resistors (dampers), whose impedances (8.334a, c) [(8.334b, d)] are due only to selfs (masses) and capacitors (springs) has lossless transmission frequency passband (8.336b, c) [(8.338a, b)] or (8.337b, c) [(8.338c, d)]:*

$$m_b k_a > m_a k_b: \qquad \underline{\omega} \equiv \sqrt{\frac{k_b}{m_b}} < \omega < \sqrt{\frac{k_a}{m_a}} \equiv \bar{\omega}, \qquad (8.338a, b)$$

$$m_a k_b > m_b k_a: \qquad \underline{\omega} \equiv \sqrt{\frac{k_a}{m_a}} < \omega < \sqrt{\frac{k_b}{m_b}} \equiv \bar{\omega}, \qquad (8.338c, d)$$

$$\omega > \sqrt{\frac{k_b + 4k_a}{m_b + 4m_a}} \equiv \omega_*, \qquad (8.338e)$$

with a cut-off frequency (8.335d)[(8.338e)]. Outside the passband a finite (8.330b) [(8.331b)] total signal (8.321c) decays (8.330c) [(8.331c)] in the upstream (8.330a) [downstream (8.331a)] direction in the absence of dissipation due to successive reflections. Thus, there are five regimes of signal transmission relating to the frequency passband $(\underline{\omega}, \bar{\omega})$ in (8.336b, c; 8.337b, c) [(8.338a–d)] and cut-off frequency (8.335c, d) [(8.338e)]: (i–iii) there is no lossless transmission outside the *frequency passband (8.339a, e) or if the cut-off frequency lies above the frequency passband (8.339d):*

$$
\text{lossless transmission}
\begin{cases}
no & \text{if} & \omega < \underline{\omega}, & (8.339a) \\
\underline{\omega} < \omega < \overline{\omega} & \text{if} & \omega_* < \underline{\omega}, & (8.339b) \\
\omega_* < \omega < \overline{\omega} & \text{if} & \underline{\omega} < \omega_* < \overline{\omega}, & (8.339c) \\
no & \text{if} & \omega_* > \overline{\omega}, & (8.339d) \\
no & \text{if} & \omega > \underline{\omega}, & (8.339e)
\end{cases}
$$

(iv) if the cut-off frequency lies below the frequency passband (8.339b) it has no effect and there is lossless transmission over the whole frequency passband; (v) if the cut-off frequency lies within the frequency passband (8.339c) it limits the lossless transmission to the upper part. A generalization of oscillations varying with time (chapters 2, 4 and 8) is waves that oscillate in space-time (notes 6.1–6.23, 7.1–7.55, 8.1–8.17).

NOTE 8.1: Isotropic Equation of Mathematical Physics

Many physical phenomena and engineering processes are described by differential equations (chapters 2, 4, 6, and 8) that may be linear or non-linear. The non-linear differential equations may be linearized by considering small perturbations of a mean state, for example, water waves in a channel (notes 7.12–7.13) or the acoustics of horns (notes 7.16–7.17). The linear differential equations have constant coefficients (sections 1.3–1.6 and 7.4–7.5) in a steady homogeneous medium using Cartesian coordinates, and have variable coefficients otherwise, that is: (i) for an inhomogeneous medium, even in one dimension (notes 7.1–7.46); (ii) for an homogeneous medium using curvilinear coordinates (notes 8.3–8.17). An example of (ii) is (chapter III.7) the generalized isotropic equation of mathematical physics with: (i) spatial dependence specified by the Laplacian; (ii) temporal dependence specified by a linear differential equation with constant coefficients:

$$
\nabla^2 F + \sum_{m=0}^{M} A_m \frac{\partial^m F}{\partial t^m} = 0. \tag{8.340}
$$

A particular case (8.341b–d) of second order (8.341a) in time is (III.7.255) ≡ (8.341e):

$$
M = 2; \quad \{A_0, A_1, A_2\} = \left\{\beta, \frac{1}{\alpha}, -\frac{1}{c^2}\right\} \equiv const; \quad \nabla^2 F - \frac{1}{c^2}\frac{\partial^2 F}{\partial t^2} + \frac{1}{\alpha}\frac{\partial F}{\partial t} + \beta F = 0,
$$

$$
\tag{8.341a–e}
$$

which is the second-order isotropic equation of mathematical physics that describes wave propagation at a speed c, in a dissipative medium with diffusivity α, in the presence of a potential β, all assumed to be constant. The general case (8.340) including, in particular, (8.341a-e) is considered next (note 8.2).

NOTE 8.2: Laplace, Wave, Diffusion, and Helmholtz Equations

The Laplace equation, adding the second (third) term in (8.321e) leads to the wave (diffusion or heat) equation; considering only the first and fourth terms leads to the Helmholtz equation. The complete equation (8.341e) with all terms, as well as its generalization (8.340), can be reduced to a Helmholtz equation by considering the Fourier transform in time (1.549c) $\equiv$ (8.342a):

$$F(\bar{x},t) = \int_{-\infty}^{+\infty} \tilde{F}(\bar{x};\omega)\, e^{-i\omega t}\, d\omega: \qquad\qquad \frac{\partial F}{\partial t} \to -i\omega \tilde{F}, \qquad\qquad \text{(8.342a, b)}$$

which implies that derivation with regards to time (8.342b) is equivalent to multiplication by $-i\omega$, where ω is the frequency. Substitution of (8.342b) in (8.340) shows that *the solution of the generalized isotropic equation of mathematical physics (8.340) has (standard CLXXIX) a Fourier transform in time (8.342a) that satisfies a Helmholtz equation (8.343b):*

$$k^2 \equiv \sum_{j=0}^{M} A_j (-i\omega)^j : \qquad\qquad \nabla^2 \tilde{F} + k^2 \tilde{F} = 0, \qquad\qquad \text{(8.343a, b)}$$

with square of the wavenumber (8.343a), which is complex in the pressure of time derivatives of odd order, for example, (8.344a) for (8.341a–e) the spectrum of the second-order isotropic equation of mathematical physics (8.344b):

$$k^2 = \beta - i\omega\alpha + \frac{\omega^2}{c^2} : \qquad\qquad \nabla^2 \tilde{F} + k^2 \tilde{F} = 0. \qquad\qquad \text{(8.344a, b)}$$

The solution of the Helmholtz equation (8.343b) $\equiv$ (8.344b) is simplest in Cartesian coordinates in N dimensions (note 8.3) when the Laplacian is a second-order partial differential operator with constant coefficients.

NOTE 8.3: Separation of Variables in Cartesian Coordinates

Using the Laplacian in N-dimensional Cartesian coordinates (8.345a) the Helmholtz equation (8.344b) becomes (8.345b):

$$\nabla^2 \tilde{F} = \sum_{n=1}^{N} \frac{\partial^2 \tilde{F}}{\partial x_n^2} = -k^2\,\tilde{F}: \qquad\qquad \tilde{F}(x_1,...,x_N\,;x_N\,;\omega) = \prod_{n=1}^{N} X_n(x_n), \qquad \text{(8.345a–c)}$$

whose solution may be sought by the method of **separation of variables,** as the product (8.345c) of N functions, one of each variable. Substituting (8.345c) in (8.345b) and dividing by $\tilde{F}$ leads to (8.346a):

$$\sum_{n=1}^{N} \frac{1}{X_n} \frac{d^2 X_n}{dx_n^2} = -k^2 = -\sum_{n=1}^{N} k_n^2; \qquad \frac{1}{X_n} \frac{d^2 X_n}{dx_n^2} = -k_n^2, \qquad \text{(8.346a–c)}$$

since each term on the l.h.s. of (8.346a) depends on a different variable, they must all be constant (8.346c) with their sum satisfying (8.346b). Thus, to the **position vector** of coordinates x_n may be associated a **wavevector** with components k_n, whose sum of squares specifies the **wavenumber** k. The differential equation (8.346c) ≡ (8.347a) has solutions (8.347b):

$$\frac{d^2 X_n}{dx_n^2} + k_n^2 X_n = 0: \qquad X_n(x_n) = B_n^+ \exp(i k_n x_n) + B_n^- \exp(-i k_n x_n), \qquad \text{(8.347a, b)}$$

which substituted in (8.345c) lead to (8.347c, d):

$$\tilde{F}(x_1,....,x_N ;\omega) = \prod_{n=1}^{N} C_n \cos(k_n x_n - \alpha_n)$$

$$= 2^{-N} \prod_{n=1}^{N} C_n \left\{ \left[\exp i(k_n x_n - \alpha_n) \right] + \exp\left[-i(k_n x_n - \alpha_n) \right] \right\},$$

$$\text{(8.347c, d)}$$

where $B_n^{\pm}$ in (8.347b) and (C_n, α_n) in (8.347c, d) are alternative pairs of arbitrary constants related (8.347b) ≡ (8.347d) by (8.348a, b) ≡ (8.348c, d):

$$2 B_n^{\pm} = C_n \exp(\mp i\alpha_n), \qquad C_n = 2|B_n^+|, \qquad \exp(2 i\alpha_n) = \frac{B_n^-}{B_n^+}. \qquad \text{(8.348a–d)}$$

Thus, *the Helmholtz equation (8.344b) in N-dimensional Cartesian coordinates (8.345a, b) has solution (standard CLXXX) in terms of sinusoidal functions alone (8.345c; 8.347b) ≡ (8.347c, d) where $B_n^{\pm}$ and (C_n, α_n) are alternative pairs of arbitrary constants (8.348a–d).* In the case of polar (spherical) coordinates in the plane (in space) the Laplacian has variable coefficients and the method of separation of variables leads to linear ordinary differential equations with variable coefficients whose solutions [note 8.4 (8.5)] involve special functions (chapter 9).

NOTE 8.4: **Cylindrical Coordinates and Bessel Functions**

The Laplacian in cylindrical coordinates (III.6.45a, b) in space adds to the Laplacian in polar coordinates (I.11.28b, c) in the plane plus an orthogonal Cartesian coordinate z, leading (8.344b) to the Helmholtz equation (8.349):

$$\frac{1}{r}\frac{\partial}{\partial r}\left(r\frac{\partial \tilde{F}}{\partial r}\right) + \frac{1}{r^2}\frac{\partial^2 \tilde{F}}{\partial \phi^2} + \frac{\partial^2 \tilde{F}}{\partial z^2} + k^2 \tilde{F} = 0,\qquad(8.349)$$

The latter can be solved by separation of variables (8.350a) leading to (8.350b):

$$\tilde{F}(r,\phi,z) = X(r)\,\Phi(\phi)\,Z(z): \quad \frac{1}{Xr}\frac{d}{dr}\left(r\frac{dX}{dr}\right) + \frac{1}{r^2\Phi}\frac{\partial^2 \Phi}{\partial \phi^2} + \frac{1}{Z}\frac{d^2 Z}{dz^2} + k^2 = 0.$$

$$(8.350a, b)$$

The first three terms of (8.350b) depend on different variables leading to the constants (8.351a, b) that must satisfy (8.351c):

$$\frac{1}{\Phi}\frac{d^2\Phi}{d\phi^2} = -m^2, \quad \frac{1}{Z}\frac{d^2 Z}{dz^2} = -K^2, \quad \frac{1}{Xr}\frac{d}{dr}\left(r\frac{dX}{dr}\right) - \frac{m^2}{r^2} + k^2 - K^2 = 0.$$

$$(8.351a–c)$$

The solutions of (8.351a) [(8.351b)] are sinusoidal functions (8.352a) [(8.352b)]:

$$\Phi(\phi) = C_+\,e^{im\phi} + C_-\,e^{-im\phi}, \qquad Z(z) = D_+\,e^{iKz} + D_-\,e^{-iKz}, \quad (8.352a, b)$$

where $C_\pm, D_\pm$ are arbitrary constants. The differential equation (8.351c) $\equiv$ (8.353b) is a **cylindrical Bessel differential equation** (standard CLXXXI):

$$\bar{k} = \left|k^2 - K^2\right|^{1/2}: \qquad r^2\frac{d^2 X}{dr^2} + r\frac{dX}{dr} + \left(\bar{k}^2 r^2 - m^2\right)X = 0. \qquad (8.353a, b)$$

whose solution is a linear combination (8.354b) of **Bessel (Neumann) functions** $J_m(Y_m)$:

$$k^2 = K^2 + \bar{k}^2: \qquad X(r) = E_+\,J_m\left(\bar{k}\,r\right) + E_-\,Y_m\left(\bar{k}\,r\right), \qquad (8.354a, b)$$

with: (i) integer order m equal to the azimuthal wavenumber m in (8.351a; 8.352a); (ii) variable $\bar{k}r$ involving the radial wavenumber $\bar{k}$ in (8.354a) $\equiv$ (8.353a); (iii) the sum of the squares of the radial wavenumber $\bar{k}$ in (8.354b) and of the axial wavenumber K in (8.351b; 8.352b) is the square of the total wavenumber k in the Helmholtz equation (8.349) $\equiv$ (8.350a, b).

Substituting (8.352a, b) and (8.354b) in (8.350a) it follows that *the solution (standard CLXXXII) of the Helmholtz equation (8.343b) ≡ (8.344b) in cylindrical coordinates (8.349) is (8.355):*

$$\tilde{F}(r,\phi,z) = \left(D_+\,e^{iKz} + D_-\,e^{-ikz}\right)\left(C_+\,e^{im\phi} + C_-\,e^{-im\phi}\right)\left[E_+\,J_m\left(\bar{k}\,r\right) + E_-\,Y_m\left(\bar{k}\,r\right)\right],$$

$$(8.355)$$

involving: (i) three pairs of arbitrary constants $\left(C_\pm, D_\pm, E_\pm\right)$; *(ii–iii) products of sinusoidal functions of the axial z and azimuthal* ϕ *coordinates by (iv) a linear combination of Bessel* J_m *and Neumann* Y_m *functions; (v) the* **azimuthal, axial, radial, and total wavenumbers** *respectively* $m, K, \bar{k}$, *and* k, *with the last three related by (8.353a) ≡ (8.354a). In the case of (standard CLXXXIII) polar coordinates in the plane: (i) the dependence on the axial coordinate z in the Laplacian operator is omitted, so that the Helmholtz equation (8.349) simplifies to (8.356a):*

$$\frac{1}{r}\frac{\partial}{\partial r}\left(r\frac{\partial \tilde{F}}{\partial r}\right) + \frac{1}{r^2}\frac{\partial^2 \tilde{F}}{\partial \phi^2} + k^2\tilde{F} = 0:$$

$$(8.356a, b)$$

$$\tilde{F}(r,\phi) = \left(C_+e^{im\phi} + C_-e^{-im\phi}\right)\left[E_+J_m\left(kr\right) + E_+\,Y_m\left(kr\right)\right],$$

(ii) the corresponding axial wavenumber is zero $K = 0$, *omitting one of the factors in the solution (8.355) when passing to (8.356b) were (8.354a) the total and radial wavenumbers coincide.* The solution of the Helmholtz equation in spherical coordinates (note 8.5) involves, besides sinusoidal and spherical Bessel functions, the associated Legendre functions.

NOTE 8.5: Spherical Coordinates and Associated Legendre Functions

The Laplace operator in spherical coordinates (III.6.46a, b) leads (8.344b) to the Helmholtz equation (8.357):

$$\frac{1}{R^2}\frac{\partial}{\partial R}\left(R^2\frac{\partial \tilde{F}}{\partial R}\right) + \frac{1}{R^2\sin\theta}\frac{\partial}{\partial \theta}\left(\sin\theta\frac{\partial \tilde{F}}{\partial \theta}\right) + \frac{1}{R^2\sin^2\theta}\frac{\partial^2 \tilde{F}}{\partial \phi^2} + k^2\,\tilde{F} = 0. \quad (8.357)$$

The solution by separation of variables (8.358a) leads to (8.358b):

$$\tilde{F}(R,\theta,\phi) = X(R)\,\Theta(\theta)\Phi(\phi): \qquad (8.358a)$$

$$\frac{1}{X}\frac{d}{dR}\left(R^2\frac{dX}{dR}\right) + \frac{1}{\Theta\sin\theta}\frac{d}{d\theta}\left(\sin\theta\frac{d\Theta}{d\theta}\right) + \frac{1}{\Phi\sin^2\theta}\frac{d^2\Phi}{d\phi^2} + k^2R^2 = 0, \quad (8.358b)$$

which is satisfied by three separate ordinary differential equations specifying the: (i) azimuthal dependence (8.351a) in terms of sinusoidal functions (8.352a); (ii) latitudinal dependence (8.359a):

$$\frac{1}{\Theta \sin \theta} \frac{d}{d\theta} \left(\sin \theta \frac{d\Theta}{d\theta} \right) - \frac{m^2}{\sin^2 \theta} = -n(n+1), \qquad (8.359a)$$

leads to an **associated Legendre differential equation** (standard CLXXXIV):

$$\frac{d^2\Theta}{d\theta^2} + \cot \theta \frac{d\Theta}{d\theta} + \left[n(n+1) - m^2 \csc^2 \theta \right] \Theta = 0, \qquad (8.359b)$$

*whose solution (8.360) is a linear combination of **associated Legendre functions** of degree n and order m of the first P_n^m and second Q_n^m kind:*

$$\Theta(\theta) = D_+ \, P_n^m \left(\cos \theta \right) + D_- \, Q_n^m \left(\cos \theta \right); \qquad (8.360)$$

(iii) radial dependence (8.361a) $\equiv$ (8.361b):

$$\frac{1}{X} \frac{d}{dR} \left(R^2 \frac{dX}{dR} \right) + k^2 R^2 - n(n+1) = 0 \Leftrightarrow R^2 \frac{d^2X}{dR^2} + 2R \frac{dX}{dR} + \left[k^2 R^2 - n(n+1) \right] X = 0,$$

$$(8.361a, b)$$

specified by a **spherical Bessel differential equation** (standard CLXXXV) *whose general integral (8.362) is a linear combination of **spherical Bessel** j_n and **Neumann** y_n functions of order n:*

$$X(R) = E_+ \, j_n \left(kR \right) + E_- \, y_n \left(kR \right), \qquad (8.362)$$

where k is the radial wavenumber. Substituting (8.352a; 8.360; 8.362) in (8.358a) it follows that *the solution (standard CLXXXVI) of the Helmholtz equation (8.344b) in spherical coordinates (8.357) is:*

$$\tilde{F}(R,\theta,\phi) = \left(C_+ \, e^{im\phi} + C_- \, e^{-im\phi} \right) \left[E_+ \, j_n \left(kR \right) + E_+ \, y_n \left(kR \right) \right]$$

$$\times \left[D_+ \, P_n^m \left(\cos \theta \right) + D_- \, Q_n^m \left(\cos \theta \right) \right], \qquad (8.363)$$

involving: (i) three pairs of arbitrary constants of integration $(C_\pm, D_\pm, E_\pm)$; (ii) sinusoidal functions of longitude (8.352a) with wavenumber m; (iii) associated Legendre functions (8.360) of two kinds of the cosine of the latitude with order m and degree n; (iv) spherical Bessel and Neumann functions (8.342) of order n and variable k R *where the radial distance is multiplied by the radial wavenumber.* The solution of the Helmholtz equation in cylindrical (spherical) coordinates in three dimensions [notes 8.4 (8.5)] can be generalized to hypercylindrical (hyperspherical) coordinates [notes 8.12 (8.6–8.11)] in any higher number of dimensions.

NOTE 8.6: Multidimensional Hyperspherical and Hypercylindrical Coordinates

The solution of the Helmholtz equation in hyperspherical or hypercylindrical coordinates (subsections III.9.7.2–3) involves six steps: (i) relation with N-dimensional Cartesian coordinates (notes 8.6–8.7); (ii) orthogonal base vectors with their moduli specifying the scale factors (note 8.8); (iii) the Laplacian operator leading to the Helmholtz equation (notes 8.9–8.10); (iv) the separation of variables leading to sinusoidal functions in the azimuthal and axial directions and Bessel functions in the radial direction (notes 8.11–8.12); (v) the associated Legendre functions appear for the first latitude and the higher-order latitudes lead to hyperspherical associated Legendre functions (notes 8.13–8.14); (vi) in the case of hypercylindrical coordinates, the last latitude is replaced by a Cartesian axial coordinate leading to sinusoidal functions (notes 8.15–8.17).

The hyperspherical (hypercylindrical) coordinates (8.364a–c) [(8.365a–d)]:

$$0 \le R < \infty, \qquad 0 \le \theta_1,...,\theta_{N-2} < \pi, \qquad 0 \le \phi < 2\pi, \qquad \text{(8.364a–c)}$$

$$0 \le r < \infty, \qquad 0 \le \theta_1,...,\theta_{N-3} < \pi, \qquad 0 \le \phi < 2\pi, \qquad -\infty < z < +\infty, \qquad \text{(8.365a–d)}$$

are defined by N relations with the N-dimensional Cartesian coordinates of which: (i) $N-3$ are similar in terms of the distance from the origin R (from the axis r), and $N-3$ latitudes $\theta_1,.....,\theta_{N-3}$ leading to (8.366a–e) [(8.366a′–e′)]:

$$x_1 = \{R,r\}\cos\theta_1, \qquad \text{(8.366a, a′)}$$

$$x_2 = \{R,r\}\sin\theta_1\cos\theta_2, \qquad \text{(8.366b, b′)}$$

$$x_3 = \{R,r\}\sin\theta_1\sin\theta_2\cos\theta_3, \qquad \text{(8.366c, c′)}$$

$$\vdots$$

$$x_n = \{R,r\}\sin\theta_1\sin\theta_2\cdots\sin\theta_{n-1}\cos\theta_n, \qquad \text{(8.366d′)}$$

$$\vdots$$

$$x_{N-3} = \{R,r\}\sin\theta_1\sin\theta_2\cdots\sin\theta_{N-4}\cos\theta_{N-3}, \qquad \text{(8.346e, e′)}$$

(ii) the hyperspherical coordinates have one more latitude θ_{N-2} and a longitude ϕ adding three equations:

$$x_{N-2} = R \sin \theta_1 \sin \theta_2 \cdots \sin \theta_{N-3} \cos \theta_{N-2}, \tag{8.366f}$$

$$x_{N-1} = R \sin \theta_1 \sin \theta_2 \cdots \sin \theta_{N-3} \cos \theta_{N-2} \cos \phi, \tag{8.366g}$$

$$x_N = R \sin \theta_1 \sin \theta_2 \cdots \sin \theta_{N-3} \sin \theta_{N-2} \sin \phi, \tag{8.366h}$$

(iii) the hypercylindrical coordinates have one axial Cartesian coordinate z and a longitude:

$$x_{N-2} = r \sin \theta_1 \sin \theta_2 \cdots \sin \theta_{N-3} \cos \phi, \tag{8.366f´}$$

$$x_{N-1} = r \sin \theta_1 \sin \theta_2 \cdots \sin \theta_{N-3} \sin \phi, \tag{8.366g´}$$

$$x_N = z. \tag{8.366h´}$$

Thus, *the transformation from hyperspherical (8.364a–c) [hypercylindrical (8.365a–d)] to Cartesian coordinates in N-dimensions is given [standard CLXXXVII (CLXXXVIII)] by (8.366a–h) [(8.366a´–h´)]. In $N = 2$ two dimensions $\left(x_1 \equiv x, \ x_2 \equiv y\right)$ this leads to polar coordinates (r, ϕ). In $N = 3$ three dimensions, $\left(x_3 \equiv z\right)$ this leads to spherical (R, θ, ϕ) [cylindrical (r, ϕ, z)] coordinates. In $N \geq 4$ dimensions, there are $N - 2(N - 3)$ latitudes $\left(\theta_1, ..., \theta_{N-2}\right) \left[\left(\theta_1, ..., \theta_{N-3}\right)\right]$. The* name hyperspherical (hypercylindrical) coordinates arises because the first coordinate hypersurface (note 8.7) is a hypersphere (hypercylinder).

NOTE 8.7: Direct and Inverse Transformation from Cartesian Coordinates

The transformations (8.366a–h) [(8.366a´–h´)] can be inverted from N-dimensional Cartesian to hyperspherical (hypercylindrical) coordinates: (i) the distance from the origin (axis) is (8.367a) [(8.367a´)]:

$$R = \left|\left(x_1\right)^2 + \left(x_1\right)^2 + \cdots + \left(x_N\right)^2\right|^{1/2} = \left|r^2 + \left(x_N\right)^2\right|^{1/2},$$
$$\tag{8.367a, a´}$$
$$r = \left|\left(x_1\right)^2 + \left(x_2\right)^2 + \cdots + \left(x_{N-1}\right)^2\right|^{1/2},$$

showing that the coordinate hypersurface R = const (r = const) is a hypersphere (hypercylinder) of radius $R(r)$; (ii) the next $(N - 3)$ relations are similar:

$$\cot \theta_1 = x_1 \left\{ \left|\left(x_2\right)^2 + \cdots + \left(x_N\right)^2\right|^{-1/2}, \ \left|\left(x_2\right)^2 + \cdots + \left(x_{N-1}\right)^2\right|^{-1/2} \right\}, \tag{8.367b, b´}$$

$$\cot\theta_2 = x_2\left\{\left|\left(x_3\right)^2+\cdots+\left(x_N\right)^2\right|^{-1/2}, \quad \left|\left(x_3\right)^2+\cdots+\left(x_{N-1}\right)^2\right|^{-1/2}\right\}, \tag{8.367c, c'}$$

$$\vdots$$

$$\cot\theta_n = x_n\left\{\left|\left(x_{n+1}\right)^2+\cdots+\left(x_N\right)^2\right|^{-1/2}, \quad \left|\left(x_{n+1}\right)^2+\cdots+\left(x_{N-1}\right)^2\right|^{-1/2}\right\}, \tag{8.367d, d'}$$

$$\cot\theta_{N-3} = x_{N-3}\left\{\left|\left(x_{N-2}\right)^2+\cdots+\left(x_N\right)^2\right|^{-1/2}, \quad \left|\left(x_{N-2}\right)^2+\left(x_{N-1}\right)^2\right|^{-1/2}\right\}. \tag{8.367e, e'}$$

(iii) the last two relations are different:

$$\cot\theta_{N-2} = x_{N-2}\left|\left(x_{N-1}\right)^2+\left(x_N\right)^2\right|^{-1/2}, \qquad x_{N-2}/x_{N-1}, \tag{8.367f, f'}$$

$$\cot\phi = x_{N-1}/x_N, \qquad z = x_N. \tag{8.367g, g'}$$

In the transformations (8.367b–g; 8.367b'–f') it would be possible to substitute the cotangent by other circular functions. *The transformations (8.367a–g) [(8.367a'–g')] from N-dimensional Cartesian coordinates to hyperspherical (hypercyindrical) coordinates are [standard CLXXXIX (CXC)] the inverses of (8.366a–h) [(8.366a'–h')], and show that (8.364b, c) [(8.365b, c)] are orthogonal coordinates on the* hypersphere (8.367a) [hypercylinder (8.367a')]. The orthogonality of the hyperspherical (hypercylindrical) coordinates is proved from the base vectors (note 8.8) leads to the scale factors.

NOTE 8.8: Base Vectors and Scale Factors

The Cartesian components of the contravariant hyperspherical base vectors (note III.9.38) follow from the transformation (8.346a–h) from hyperspherical to Cartesian coordinates (8.368a–f):

$$\vec{e}_R \equiv \frac{\partial x_m}{\partial R} = \left\{\cos\theta_1, \sin\theta_1\cos\theta_2, \sin\theta_1\sin\theta_2\cos\theta_3, \ldots, \sin\theta_1\sin\theta_2\ldots\sin\theta_{n-1}\cos\theta_n,\right.$$

$$\left.\ldots, \sin\theta_1\sin\theta_2\ldots\sin\theta_{N-2}\cos\phi, \sin\theta_1\sin\theta_2\ldots\sin\theta_{N-2}\sin\phi\right\}, \tag{8.368a}$$

$$\vec{e}_1 \equiv \frac{\partial x_m}{\partial\theta_1} = R\left\{-\sin\theta_1, \cos\theta_1\cos\theta_2, \cos\theta_1\sin\theta_2\cos\theta_3,\right.$$

$$\ldots, \cos\theta_1\sin\theta_2\sin\theta_3\ldots\sin\theta_{n-1}\cos\theta_n,$$

$$\left.\ldots, \cos\theta_1\sin\theta_2\ldots\sin\theta_{N-2}\cos\phi, \cos\theta_1\sin\theta_2\ldots\sin\theta_{N-2}\sin\phi\right\}, \tag{8.368b}$$

$$\vec{e}_2 \equiv \frac{\partial x_m}{\partial \theta_2}$$

$$= R \sin \theta_1 \{ 0, -\sin \theta_2, \cos \theta_2 \cos \theta_3, \cos \theta_2 \sin \theta_3 \cos \theta_4,$$

$$\cdots, \cos \theta_2 \sin \theta_3 \cdots \sin \theta_{n-1} \cos \theta_n,$$

$$\cdots, \cos \theta_2 \sin \theta_3 \sin \theta_4 \sin \theta_{N-2} \cos \phi, \cos \theta_2 \sin \theta_3 \sin \theta_4 \sin \theta_{N-2} \sin \phi \}$$

$$\vdots$$

$$(8.368c)$$

$$\vec{e}_n \equiv \frac{\partial x_m}{\partial \theta_n} = R \sin \theta_1 \cdots \sin \theta_{n-1} \{ 0, 0, \cdots, 0, -\sin \theta_n, \cos \theta_n \sin \theta_{n+1}, \dots,$$

$$\cos \theta_n \sin \theta_{n+1} \dots \sin \theta_{N-2} \cos \phi, \cos \theta_n \sin \theta_{N+1} \cdots \sin \theta_{N-2} \sin \phi \},$$

$$\vdots$$

$$(8.368d)$$

$$\vec{e}_{N-2} \equiv \frac{\partial x_m}{\partial \theta_{N-2}} = R \sin \theta_1 \sin \theta_2 \dots \sin \theta_{N-3} \{ 0, 0, \dots, 0,$$

$$\cos \theta_{N-2} \cos \phi, \cos \theta_{N-2} \sin \phi \},$$

$$(8.368e)$$

$$\vec{e}_\phi \equiv \frac{\partial x_m}{\partial \phi} = R \sin \theta_1 \sin \theta_2 \dots \sin \theta_{N-2} \{ 0, 0, \dots, 0, -\sin \phi, \cos \phi \}. \quad (8.368f)$$

showing that:

$$n = 1, \dots, N-2: \qquad\qquad 0 = \vec{e}_r . \vec{e}_n = \vec{e}_\phi . \vec{e}_n = \vec{e}_r . \vec{e}_\phi, \qquad (8.369a\text{–}c)$$

all base vectors are orthogonal.

 The hyperspherical coordinates are an orthogonal curvilinear coordinate system in N dimensions, and the modulus of the base vectors specify the scale factors (8.350a, b):

$$n = 1, \cdots, N: \quad h_n \equiv |\vec{e}_n| = \{ 1, R, R \sin \theta_1, R \sin \theta_1 \sin \theta_2, \cdots,$$

$$R \sin \theta_1 \sin \theta_2 \cdots \sin \theta_{n-2}, \cdots, R \sin \theta_1 \sin \theta_2 \cdots \sin \theta_{N-2} \};$$

$$(8.370a, b)$$

$$h_n \equiv \begin{cases} 1, r, r \sin \theta_1, r \sin \theta_1 \sin \theta_2, \dots, r \sin \theta_1 \sin \theta_2, \\ \dots, r \sin \theta_n, \dots, r \sin \theta_1 \sin \theta_2, \dots, r \sin \theta_{N-3}, 1 \end{cases},$$

$$(8.370a', b')$$

the scale factors in hypercylindrical coordinates (8.370a, b') are: (i) similar for the first $N-1$ with (8.370b) $\equiv$ (8.370b') with the distance from the origin (8.367a) replaced by the distance from the axis (8.367a'); (ii) the last is unity because it corresponds to a Cartesian coordinate (8.366h') $\equiv$ (8.367g'); (iii) the first scale factor is unity because it corresponds to a distance, namely the distance from the origin (8.367a) [z-axis (8.367a′)]. The scale factors for the orthogonal curvilinear coordinate system specify through their square (inverse square) the diagonal of the covariant (contravariant) metric tensor (III.9.450b) ≡ (8.371a) [(III.9.450) ≡ (8.371b)] and its determinant (8.371c):

$$g_{nm} = (h_n)^2 \, \delta_{nm} \, , \qquad g^{nm} = h_n^{-2} \, \delta_{nm} \, ; \qquad g = Det(g_{nm}) = \prod_{n=1}^{N} (h_n)^2 \, ; \qquad (8.371a\text{–}c)$$

the determinant of the covariant metric tensor (8.371c) is given for hyperspherical (8.370a, b) [hypercylindrical (8.370a, b′)] coordinates by (8.372) [(8.372′)]:

$$h \equiv |g|^{1/2} = \prod_{n=1}^{N} h_n = R^{N-1} \, \sin^{N-2} \theta_1 \sin^{N-3} \theta_2 \dots \ \sin^{N-n} \theta_{n-1} \dots \sin^2 \theta_{N-3} \sin \theta_{N-2} \, ,$$

$$(8.372)$$

$$h \equiv |g|^{1/2} = \prod_{n=1}^{N} h_n = r^{N-2} \, \sin^{N-3} \theta_1 \sin^{N-3} \theta_2 \dots \ \sin^{N-n} \theta_{n-2} \dots \sin^2 \theta_{N-4} \sin \theta_{N-3} \, ,$$

$$(8.372′)$$

Thus, the *N-dimensional hyperspherical (8.364a–c) [hypercylindrical (8.365a–d)] coordinates [standard CXCI(CXCII)] base vectors (8.368a–f), which are mutually orthogonal (8.369a–c) and whose moduli are the scale factors (8.370a, b) [(8.370a′, b′)], appearing in the metric tensor (8.371a–c) whose determinant is (8.372) [(8.372′)]. The* scale factors of an orthogonal curvilinear coordinate system in *N*-dimensions specify the Laplacian operator (note III.9.44) and hence the Helmholtz equation in hyperspherical (hypercylindrical) coordinates (note 8.9).

NOTE 8.9: **Helmholtz Equation in Hyperspherical Coordinates**

The contravariant metric tensor (8.371b) and the determinant of the covariant metric tensor (8.371c) can be used to write any invariant differential operator (note III.9.43), for example, the scalar Laplacian (III.9.469a) ≡ (8.373a):

$$\nabla^2 \equiv \frac{1}{h} \frac{\partial}{\partial x_i} \left(g^{ij} h \frac{\partial}{\partial x_j} \right) = \frac{1}{h} \frac{\partial}{\partial x_i} \left(\frac{h}{h_i^2} \frac{\partial}{\partial x_i} \right), \qquad (8.373a, b)$$

which simplifies to (8.373b) in orthogonal curvilinear coordinates (8.371a, b). Using the scale factors (8.370a, b) for hyperspherical coordinates (8.364a–c) the successive terms are: (i) in the radius:

$$\frac{1}{\sqrt{g}} \frac{\partial}{\partial R} \left[\sqrt{g} \, (h_1)^{-2} \frac{\partial}{\partial R} \right] = \frac{1}{R^{N-1}} \frac{\partial}{\partial R} \left(R^{N-1} \frac{\partial}{\partial R} \right) = \frac{\partial^2}{\partial R^2} + \frac{N-1}{R} \frac{\partial}{\partial R} \, , \qquad (8.374a)$$

which coincides with the radial part of the Laplacian in polar (8.349) [spherical (8.357)] coordinates for $N = 2$ ($N = 3$); (ii) in the first latitude:

$$\frac{1}{\sqrt{g}} \frac{\partial}{\partial \theta_1} \left[\sqrt{g} \, (h_2)^{-2} \frac{\partial}{\partial \theta_1} \right] = \frac{1}{R^2 \sin^{N-2} \theta_1} \frac{\partial}{\partial \theta_1} \left(\sin^{N-2} \theta_1 \frac{\partial}{\partial \theta_1} \right); \quad (8.374b)$$

(iii) in the second latitude:

$$\frac{1}{\sqrt{g}} \frac{\partial}{\partial \theta_2} \left[\sqrt{g} \, (h_3)^{-2} \frac{\partial}{\partial \theta_2} \right]$$

$$= \frac{1}{R^2 \sin^2 \theta_1 \sin^{N-3} \theta_2} \frac{\partial}{\partial \theta_2} \left(\sin^{N-3} \theta_2 \frac{\partial}{\partial \theta_2} \right); \quad (8.374c)$$

(iv) for the *n*-th latitude:

$$n = 1, \ldots, N - 2: \quad \frac{1}{\sqrt{g}} \frac{\partial}{\partial \theta_n} \left[\sqrt{g} \, (h_{n+1})^{-2} \frac{\partial}{\partial \theta_n} \right]$$

$$= \frac{1}{R^2 \sin^2 \theta_1 \ldots \sin^2 \theta_{n-1} \sin^{N-n-1} \theta_n} \frac{\partial}{\partial \theta_n} \left(\sin^{N-n-1} \theta_n \frac{\partial}{\partial \theta_n} \right); \quad (8.374d)$$

(v) for the last or $(N - 2)$-th latitude:

$$\frac{1}{\sqrt{g}} \frac{\partial}{\partial \theta_{N-2}} \left[\sqrt{g} \, (h_{N-1})^{-2} \frac{\partial}{\partial \theta_{N-2}} \right]$$

$$= \frac{1}{R^2 \sin^2 \theta_1 \ldots \sin^2 \theta_{N-3} \sin \theta_{N-2}} \frac{\partial}{\partial \theta_{N-2}} \left(\sin \theta_{N-2} \frac{\partial}{\partial \theta_{N-2}} \right); \quad (8.374e)$$

(vi) for the longitude:

$$\frac{1}{\sqrt{g}} \frac{\partial}{\partial \phi} \left[\sqrt{g} \, (h_N)^{-2} \frac{\partial}{\partial \phi} \right] = \frac{1}{R^2 \sin^2 \theta_1 \ldots \sin^2 \theta_{N-2}} \frac{\partial^2}{\partial \phi^2}, \quad (8.374f)$$

which is again familiar for cylindrical ($N = 2$) [spherical ($N = 3$)] coordinates (8.349) [(8.357)]. Substituting (8.374a–f) in the Laplacian (8.373b) and then in (8.343b) ≡ (8.344b) specifies *the Helmholtz equation (8.344b) ≡ (8.375a)* in *(standard CXCIII) hyperspherical coordinates (8.364a–c; 8.366a–h) where the each coordinate has been separated in (8.375b):*

$$-k^2 \tilde{F} = \nabla^2 \tilde{F} = \frac{1}{R^{N-1}} \frac{\partial}{\partial R}\left(R^{N-1} \frac{\partial \tilde{F}}{\partial R} \right)$$

$$+ \frac{1}{R^2 \sin^{N-2} \theta_1} \frac{\partial}{\partial \theta_1}\left(\sin^{N-2} \theta_1 \frac{\partial \tilde{F}}{\partial \theta_1} \right)$$

$$+ \frac{1}{R^2 \sin^2 \theta_1 \sin^{N-3} \theta_2} \frac{\partial}{\partial \theta_2}\left(\sin^{N-3} \theta_2 \frac{\partial \tilde{F}}{\partial \theta_1} \right) + \ldots$$

$$+ \frac{1}{R^2 \sin^2 \theta_1 \ldots \sin^2 \theta_{n-1} \sin^{N-n-1} \theta_n} \frac{\partial}{\partial \theta_n}\left(\sin^{N-n-1} \theta_n \frac{\partial \tilde{F}}{\partial \theta_n} \right)$$

$$+ \ldots + \frac{1}{R^2 \sin^2 \theta_1 \ldots \sin^2 \theta_{N-2} \sin \theta_{N-2}} \frac{\partial}{\partial \theta_{N-2}}\left(\sin \theta_{N-2} \frac{\partial \tilde{F}}{\partial \theta_{N-2}} \right)$$

$$+ \frac{1}{R^2 \sin^2 \theta_1 \sin^2 \theta_2 \ldots \sin^2 \theta_{N-2}} \frac{\partial \tilde{F}}{\partial \phi^2}.$$

$$(8.375a, b)$$

In space ($N = 3$) the Helmholtz equation in hyperspherical coordinates (8.375b) simplifies to (8.357) in spherical coordinates, and in any dimension, it can be written in a "nested form" (note 8.10) that facilitates the subsequent solution by separation of variables (note 8.11).

NOTE 8.10: Nested Form of the Helmholtz Equation

Multiplying by R^2 the Helmholtz equation (8.375b) is rewritten (8.376):

$$-k^2 R^2 \tilde{F} = R^2 \partial^2 \tilde{F}/\partial R^2 + (N-1) R \partial \tilde{F}/\partial R$$

$$+ \csc^{N-2} \theta_1 \{(\partial/\partial \theta_1)[\sin^{N-2} \theta_1 (\partial \tilde{F}/\partial \theta_1)]$$

$$+ \csc^2 \theta_1 \{\csc^{N-3} \theta_2 (\partial/\partial \theta_2)[\sin^{N-3} \theta_2 (\partial \tilde{F}/\partial \theta_2)]$$

$$+ \csc^2 \theta_2 \{\csc^{N-4} \theta_3 (\partial/\partial \theta_3)[\sin^{N-4} \theta_3 (\partial \tilde{F}/\partial \theta_3)] + \cdots \qquad (8.376)$$

$$+ \csc^2 \theta_{n-1} \{\csc^{N-n-1} \theta_n (\partial/\partial \theta_n)[\sin^{N-n-1} \theta_n (\partial \tilde{F}/\partial \theta_n)] + \cdots$$

$$+ \csc^2 \theta_{N-3} \{\csc \theta_{N-2} (\partial/\partial \theta_{N-2})[\sin \theta_{N-2} (\partial \tilde{F}/\partial \theta_{N-2})]$$

$$+ \csc^2 \theta_{N-2} \partial^2 \tilde{F}/\partial \phi^2\}\} \cdots \}\}\}.$$

in a "nested form," taking factors out of the brackets as early as possible. This facilitates the solution by separation of variables, as shown next. The solution of the Helmholtz equation in hyperspherical coordinates is obtained by separation of variables:

$$\tilde{F}\left(r,\theta_1,\cdots,\theta_{N-2},\phi,\omega\right) = X(R)\,\Phi(\phi)\prod_{n=1}^{N-2}\Theta_n(\theta_n).\qquad(8.377)$$

with substitution (8.377) in (8.376) and division by $\tilde{F}$ leading to (8.378):

$$-k^2R^2 = X^{-1}\Big[R^2\,d^2X/dR^2 + (N-1)\,R\,dX/dR\Big]$$

$$+\Theta_1^{-1}\Big[d^2\Theta_1/d\theta_1^2 + (N-2)\,\cot\theta_1\,d\Theta_1/d\theta_1\Big]$$

$$+\csc^2\theta_1\Big\{\Theta_2^{-1}\Big[d^2\Theta_2/d\theta_2^2 + (N-3)\,\cot\theta_2\,d\Theta_2/d\theta_2\Big]$$

$$+\csc^2\theta_2\Big\{\Theta_3^{-1}\Big[d^2\Theta_3/d\theta_3^2 + (N-4)\,\cot\theta_3\,d\Theta_3/d\theta_3\Big]+\cdots$$

$$\qquad\qquad(8.378)$$

$$+\csc^2\theta_{n-1}\Big\{\Theta_n^{-1}\Big[d^2\Theta_n/d\theta_n^2 + (N-n-1)\cot\theta_n\,d\Theta_n/d\theta_n\Big]+\cdots$$

$$+\csc^2\theta_{N-1}\Big\{\Theta_{N-2}^{-1}\Big[d^2\Theta_{N-2}/d\theta_{N-2}^2 + \cot\theta_{N-2}\,d\,\Theta_{N-2}/d\theta_{N-2}\Big]$$

$$+\csc^2\theta_n\Phi^{-1}d^2\Phi/d\phi^2\ \}\cdots\}\cdots\}\ \},$$

separating the variables $(R,\theta_1,\theta_2,\cdots,\theta_n,\cdots\theta_{N-2},\phi)$ as much as possible, for the next step (note 8.11). Thus, *the Helmholtz equation in hyperspherical coordinates (8.375a, b) written (standard CXCIV) in "nested form" (8.376) has a solution by separation of variables (8.377) leading (8.378) to a set of N separate ordinary differential equations,* which are considered next (note 8.11).

NOTE 8.11: **Separation of Variables and Set of Ordinary Differential Equations**

The solution of the Helmholtz equation in hyperspherical coordinates (8.375b) ≡ (8.376) by separation of variables (8.377) leads (8.378) to a set of N-independent ordinary differential equations: (i) the first term on the r.h.s. of (8.378) is the only one depending on the radius, so it equals R^2 multiplied by a constant, and denoting the latter by $q_1(1+q_1)$ leads to (8.379a, b):

$$q_1 \equiv n:\qquad R^2\frac{d^2X}{dR^2}+(N-1)R\frac{dX}{dR}+\Big[k^2R^2-n(n+1)\Big]X=0,\qquad(8.379a, b)$$

which simplifies to (8.361b) for $N = 3$; the last factor on the r.h.s. of (8.378) is the only one depending on the longitude, so it must be a constant $-m^2$, leading to (8.351a; 8.352a); (iii) the last latitude θ_{N-2} appears only in the last two terms on the r.h.s. of (8.378) and must be a constant leading to (8.380a):

$$\Theta_{N-2}^{-1} \, d^2 \, \Theta_{N-2}/d\theta_{N-2}^2 + \cot\theta_{N-2} \, \Theta_{N-2}^{-1} \, d\Theta_{N-2}/d\theta_{N-2}$$
$$+ \csc^2\theta_{N-2} \, \Phi^{-1} \, d^2\Phi/d\phi^2 = - \, q_{N-2} \left(1 + q_{N-2}\right), \tag{8.380a}$$

which on account of (8.351b) is equivalent to (8.380b):

$$d^2\Theta_{N-2}/d\theta_{N-2}^2 + \cot\theta_{N-2} \, d\Theta_{N-2}/d\theta_{N-2}$$
$$+ \left[q_{N-2}\left(1 + q_{N-2}\right) - m^2 \csc^2\theta_{N-2} \right]\Theta_{N-2} = 0; \tag{8.380b}$$

(iv) a similar reasoning for θ_{N-3} leads to (8.381):

$$d^2\Theta_{N-3}/d\theta_{N-3}^2 + 2\cot\theta_{N-3} \, d\Theta_{N-3}/d\theta_{N-3}$$
$$+ \left[q_{N-3}\left(1 + q_{N-3}\right) - q_{N-2}\left(1 + q_{N-2}\right) \csc^2\theta_{N-3} \right]\Theta_{N-3} = 0; \tag{8.381}$$

(v) the corresponding ordinary differential equation for θ_n is:

$$n = 3, \ldots, N-2: \quad d^2 \, \Theta_{N-n}/d\theta_{N-n}^2 + (n-1) \, \cot\theta_{N-n} \, d\Theta_{N-n}/d\theta_{N-n}$$
$$+ \left[q_{N-n}\left(1 + q_{N-n}\right) - q_{N-n+1}\left(1 + q_{N-n+1}\right) \csc^2\theta_{N-n} \right]\Theta_{N-n} = 0;$$
$$\tag{8.382a, b}$$

(vi) the ordinary differential equation for the first latitude is (8.382b) ≡ (8.383b) with (8.379a) ≡ (8.383a):

$$n = 1: \frac{d^2\Theta}{d\theta_1^2} + (N-2)\cot\theta_1 \frac{d\Theta}{d\theta_1} + \left[n(n+1) - q_2\left(1 + q_2\right)\csc^2\theta_1 \right]\Theta_1 = 0. \tag{8.383a, b}$$

Thus, *the solution by separation of variables (8.377) of the Helmholtz equation (8.344b) in hyperspherical coordinates (8.375b) ≡ (8.376) leads to (standard CXCV) a, set of N-separate ordinary differential equations (8.379a, b; 8.351a; 8.380b; 8.381; 8.382a, b; 8.383b)*, which are considered next in two sets: (i) the Bessel and associated Legendre differential equations that appeared before (note 8.5) in spherical coordinates (note 8.12); (ii) the generalization to hyperspherical associated Legendre functions needed for hyperspherical coordinates (note 8.13) of higher dimension $N \geq 4$.

NOTE 8.12: Dependences on Longitude, Radius, and Latitudes

The simplest dependence is on longitude, which leads to (8.351a; 8.352a) as in the cases of cylindrical (spherical) coordinates [note 8.4 (8.5)]. The radial dependence (8.379a) for space $N = 3$ is specified by a spherical Bessel equation (8.361b) of order $q_1 = n$, which is reducible to a cylindrical Bessel equation (8.353b) via a change of the dependent variable that involves multiplication by $\sqrt{R} = R^{1-N/2}$ when $N = 3$. This suggests the change of the dependent variable (8.384a) in the N-dimensional case that transforms (8.379b) to (8.384b):

$$X(R) = R^{1-N/2}\, S(R): \qquad R^2 \frac{d^2 S}{dR^2} + R \frac{dS}{dR} + \left[k^2 R^2 - \left(\frac{N}{2} - 1 \right)^2 - n(n+1) \right] S = 0.$$

$$(8.384a, b)$$

The latter (8.384b) is (subsection 9.5.22), a Bessel equation (8.353b) of order ν in (8.385a) so that the radial dependence (8.354b) is specified by (8.385b) in terms of Bessel and Neumann functions:

$$\nu^2 = n(n+1) + \left(\frac{N}{2} - 1 \right)^2 : \qquad X(R) = R^{1-N/2} \left[E_+ J_\nu(kR) + E_- Y_\nu(kR) \right]. \quad (8.385a, b)$$

In three dimensions (8.386a) from (8.385a) follows (8.386b) and in (8.385b) appear the spherical Bessel functions (8.386c):

$$N = 3: \;\; \nu^2 = n^2 + n + \frac{1}{4} = \left(n + \frac{1}{2} \right)^2, \;\; X(R) = R^{-1/2} \left[E_+ J_{n+1/2}(kR) + E_- Y_{n+1/2}(kR) \right];$$

$$(8.386a\text{–}c)$$

the agreement of (8.362) with (8.386c) shows (8.387a) that the spherical (8.362) and cylindrical (8.386c) Bessel (Neumann) functions are related by (8.387a) [(8.387b)]:

$$\left\{ j_n(kR), y_n(kR) \right\} = \sqrt{\frac{\pi}{2kR}} \left\{ J_{n+1/2}(kR), \Psi_{n+1/2}(kR) \right\}, \quad (8.387a\text{–}c)$$

where the constant factor $\sqrt{\pi/2}$ was inserted for agreement with the literature (subsection 9.5.24) and can be absorbed into the arbitrary constants $E_\pm$ in (8.386c) $\equiv$ (8.362). It has been shown that *the solution (8.377) of the Helmholtz equation (8.375a, b) $\equiv$ (8.376) in hyperspherical coordinates (8.364a–c) in N dimensions (8.366a–h) has radial dependence (8.379b) specified (standard CXCVI) by a Bessel differential equation (8.384a, b) of order (8.385a). The solution in N-dimensions in terms of Bessel and Neumann functions (8.386c) simplifies in two (three) dimensions to cylindrical (8.353b; 8.354b) [spherical*

(8.361b; 8.362) ≡ (8.386a–c; 8.387a, b)] Bessel and Neumann functions of order m $(m = n + 1/2)$ *and variable $\bar{k}\,r$ (kR). The remaining dependence on the first (other) latitudes leads to associated Legendre (hyperspherical-associated Legendre) functions as for (generalizing) the case (note 8.5) of spherical to hyperspherical coordinates (note 8.13).*

NOTE 8.13: Hyperspherical Associated Legendre Functions

The last latitude (8.380b) satisfies an associated Legendre differential equation (8.359b) with order m and degree q_{N-2}, thus leading to (8.360) ≡ (8.388):

$$\Theta_{N-2}\left(\theta_{N-2}\right)=D_{N-2}^{+}\,P_{q_{N-2}}^{m}\left(\theta_{N-2}\right)+D_{N-2}^{-}\,Q_{q_{N-2}}^{m}\left(\theta_{N-2}\right); \qquad (8.388)$$

the dependence of the solution of the Helmholtz equation in hyperspherical coordinates on the last latitude (8.388) ≡ (8.360) is similar to spherical harmonics (8.380b) ≡ (8.359b) with $\theta = \theta_{N-2}$ and $n = q_{N-2}$. For the remaining co-latitudes (8.381; 8.382a, b; 8.383a, b) a more general ordinary differential equation appears (8.389) that may be designated the **hyperspherical-associated Legendre differential equation**:

$$\frac{d^{2}\Theta}{d\theta^{2}}+(1+\ell)\cot\theta\,\frac{d\Theta}{d\theta}+\Big[n(n+1)-m^{2}\csc^{2}\theta\Big]\Theta=0; \qquad (8.389)$$

its solution in terms of hyperspherical-associated Legendre functions of two kinds and degree n, *order m, and dimension* ℓ:

$$\Theta(\theta)=D_{+}\,P_{n,\ell}^{m}\left(\cos\theta\right)+D_{-}\,P_{n,\ell}^{m}\left(\cos\theta\right), \qquad (8.390)$$

specifies (standard CXCVII) also the dependence (8.382a, b) ≡ (8.391a) of the solution (8.390) of the Helmholtz equation (8.344b) in hyperspherical coordinates (8.375b) on the n-th latitude:

$$\ell = N-n: \qquad \frac{d^{2}\Theta_{\ell}}{d\theta_{\ell}^{2}}+(N-\ell-1)\cot\theta_{\ell}\,\frac{d\Theta_{\ell}}{d\theta_{\ell}}$$

$$\hspace{3cm} +\Big[q_{\ell}\left(1+q_{\ell}\right)-q_{\ell+1}\left(1+q_{\ell+1}\right)\csc^{2}\theta_{\ell}\Big]\Theta_{\ell}=0; \qquad (8.391a, b)$$

the solution of (8.382b) ≡ (8.389) is (8.390) ≡ (8.392a, b):

$$\ell = 1,...,N-3: \qquad \Theta_{\ell}\left(\theta_{\ell}\right)=D_{\ell}^{+}\,P_{q_{\ell},\nu_{\ell}}^{\mu_{\ell}}\left(\cos\theta_{\ell}\right)+D_{\ell}^{-}\,Q_{q_{\ell},\nu_{\ell}}^{\mu_{\ell}}\left(\cos\theta_{\ell}\right), \qquad (8.392a, b)$$

where the degree is q_m, *the order is (8.392c), and the dimension is (8.392d):*

$$\mu_\ell = \left| q_\ell \left(1 + q_\ell \right) \right|^{1/2}, \qquad \nu_\ell = N - \ell - 2. \qquad (8.392c,\ d)$$

The simplest case of solution of the Helmholtz equation in hyperspherical coordinates beyond spherical harmonics (note 8.5) is four-dimensional (note 8.14).

NOTE 8.14: Hyperspherical Harmonics in Four Dimensions

The simplest case beyond spherical harmonics (note 8.5) is four-dimensional, and is reviewed next: (i) the four-dimensional hyperspherical coordinates $(r,\ \theta,\ \Psi,\ \phi)$ are related to the Cartesian coordinates (8.364a–c) ≡ (8.393a) by (8.366a–h) ≡ (8.393b):

$$0 \le r < \infty,\ 0 \le \theta, \psi \le \pi,\ 0 \le \phi < 2\pi: \qquad (8.393a)$$

$$\{x_1, x_2, x_3, x_4\} = R\{\cos\theta, \sin\theta\cos\psi, \sin\theta\sin\psi\cos\phi, \sin\theta\sin\psi\sin\phi\}; \qquad (8.393b)$$

(ii) the inverse coordinate transformation from four-dimensional Cartesian to hyperspherical is (8.367a–g) ≡ (8.394a–d):

$$R = \left| x_1^2 + x_2^2 + x_3^2 + x_4^2 \right|^{1/2},\ \cot\theta = z \left| x_4^2 + x_2^2 + x_3^2 \right|^{-1/2},$$

$$\cot\psi = x_3 \left| x_1^2 + x_2^2 \right|^{-1/2},\ \cot\phi = x_2 / x_1\ ; \qquad (8.394a\text{–}d)$$

(iii) the hyperspherical base vectors (8.368a–f) ≡ (8.395a–d) are:

$$\bar{e}_R \equiv \partial\bar{x}/\partial R = \{\cos\theta, \sin\theta\cos\psi, \sin\theta\sin\psi\cos\phi, \sin\theta\sin\psi\sin\phi\},$$

$$\bar{e}_\theta \equiv \partial\bar{x}/\partial\theta = R\{-\sin\theta, \cos\theta\cos\psi, \cos\theta\sin\psi\cos\phi, \cos\theta\sin\psi\sin\phi\},$$

$$\bar{e}_\psi \equiv \partial\bar{x}/\partial\psi = R\sin\theta\{0, -\sin\psi, \cos\psi\cos\phi, \cos\psi\sin\phi\},$$

$$\bar{e}_\phi \equiv \partial\bar{x}/\partial\phi = R\sin\theta\sin\psi\{0, 0, -\sin\phi, \cos\phi\}; \qquad (8.395a\text{–}d)$$

(iv) they are mutually orthogonal and their moduli specify the scale factors (8.370b) ≡ (8.396a–d):

$$h_R = 1,\ h_\theta = R,\ h_\psi = R\sin\theta,\ h_\phi = R\sin\theta\sin\psi: \qquad |g|^{1/2} = R^3 \sin^2\theta\sin\psi,$$

$$(8.396a\text{–}e)$$

as well as the determinant of the covariant metric tensor (8.372) ≡ (8.396e); (v) the four-dimensional Helmholtz equation in hyperspherical coordinates is (8.375b) ≡ (8.397a, b):

$$
-k^2 \tilde{F} = \nabla^2 \tilde{F} \equiv \frac{1}{R^3} \frac{\partial}{\partial R}\left(R^3 \frac{\partial \tilde{F}}{\partial R}\right) + \frac{1}{R^2 \sin^2 \psi} \frac{\partial}{\partial \psi}\left(\sin^2 \psi \frac{\partial \tilde{F}}{\partial \psi}\right)
$$

$$
+ \frac{1}{R^2 \sin^2 \psi \sin \theta} \frac{\partial}{\partial \theta}\left(\sin \theta \frac{\partial \tilde{F}}{\partial \theta}\right) + \frac{1}{R^2 \sin^2 \psi \sin^2 \theta} \frac{\partial^2 \tilde{F}}{\partial \phi^2};
$$

(8.397a, b)

(vi) the solution by separation of variables (8.377) is (8.398):

$$
\tilde{F}(r,\theta,\psi,\phi,t) = X(R)\,\Theta(\theta)\,\Psi(\psi)\,\Phi(\phi),
$$

(8.398)

where (8.378) ≡ (8.399):

$$
-k^2 R^2 = X^{-1}\left(R^2 d^2 X/dR^2 + 3\,R\,dX/dR\right) + \Psi^{-1}\left[d^2\Psi/d\psi^2 + 2\cot\psi\,d\Psi/d\psi\right]
$$

$$
+ \csc^2 \psi\,\Theta^{-1}\left[d^2\Theta/d\theta^2 + \cot\theta\,d\Theta/d\theta + \csc^2\theta + \Phi^{-1}d^2\Phi/d\phi^2\right];
$$

(8.399)

(vii) this leads to a set of four ordinary differential equations, with the first specifying the dependence on longitude (8.351a; 8.352a); (viii) the second specifies the dependence on the radius (8.379a, b) ≡ (8.400a, b):

$$
N = 4: \qquad R^2 \frac{d^2 X}{dR^2} + 3\,R\,\frac{dX}{dR} + \left[k^2 R^2 - n(n+1)\right] X = 0,
$$

(8.400a, b)

whose solution is specified by Bessel functions (8.385b) ≡ (8.401b) of order ν in (8.385a) ≡ (8.401a) with (8.400a):

$$
\nu^2 = n^2 + n + 1: \qquad X(R) = R^{-1}\left[E_+ J_\nu(kR) + E_- Y_\nu(kR)\right];
$$

(8.401a, b)

(ix) on the last latitude (8.402a–d) that leads to (8.402e) ≡ (8.359b):

$$
\ell = 2,\ \theta_1 \equiv \theta,\ \ \Theta_2 \equiv \Theta,\ \ q_2 \equiv q: \quad \frac{d^2\Theta}{d\theta^2} + \cot\theta \frac{d\Theta}{d\theta} + \left[q(q+1) - m^2 \csc^2\theta\right]\Theta = 0,
$$

(8.402a–e)

whose solution is (8.360) ≡ (8.403) involves the original associated Legendre functions of two kinds:

$$\Theta(\theta) = D_+ \, P_q^m(\cos\theta) + D_- \, Q_q^m(\cos\theta);\qquad(8.403)$$

(xi) on the first latitude (8.404a–d) that leads (8.404e) ≡ (8.391b) to (8.404e) ≡ (8.391b):

$\ell = 1,\ \theta_1 \equiv \psi,\ \Theta_1 \equiv \Psi,\ q_1 \equiv n:$

$$\frac{d^2\Psi}{d\psi^2} + 2\cot\psi\,\frac{d\Psi}{d\psi} + \left[n(n+1) - q(q+1)\csc^2\psi \right]\Psi = 0,\qquad\text{(8.404a–e)}$$

whose solution involves (8.392b, c) ≡ (8.405a, b) the hyperspherical-associated Legendre functions of two kinds:

$$\mu \equiv |q(1+q)|^{1/2}:\qquad \Psi(\psi) = B_+ \, P_{n,1}^{\mu}(\cos\psi) + B_- \, Q_{n,1}^{\mu}(\cos\psi);\qquad\text{(8.405a, b)}$$

(xi) substituting (8.352b; 8.401b; 8.403; 8.405b) in (8.398) follows that:

$$\tilde{F}(R,\theta,\psi,\phi) = \frac{1}{R}\left(C_+ e^{im\phi} + C_- e^{im\phi}\right)\left[E_+ \, J_\nu(kR) + E_- \, Y_\nu(kR)\right]$$

$$\left[D_+ \, P_q^m(\cos\theta) + D_- \, P_q^m(\cos\theta)\right]\left[B_+ \, P_{n,1}^{\mu}(\cos\psi) + B_- \, Q_{n,1}^{\mu}(\cos\phi)\right],$$

$$\text{(8.406)}$$

the solution (8.406) of the Helmholtz equation (8.397a, b) in hyperspherical coordinates in four dimensions (8.393a, b) is obtained by separation of variables (8.398) as (standard CXCVIII) the product of dependences on: (a) the longitude (8.352b) specified by sinusoidal functions; (b) on the radius (8.400b) specified by Bessel and Neumann functions (8.401b) of order (8.401a); (c) on the last latitude (8.402e) by associated Legendre functions of two kinds (8.403); (d) on the first latitude (8.404e) by hyperspherical-associated Legendre functions (8.405b) of dimension one. The constants azimuthal m, radial n, and latitudinal q wavenumbers are arbitrary as well as the coefficients $B_\pm, C_\pm, D_\pm, B_\pm$. The hyperspherical-associated Legendre functions appear only in the dimension $\ell = 1$ because the hyperspherical coordinates are of dimension four in (8.394a–d), as confirmed by the base vectors (8.395a–d), scale factors (8.396a–d) determinant of the metric tensor (8.396e) and Laplacian in (8.397b). Keeping the dimension N = 4 but using hypercylindrical coordinates only the original associated Legendre functions of dimension zero appear (note 8.15).

NOTE 8.15: Hypercylindrical Harmonics in Four Dimensions

The four-dimensional case in hypercylindrical coordinates is similar to the three-dimensional case in spherical coordinates because: (i) the relation to Cartesian coordinates (8.366a′–h′) ≡ (8.407b) involves an orthogonal Cartesian coordinate instead of second latitude (8.365a–d) ≡ (8.407a):

$$0 \le r < \infty, 0 \le \theta < \pi, 0 \le \phi \le 2\pi, -\infty < z < +\infty:$$

$$\{x_1, x_2, x_3, x_4\} = \{r\cos\theta, r\sin\theta\cos\phi, r\sin\theta\sin\phi, z\};$$

(8.407a, b)

(ii) the inverse coordinate transformation from four-dimensional Cartesian to hypercylindrical is (8.367a′–g′) ≡ (8.408a–d):

$$r = \left|x_1^2 + x_2^2 + x_3^2\right|^{1/2}, \ \cot\theta = x_1\left|x_2^2 + x_3^2\right|^{-1/2}, \ \cot\phi = x_2/x_3, \ z \equiv x_4; \quad (8.408a\text{–}d)$$

(iii) the hypercylindrical base vector are (8.409a–d):

$$\vec{e}_r \equiv \partial\vec{x}/\partial r = \{\cos\theta, \ \sin\theta\cos\phi, \sin\theta\sin\phi, 0\}, \quad (8.409a)$$

$$\vec{e}_\theta \equiv \partial\vec{x}/\partial\theta = r\{-\sin\theta, \ \cos\theta\cos\phi, \cos\theta\sin\phi, 0\}, \quad (8.409b)$$

$$\vec{e}_\phi \equiv \partial\vec{x}/\partial\phi = r\sin\theta\{0, -\sin\phi, \ \cos\phi, 0\}, \ \vec{e}_z \equiv \partial\vec{x}/\partial z = (0,0,0,1); \quad (8.409c, d)$$

(iv) they are mutually orthogonal and their modulus specifies the scale factors (8.410a–d):

$$h_r = 1 = h_z, \quad h_\theta = r, \quad h_\phi = r\sin\theta, \quad |g|^{1/2} = r^2\sin\theta, \quad (8.410a\text{–}e)$$

as well as the determinant of the covariant metric tensor (8.410e); (v) the four dimensional Helmholtz equation (8.411a):

$$-k^2\tilde{F} = \nabla^2\tilde{F} = \frac{1}{r^2}\frac{\partial}{\partial r}\left(r^2\frac{\partial\tilde{F}}{\partial r}\right) + \frac{1}{r^2\sin\theta}\frac{\partial}{\partial\theta}\left(\sin\theta\frac{\partial\tilde{F}}{\partial r}\right) + \frac{1}{r^2\sin^2\theta}\frac{\partial^2\tilde{F}}{\partial\phi^2} + \frac{\partial^2\tilde{F}}{\partial z^2},$$

(8.411a, b)

where the Laplacian (8.411b) is similar to the spherical (8.357) replacing R by r and adding the last term of the cylindrical (8.349); (vi) the solution by separation of variables (8.412):

$$\tilde{F}(r,\theta,\phi,z) = X(r)\,\Theta(\theta)\,\Phi(\phi)\,Z(z), \quad (8.412)$$

is (8.413) the product of (8.363) by (8.352a):

$$\tilde{F}(r,\theta,\phi,z) = \left(B_+ e^{ikz} + B_- e^{-ikz}\right)\left(C_+ e^{im\phi} + C_- e^{im\phi}\right)$$

$$\left[E_+ j_n(kR) + E_- y_n(kR)\right]\left[D_+ P_n^m(\cos\theta) + D_- Q_n^m(\cos\theta)\right].$$

(8.413)

It has been shown that *the solution of the Helmholtz equation (8.397a, b) [(8.411)] in four-dimensional hyperspherical (8.393a, b; 8.394a–d) [hypercylindrical (8.407a, b; 8.408a–d)] coordinates [standard CXCVIII (CXCIX)] is (8.406) [(8.413)] with arbitrary azimuthal m, radial $n(\bar{k})$ and latitudinal q (axial k) wavenumbers, corresponding to the base vectors (8.395a–d) [(8.409a–d)], scale factors (8.396a–d) [(8.410a–d)], determinant of the metric tensor (8.396e) [(8.410e)] and Laplacian (8.397b) [(8.411b)]. The superposition of solutions is valid* and is used to specify the general integral of the equation of mathematical physics (8.340) in hyperspherical (hypercylindrical) coordinates (notes 8.16 (8.17)].

NOTE 8.16: **Linear Superposition of Hyperspherical Harmonics**

When substituting the solution (8.377) of the Helmholtz equation (8.343b) in the generalized isotropic equation of mathematical physics (8.340) using (8.343a) the following two changes are made: (i) a general superposition of solutions is used with integer parameters; (ii) only one function in each coordinate is used to simplify the formuli. Thus *generalized isotropic equation of mathematical physics (8.340) in hyperspherical coordinates (8.375a, b) ≡ (8.376) has solution (standard CC) as a superposition of* **hyperspherical harmonics** (8.414):

$$\tilde{F}(R,\theta_1,\cdots,\theta_{N-2},\phi,t) = \int_{-\infty}^{+\infty} d\omega\, B_{m,n,q_1,\cdots,q_{N-2}}(\omega) \sum_{m=-\infty}^{+\infty} e^{i(m\phi-\omega t)} J_\nu(kR)$$

(8.414)

$$\sum_{q_{N-2}=1}^{\infty} P_{q_{N-2}}^m(\cos\theta_{N-2}) \sum_{q_{N-3},\cdots,q_1=1}^{\infty} \prod_{\ell=1}^{N-3} P_{q_\ell,\nu_\ell}^{\mu_\ell}(\cos\theta_\ell),$$

involving: (i) an integration over frequency and arbitrary coefficients B depending not only on frequency but also on the azimuthal m, radial q_1, and latitudinal $\left(q_1,....,q_{N-2}\right)$ wavenumbers; (ii) the dependence on longitude ϕ is specified (8.352b) by sinusoidal functions with azimuthal wavenumber m; (iii) the dependence on the radius R is specified (8.379b) by Bessel functions (8.385b) of order (8.385a) and variable k R where k is the wavenumber (8.343a); (iv) the dependence of the last latitude θ_{N-2} is specified (8.380b) by associated Legendre functions (8.388) of order m and degree q_{N-2}; (iv) the dependence on the remaining N − 3 latitudes $\theta_1,\cdots,\theta_{N-3}$ is specified (8.382a, b) by hyperspherical-associated Legendre functions (8.392b) with *degree q_ℓ, order (8.392c), and dimension (8.392d) up (8.392a) to $N-2$; the sums over the wavenumbers $m,n,q_1,...,q_{N-2}$ could be replaced by integrals.* Similar results apply in hypercylindrical coordinates with one latitude less and adding one axial Cartesian coordinate, thus relating hyperspherical (hypercylindrical) harmonics [notes 8.16 (8.17)].

NOTE 8.17: Relation between Hyperspherical and Hypercylindrical Coordinates

In the case of hypercylindrical coordinates, the Laplacian (8.375a, b) has one latitude less replaced by an axial Cartesian coordinate in the generalized equation of mathematical physics (8.340) leading to (8.415):

$$0 = \sum_{j=0}^{M} A_j \, \partial_j \tilde{F} / \partial t^j + \frac{1}{r^{N-1}} \frac{\partial}{\partial r}\left(r^{N-1} \frac{\partial \tilde{F}}{\partial r} \right)$$

$$+ \frac{\partial^2 \tilde{F}}{\partial z^2} + \frac{1}{r^2 \sin^{N-3}\theta_1} \frac{\partial}{\partial \theta_1}\left(\sin^{N-3}\theta_1 \frac{\partial \tilde{F}}{\partial \theta_1} \right) + \cdots$$

$$+ \frac{1}{r^2 \sin^{N-3}\theta_1 \cdots \sin^2\theta_{n-1} \sin^{N-n-2}\theta_n} \frac{\partial}{\partial \theta_n}\left(\sin^{N-n-3}\theta_n \frac{\partial \tilde{F}}{\partial \theta_n} \right) \quad (8.415)$$

$$+ \cdots + \frac{1}{r^2 \sin^2\theta_1 \cdots \sin^2\theta_{n-4} \sin\theta_{N-3}} \frac{\partial}{\partial \theta_{N-3}}\left(\sin\theta_{N-3} \frac{\partial \tilde{F}}{\partial \theta_{N-3}} \right)$$

$$+ \frac{1}{r^2 \sin^2\theta_1 \sin^2\theta_2 \cdots \sin^2\theta_{N-3}} \frac{\partial^2 \tilde{F}}{\partial \phi^2}.$$

The solution is similar to (8.414) with one latitude θ_{N-2} less replaced by (8.351b; 8.352b) an axial Cartesian coordinates leading to (8.416):

$$\tilde{F}(r,\theta_1,\cdots,\theta_{N-3},\phi,t) = \int_{-\infty}^{+\infty} d\omega \int_{-\infty}^{+\infty} dk \, B_{m,n,q_1,\cdots,q_{N-3}}(k,\omega) \sum_{m=-\infty}^{+\infty} e^{i(kz+m\phi-\omega t)} J_\nu(\overline{k}R)$$

$$\sum_{q_{N-3}=1}^{+\infty} P_{q_{N-3}}^m(\cos\theta_{N-3}) \sum_{q_1,\cdots,q_{N-4}=1}^{\infty} \prod_{\ell=1}^{N-4} P_{q_\ell,\nu_\ell}^{\mu_\ell}(\cos\theta_\ell).$$

$$(8.416)$$

Thus, the solution (8.414) [(8.416)] of the generalized isotropic equation of mathematical physics (8.340) in hyperspherical (8.375a, b) [hypercylindrical (8.415)] coordinates is [standard CC (CCI)] similar, with the following distinctions: (i) they are $N-2(N-3)$ latitudes and thus, in the degree q_ℓ, order (8.392c), and dimension

(8.392d) of the hyperspherical associated Legendre functions are used (8.417a, b) instead of (8.392a, d):

$$\ell = 1, \cdots, N-3; \qquad v_\ell = N - \ell - 3; \qquad v \equiv q_1(q_1 + 1) - \left(\frac{N}{2} - \frac{3}{2}\right)^2, \qquad (8.417a\text{--}c)$$

(ii) there is integration of frequency ω (and also on the axial wavenumber k) and the coefficient B is a function of one (two) variables with azimuthal m, radial q_1, and $N - 3$ ($N - 4$) latitudinal $q_2, ..., q_{N-2}$ ($q_2, ..., q_{N-3}$) latitudinal wavenumbers; (iii) the radial dependence is specified by Bessel functions of order (8.385a) [(8.414c)] and variable $k R (\bar{k} r)$ involving the distance from the origin R (from the axis r) and the total (8.343a) [axial (8.353a)] wavenumber. These results involve **special functions**, for example, Bessel and hyperspherical-associated Legendre functions that are solutions of linear differential equations with variable coefficients and are considered next (chapter 9), together with some general properties of non-linear differential equations.

Conclusion 8

The analogy between mass m (self L), damper b (resistor R), spring k (capacitor 1/C), and applied F(t) [electromotive E(t)] force (Figure 8.1b) leads to the simulation of mechanical (electrical) circuits [Figure 8.1a(c)], for example, two-dimensional oscillators consisting of two masses (selfs) supported by springs (in series with capacitors), and connected (coupled) by an intermediate spring k_3 (capacitor C_3), plus the corresponding dampers (μ_1, μ_2, μ_3) [resistors (R_1, R_2, R_3)]. Another mechanical circuit with two degrees-of-freedom, namely translation z and rotation θ, is a plane rigid body supported on unequal springs and dampers (Figure 8.2a), including as particular cases two point masses (Figure 8.2b) or a homogeneous rod (Figure 8.2c). The vibration absorber applies to a damped forced mechanical (electrical) circuit [Figure 8.3a (b)] primary circuit, by adding an undamped unforced secondary circuit with natural frequency tuned to the applied frequency.

The Markov chains applies to a radioactive disintegration chain (Figure 8.4a), which is described by a system of first-order differential equations in which each element depends only on the preceding; the system has resonant solutions in the cases of coincident disintegration rates (Diagram 8.2). An N-dimensional mechanical (electrical) oscillator [Figure 8.4b(c)], consisting of circuits in series, is described by a system of second-order differential equations in which each circuit depends both on the preceding and following; resonant solutions occur for forcing at an applied frequency coincident with an oscillation frequency (Diagram 8.1). An infinite transmission line made of mechanical (electrical) circuits [Figure 8.4b(c)] can have six distinct types of cells, illustrated in the electrical case, namely having in the connecting branch no (only) self [Figure 8.7a (8.8a)], resistor [Figure 8.7b (8.8b)] or capacitor [Figure 8.7c (8.8c)]. A signal travels without loss along a transmission line when the elements are electrical (mechanical) impedances of circuits with self (mass) and capacitor (springs) but no resistor (damper). A transmission line (Figure 8.6) is an infinite sequence of electrical (mechanical) circuits [Figure 8.5a(c)] represented by impedances [Figure 8.5b(d)] in series Z_b and parallel Z_a. As an example is an electrical (mechanical) transmission line [Figure 8.4c(b)] with selfs (masses) and capacitors (springs) but no resistors (dampers); lossless transmission is possible if the frequency passband lies at least partially above a cut-off frequency.

The mechanical and electrical oscillations (waves) are described by ordinary (partial) differential equations with time (and position) as independent variables. Linear dissipative waves of second-order in space are described by the generalized equation of mathematical physics, with the spatial dependence specified by the Laplacian operator. The solution reduces to ordinary differential equations if the Laplacian is separable, for example, (Diagram 8.3) for:

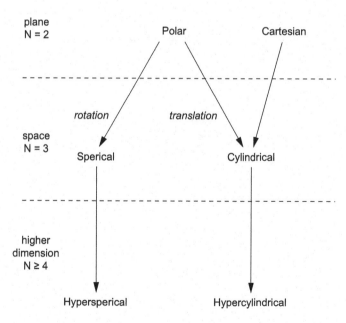

COORDINATE SYSTEMS

DIAGRAM 8.3
The two most common coordinate systems in the plane are Cartesian and polar. The polar coordinates yield cylindrical (spherical) coordinates by translation perpendicular to the plane (rotation around an axis passing through the center). The hyperspherical (hypercylindrical) coordinates in N dimensions add $N - 2$ rotational coordinates to the spherical (cylindrical) coordinates.

(i) Cartesian coordinates in any dimension; (ii) polar coordinates in the plane, which extend by translation (rotation) to cylindrical (spherical) coordinates in space; (iii) adding $N - 2$ Cartesian coordinates leads to hyperspherical (hypercylindrical) coordinates. The separation of variables in the Laplacian for these (i) to (iii) and some other orthogonal coordinate systems lead to linear ordinary differential equations with variable coefficients whose solutions are special functions.

Bibliography

The bibliography of *"Simultaneous Differential Equations and Multi-dimensional Vibrations,"* which is the fourth book of Volume IV *Ordinary Differential Equations with Applications to Trajectories and Oscillations,* and the seventh book of the series *"Mathematics and Physics for Science and Technology,"* adds the subject of basic mechanics of "Material Particles." The books in the bibliography that have influenced the present volume the most are marked with one, two, or three asterisks.

Material Particles

* Appell, P. *Traité de Mécanique Rationelle,* **5** vols., Gauthier-Villars, Paris, 1900–1904, 4éme édition, 1919–1923.

*Ames, J. S. and Murnaghan, F. D. *Theoretical Mechanics.* Gin, London, 1929, reprinted Dover, New York, 1957.

Axisa, F. V., Trompette, F., and Antunes, J. *Modelling of Mechanical Systems,* **3** vols. Butterworth Heineman, London, 2007.

Beckers, M. *Introduction to Theoretical Mechanics.* McGraw-Hill, New York, 1970.

Beer, F. P. and Johnston, E. R. *Vector Mechanics for Engineers: Statics.* McGraw-Hill, New York, 1966.

Beer, F. P. and Johnston, E. R. *Vector Mechanics for Engineering: Dynamics.* McGraw-Hill, New York, 1966.

Bullen, K. E. *Theory of Mechanics.* Cambridge University Press, Cambridge, 1977.

** Cabannes, H. *Mécanique.* Dunod, Paris, 1968.

*** Campos, L. M. B. C. *Mecanica Aplicada I: Estatica, Cinematica e Dinamica Tensorial.* Escolar Editora, Lisbon, 2003.

*** Campos, L. M. B. C. *Mecânica Aplicada II: Dinamica Variacional e Gemetria Tensorial.* Escolar Editora, Lisbon, 2004.

D'Alembert, J. R. *Traité de dynamique.* David, Paris, 1743.

D'Alembert, J. R. *Recherches sur le system du monde.* 3 vols., David, Paris, 1754–1759.

Fogiel, M. *Mechanics: Statics and Dynamics.* Research and Education Association, Piscataway, New Jersey, 1965.

Gariel, M. *Recueil de Travaux Scientifiques de L. Foucault.* Gauthier-Villars, Paris, 1878.

Goldstein, H. *Classical Mechanics.* Addison-Wesley, Reading, MA, 1950.

Hamel, G. *Mechanik.* Teubner, Leipzig, 1904.

Hand, L. R. and Finch, J. D. *Analytical Mechanics.* Cambridge University Press, Cambridge, 1998.

* Hertz, H. *The Principles of Mechanics.* MacMillan, London, 1956, reprinted Dover, New York, 1960.

Jacobi, C. G. J. *Gesammelte Werke: VIII: Vorlesungen über Dynamik*. Berlin 1881–1891, acht band, 1866, zweite fassung, 1884, reprinted Chelsea, New York, 1969.

Jeans, J. H. *An Elementary Treatise on Theoretical Mechanics*. Ginn, London, 1907, reprinted Dover, New York, 1967.

Kosmodem'yanskii, A. A. *A Course of Theoretical Mechanics*. Translation National Science Foundation, Washington, DC, 1963.

Krysinski, T. and Malburet, F. *Mechanical Instability*. Wiley, New Jersey, 2011.

** Kuypers, F. *Klassiche Mechanik*. Wiley-VCH, Regensburg, Germany, 2016.

* Laplace, P. S. *Mécanique Céleste*. 5 vols, Gauthier-Villars, Paris, 1820, reprinted Chelsea Publications, New York. 1950.

Laurent, H. *Traite de Mécanique Rationelle*. Gauthier-Villars, Paris, 1876.

MacMillan, W. D. *Statics and Dynamics of a Particle*. MacMillan, London, 1927, reprinted Dover, New York, 1958.

Mathieu, E. *Dynamique Analytique*. Gauthier-Villars, Paris, 1878.

Maxwell, J. C. *Matter and Motion*. MacMillan, New York, 1920.

Margin, G. A. *Configurational Forces*. CRC Press, Boca Raton, FL, 2011.

** Newton, I. *Principia*, 2 vols, 1686, translation, Dover, New York, 1934, reprinted Cambridge University Press, 5 vols, Cambridge, 1972.

O' Donnell, P. J. *Essential Dynamics and Relativity*. CRC Press, Boca Raton, FL, 2015.

Osgood, W. F. *Mechanics*. MacMillan, London, 1937.

Painlevé, P. *Cours de Mécanique*. Gauthier-Villars, Paris, 2 vols., 1929–1936.

Painlevé, P. and Platrier, C. *Cours de Mécanique*. Gauthier-Villars, Paris, 3 vols., 1922–1929.

Platrier, C. *Mécanique Rationelle*, 2 vols., Dunod, Paris, 1955.

Poinsot, J. *Elements de Statique*. Gauthier-Villars, Paris, 1877.

Rao, A. V. *Dynamics of Particles and Rigid Bodies*. Cambridge University Press, Cambridge, 2006

* Routh, E. J. *Dynamics of a Particle*. Cambridge University Press, 1898, Cambridge, reprinted Dover, New York, 1960.

** Routh, E. J. *Dynamics of a System of Rigid Bodies*. MacMillan, London, 1905, reprinted Dover, New York, 2 vols., 1960.

* Rutherford, D. E. *Classical Mechanics*. Oliver & Boyd, London, 1951, 3rd ed., 1967.

Slater, L. J. and Frank, N. *Mechanics*. McGraw-Hill, New York, 1965.

Starjingki, V. M. *Mecanica Teorica*. Editora Mir, Moscow, 1986.

Strauchs, D. *Classical Mechanics: An Introduction*. Springer, Berlin, 2009.

Sturm, J. C. F. *Cours de Mécanique*. Gauthier Villars, Paris, 1978.

Symon, K. R. *Mechanics*. Addison-Wesley, New York, 1960.

Synge, J. L. and Griffith, E. A. *Principles of Mechanics*. McGraw-Hill, New York, 1942, 3rd ed., 1959.

Tenenbaum, R. A. *Dinâmica*. Editora UFRJ, Rio de Janeiro, 1997.

Webster, A. G. *The Dynamics of Particles and of Rigid, Elastic and Fluid bodies*. 1904, 2nd edition, 1912, reprinted Dover, New York, 1959.

* Whittaker, E. T. *Analytical Dynamics of Particles and Rigid Bodies*. Cambridge University Press, Cambridge, 1904, 4th ed., 1937.

References

1916 Rayleigh, J. W. S. On the Propagation of Sound in Narrow Tubes of Variable Cross-section. *Philosophical Magazine* **31**, 89–96.

1919 Webster, A. G. Acoustical Impedance and the Theory of Horns and the Phonograph. *Proceedings of the National Academy of Sciences* **5**, 275–282.

1927 Ballantine, S. On the Propagation of Sound in the General Bessel Horn of Infinite Length. *Journal of the Franklin Institute* **203**, 85–101.

1930 Olson, H. F. A. Sound Concentrator for Microphones. *Journal of the Acoustical Society of America* **1**, 410–417.

1946 Salmon, V. A. New Family of Horns. *Journal of the Acoustical Society of America* **17**, 212–218.

1962 Biees, D. A. Tapering Bars of Uniform Stress in Longitudinal Oscillations. *Journal of the Acoustical Society of America* **34**, 1567–1572.

1967 Pyle, R. W. Duality Principle for Horns. *Journal of the Acoustical Society of America* **37**, 1178A.

1971 Nagarkar, B. N. and Finch, R. D. Sinusoidal Horns. *Journal of the Acoustical Society of America* **50**, 23–31.

1984 Campos, L. M. B. C. On Some General Properties of the Exact Acoustic Fields in Horns and Baffles. *Journal of Sound and Vibration* **95**, 177–201.

1985 Campos, L. M. B. C. On the Fundamental Acoustic Mode in Variable Area Low Mach Number Nozzles. *Progress in Aerospace Sciences* **22**, 1–27.

1986 Campos, L. M. B. C. On Waves in Gases. Part I: Acoustics of Jets, Turbulence and Ducts. *Reviews of Modern Physics* **58**, 117–182.

References

Index

Printed in the United States
by Baker & Taylor Publisher Services